Caring for Older Adults

BASIC NURSING SKILLS AND CONCEPTS

Joan Carson Breitung, RN, MA, MSN

Director, Practical Nursing Program
Roger L. Putnam Vocational Technical High School
Springfield, Massachusetts

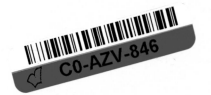
1987

W. B. SAUNDERS COMPANY

PHILADELPHIA   LONDON   TORONTO   SYDNEY   TOKYO   HONG KONG

W. B. Saunders Company: West Washington Square
                          Philadelphia, PA 19105

Library of Congress Cataloging-in-Publication Data

Breitung, Joan Carson.
  Caring for older adults.

  1. Geriatric nursing. I. Title. [DNLM: 1. Aging.
2. Geriatric Nursing.   WY 152 B835ca]
RC954.B75   1987   610.73'65   86-27982
ISBN 0-7216-1576-7

Editor: Ilze Rader
Designer: Karen O'Keefe
Production Manager: Peter Faber
Manuscript Editor: Patrice Smith
Illustrator: Risa Kornhauser and Sharon Iwanczuk
Illustration Coordinator: Walt Verbitski
Indexer: Alexandra Weir

Caring for Older Adults: Basic Nursing
Skills and Concepts   ISBN   0-7216-1576-7

Last digit is the print number: 9   8   7   6   5   4   3   2   1

To the elderly, who deserve nursing care that is given with skill and sensitivity.

Preface

The purpose of this book is to encourage productive and meaningful nursing care of the most rapidly increasing segment of our population—adults over age 65. In 1900, this group made up 4 per cent of the population. Today, the figure is between 11 and 12 per cent. Fifty years from now it is expected to have risen to 18 per cent.

Care of the Older Adult is written primarily for first level nursing students and for caregivers working in long-term-care settings. The book should be integrated with the student's study of anatomy and physiology, growth and development, fundamental skills, nutrition, and medical-surgical nursing. It is useful for any discipline associated with elderly clients: nursing assistant, nursing home administration, physical therapy, dietetics, and social services. Others who have responsibility for care of elderly clients (home health aides and mental health workers) will find that *Care of the Older Adult* is a useful resource.

Instructors in courses that cover comprehensive medical-surgical nursing care will discover that this book is a valuable addition to help focus their students' knowledge in a field in which the greatest number of career opportunities will exist in coming years.

Taking care of the elderly is challenging and complex. As a result, today's nurse needs highly developed theoretical and clinical nursing skills. The foundation of gerontologic nursing is *a knowledge of the aging process,* that universally shared experience that begins at birth. Identification of the characteristics of the aging process enables the nurse to

- explain the implications for nursing care of the older client
- combine sensitivity to and respect for the elderly with clinical skills

Part One introduces the student to geriatrics; explores myths and facts of aging; discusses nursing home placement and alternatives to placement; examines the mental disorders of old age; promotes an understanding of the mental anguish of aphasia; and discusses incontinence and constipation, sexuality and aging, and care of the dying. It also contains a chapter on nutrition, with a survey by the author on the nutritional practices of the well adult over 65.

The book is unique not only for its range of subject matter but also for the way in which the nine chapters of the body systems (Part Two) are presented. For each body system, the book
- reviews in simple terms the anatomy of the system
- describes the age-related changes that can occur
- gives related nursing procedures

It is hoped that this book will contribute to an understanding of the aging process and that it will encourage superior care that will add to the health and comfort of our elders.

Acknowledgements

I want to thank the administrators and nurses at Crescent Hill Nursing Center, East Longmeadow Nursing Home, Heritage Hall Retirement and Nursing Home, The Jewish Nursing Home of Western Massachusetts, Kendall Commons, and Mountain View Nursing Home for their assistance. Thanks also to Mary Lou DiGiacomo, vice president of nursing affairs, Mercy Hospital; Morrill Stone Ring of The Ring Nursing Home; and Teresa Theroux, administrator, Teresa Sherman, director of nursing, and Leslie Mackler, pharmacologist, Springfield Municipal Hospital, for their valuable help.

I also want to express my appreciation to Hebe Chestnutt, R.N., B.S.N., Great Falls Vo-Tech, Great Falls, MT; Shirley Czuba, R.N., and Mary Holmberg, R.N., of Platte Community College, Columbus, NE; Elizabeth J. Guy, Milwaukee, WI; Judith Lott, Hillsborough Co-Erwin VT Center, Tampa, FL; Annitta Love, R.N., B.S.N., Trenholm State Technical College, Montgomery, AL; Dianne Reed, Cossat Vo-Tech, DeQueen, AR; Joyce Terry, R.N., M.S.N., Concord, CA; and Frieda Thielman, R.N., Hawkeye Institute of Technology, Waterloo, IA, for their reviews of manuscript and helpful suggestions.

Table of Contents

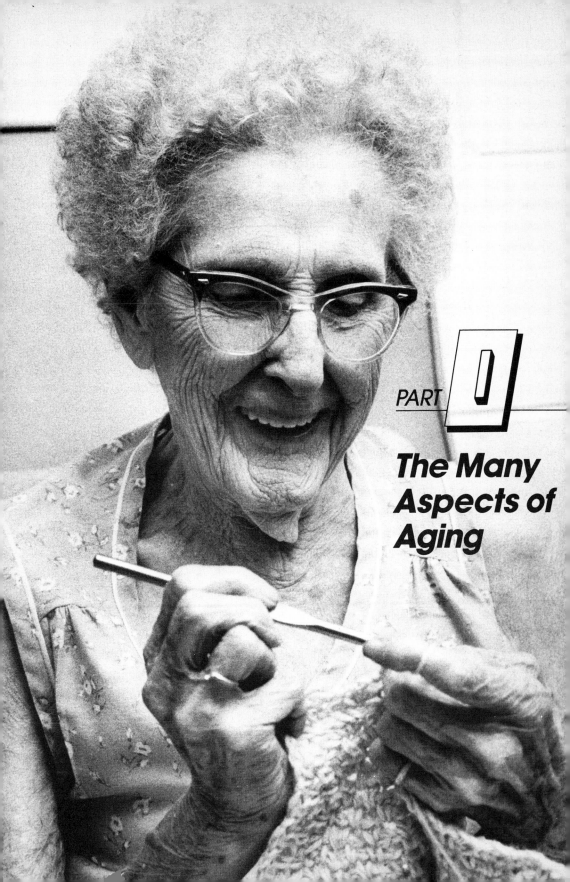

PART 0

The Many Aspects of Aging

Objectives

After completing this chapter, the student should be able to

- [ ] explain why elders have an increasing need for supportive social and health care services
- [ ] describe the significance of the Older Americans Act
- [ ] list factors that influence the aging process
- [ ] describe ways to maintain elderly persons in their own homes
- [ ] give examples of community services that provide home care and assistance for older adults
- [ ] separate the myths from the facts of aging

Vocabulary

atrophy
demographics
homeostasis
neuron
osteoporosis
proprietary
respite care
tactile
turgor

CHAPTER 1

Introduction to Aging

Chapter Outline

☐ Social and Political Aspects

The largest pool of human need and illness in today's United States is that of the elderly. While many elders are vigorous and healthy and financially secure, others are frail and in poor health. The problems are complex: poverty, malnutrition, inadequate housing compounded by physical impairments, and loss of family and friends. These problems are shared by all of us, since old people are increasing in the greatest numbers history has ever seen. As the population of elderly has expanded and the population of younger workers has declined, there has been increased dependence on government for health services, income assistance, and other supports.

☐ DEMOGRAPHICS

Demography is the study of human populations. It reveals population counts, growth estimates, vital health statistics, and economic information. With these data, health professionals can learn current and future health needs. Demographers studying the elderly use the chronologic age of 65 as an arbitrary number. In society and in this chapter, when the general term "older adults" is used, it refers to those over age 65. Actually, it is about ten years later—at age 75—when frailty and dependence start for many. It is always important to remember individual differences. Those over the age of 65 have great differences in both psychologic and physiologic characteristics. If you think about how large the number of people over 65 is, as shown in Table 1–1 and Figures 1–1 and 1–2, you can begin to realize what enormous re-

Table 1–1 ☐ **Numbers and Proportions of Older People in the United States: 1900–2040**

Year	Number of Persons 65 and Older	Per cent of Total Population 65 and Older	Number of Persons 75 and Older	Per cent of Total Population 75 and Older
1900	3.1 million	4.1	0.9 million	1.2
1940	9.0 million	6.8	2.7 million	2.0
1960	16.7 million	9.2	5.6 million	3.1
1980[a]	24.9 million	11.2	9.4 million	4.2
2000[b]	31.8 million	12.2[c]	14.4 million	5.5[c]
2020[b]	45.1 million	15.5[c]	16.9 million	5.9[c]
2030[b]	55.0 million	18.3[c]	23.2 million	7.7[c]
2040[b]	55.0 million	17.8[c]	27.9 million	9.0[c]

[a]estimate
[b]projection (base data of projection is July 1, 1976)
[c]projections based on an intermediate fertility assumption (Series II) by the U.S. Census Bureau, and one immigration assumption (see text)
From Schrier, R. W.: Clinical Internal Medicine in the Aged. Philadelphia, W. B. Saunders, 1982, p. 2; based on U.S. Bureau of the Census data.

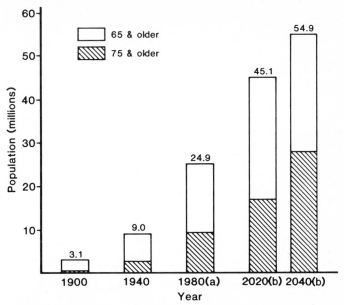

Figure 1–1 □ Growth of the older population in the United States: 1900 to 2040. (a), Estimate; (b), projections (base date of projections is July 1976). (From Schrier, R. W.: Clinical Internal Medicine in the Aged. Philadelphia, W. B. Saunders, 1982, p. 3; based on U. S. Bureau of the Census data.)

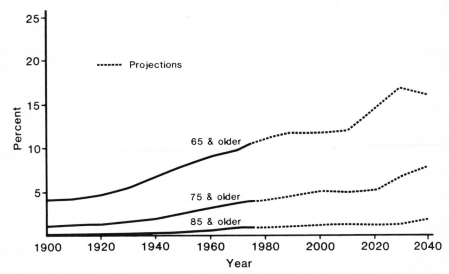

Figure 1–2 □ Percentage of the total population in the older age groups: 1900 to 2040. (From Schrier, R. W.: Clinical Internal Medicine in the Aged. Philadelphia, W. B. Saunders, 1982, p. 3; based on U. S. Bureau of the Census data.)

sources and effort will be required to meet the health care challenge in the coming decades.

It is the group of older adults *age 75 and over* who have increased in numbers the fastest (National Institutes on Aging, 1980). Presently 38 per cent of older adults are 75 and over and 9 per cent are past 85. By the year 2000, 45 per cent will be more than 75 and 12 per cent will be over 85. Most of these older adults are women.

□ ECONOMIC ASPECTS

Almost 65 per cent of the elderly live at home with family, spouse, or friends. Thirty per cent live alone; less than 5 per cent live in institutions. Most men 65 and over are married; most women who reach that same milestone are widows.

Poverty and the resulting economic consequences are among the major problems of older adults. Compulsory and voluntary retirement practices coupled with age discrimination have reduced the participation of older persons in the work force (Butler, 1977). In 1900, two thirds of men 65 and over were working. Today, only one man in five over the age of 65 is working. There is a definite trend toward earlier retirement that will probably continue for many more years. All these factors indicate a larger requirement of the elderly for supportive social services and health care services.

□ THE IMPACT OF CHRONIC DISEASE

The elderly have fewer acute illnesses than younger adults have. Rather, *chronic disease* and decline of function of sense organs set the pattern for the aging process. About 85 per cent of people over age 65 have some type of chronic health problem; about half of those with a chronic problem say that the problem interferes with their activity level.

The most common chronic afflictions are arthritis, hearing impairment, heart disease, and hypertension. Other chronic problems responsible for disability are orthopedic problems, visual impairments, diabetes, and chronic respiratory disease. Multiple health problems are often encountered.

The ability to take care of oneself, to get around independently, and to participate in the activities of daily life is often severely limited as chronic health problems progress. The help of family, friends, or public services is needed to allow the elderly person to maintain as much independence as possible.

□ *Social Services and Legislation*

There are more than 130 federal programs designed to assist the aged. Some of these services include transportation, housing, legal assistance, and home health care. In 1980, all health and welfare benefits for older adults made up one quarter of the federal budget (Developments in Aging, 1981). Unfortunately, not all needy elders receive the necessary aid, as poor coordination and inefficiency have characterized many governmental efforts.

□ LEGISLATION RELATING TO THE ELDERLY

The Social Security Act was implemented in 1935 to provide for federally administered old age, survivors', and disability insurance payments. The Social Security system is supported by employee paycheck deductions and by employer contributions. The Social Security fund does not receive money from general federal taxes. Currently, retired workers are eligible to receive 80 per cent of full monthly old-age benefits at age 62 and full benefits at age 65. People between 65 and 72 can earn up to $3000 a year and still receive these benefits. At age 72, a person may work full time and collect full benefits.

There was little national action about the problems of older adults after the enactment of the Social Security Act until the 1950's. In 1950, the first national conference on aging was convened in Washington. A federal committee was an outgrowth of this conference—the Committee on Aging. During that same year a large voluntary agency committed to social reform also formed a Committee on the Aging. Its focus was work in the areas of employment and health care. By 1961, that committee became known as the National Council on the Aging. The NCOA offers counseling services, develops programs for older adults, and publishes important information about aging.

Efforts to provide information regarding older citizens and their many needs grew more and more successful over the years.

The 1960's ushered in an era of legislation and programs for the elderly. The Older Americans Act became law in 1965. Its effect was to foster programs for older adults in community service, research, employment, and nutrition. Title I of the Older Americans Act contains the Senior Citizen's Charter (or Bill of Rights). The important effect of the Older Americans Act was the creation of the Administration on Aging (AOA) at the federal level and the individual state offices on aging. The state offices are the federally mandated Area Agencies on Aging (AAA). The AAA is an umbrella agency responsible for the planning, coordination, and funding of programs.

Medicare and Medicaid are federal health care insurance programs that

---

Senior Citizen's Bill of Rights*

Each of our senior citizens, regardless of race, color, or creed, is entitled to:

The right to be useful.
The right to freedom from want in old age.
The right to obtain employment, based on merit.
The right to a fair share of the community's recreational, educational, and medical resources.
The right to obtain decent housing suited to the needs of later years.
The right to the moral and financial support of one's family so far as is consistent with the best interests of the family.
The right to live independently, as one chooses.
The right to live and die with dignity.
The right to access to all knowledge as available to improve the later years of life.

*Prelude to A Senior Citizen's Bill of Rights, adopted at the 1961 White House Conference on Aging.

Senior Citizen's Bill of Rights. (From Care of the Older Adult, 1st ed., p. 34.)

have been available to elders since 1965. These programs are administered by the Social Security Administration.

Medicare covers *all elders who are eligible for Social Security benefits*, yet it pays only about half of the medical expenses of the elderly. The remainder must come from personal savings, private medical insurance, or other sources. *Medicaid* was designed for persons of any age whose income is too low to pay for private health insurance. Eligibility for Medicaid is determined separately by each state. Medicaid benefits come from federal grants to states and cover 50 to 80 per cent of medical care. In order to be eligible for Medicaid benefits, a person must demonstrate financial need. In general, those who are eligible for state old age assistance or welfare are also eligible for Medicaid.

☐ The Aging Process

Aging is a natural, normal process. No one known factor causes it, and, of course, there is no cure. Researchers do know that aging is influenced by several factors. When describing these factors, it is important to remember that not all things apply to all people at the same time. Genetic programming, cellular mutation, and autoimmune reactions all influence the rate of aging. In addition, environmental components such as diet and exposure to the elements play a part. Stress is a major consideration because the body is less able to resist stress as it ages. *Homeostasis*, the ability of the body to maintain equilibrium while continually adjusting to conditions that affect it, becomes impaired.

There is a decline of all responses that affect all systems of the body, especially the cardiovascular and musculoskeletal systems. Decline in the functioning of the special senses is common in the elderly. Hearing loss, particularly inability to hear high-pitched sounds, is common. There is a decline in visual perception and a decrease in sensitivity of the taste buds. Pain sensation is diminished. This is potentially dangerous, since pain is a primary warning signal of illness or injury.

More discussion of the aging process and its effect on the body's systems is presented in Part 2 of this book. However, to help you begin your understanding of how systems are affected by old age, the following gives an overview of physical changes:

1. *Integumentary system changes*

Reduced gland secretions, decreased elastic fibers, and subcutaneous tissue contribute to dryness and thinning of epithelial and subcutaneous skin layers. Skin of the elderly lacks turgor (springiness). Wrinkles appear; hair grays and thins.

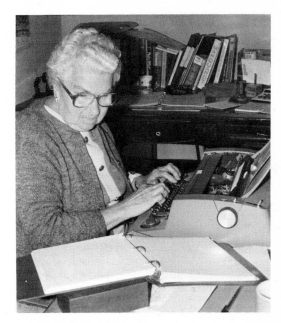

Aging varies with the individual. Some older adults at age 74 years need assistance with basic activities of living, whereas this woman is working productively part-time in an office.

2. *Musculosketal system changes*

Muscles become smaller and bones become lighter. This contributes to loss of strength and stamina of elders. Osteoporosis (loss of bone mass) is a universal phenomenon but occurs to a greater extent in women than in men. Loss of bone mass means bones are weaker, and thus the elderly person is at greater risk for fractures. Osteoporosis also contributes to changes in the curvature of the spine and the resulting decrease in height in older adults. Joints gradually degenerate with age, characteristically becoming stiffer.

3. *Cardiovascular system changes*

There is reduced cardiac output, which contributes to fatigue. The heart also reacts poorly to sudden stress. *Arteriosclerosis* (thickening, hardening of arterial walls) and *atherosclerosis* (accumulation of fatty deposits on arterial walls) can contribute to diminished circulatory function.

4. *Digestive system changes*

Changes take place in the teeth, gums, taste buds, and saliva. Appetite may decrease because of diminished function of the taste buds and decreased saliva secretion. Loss of teeth interferes with proper chewing of food. Stomach atrophy (shrinkage) and slowdown in peristalsis (wavelike movements in the hollow tubes of the body) affect digestion negatively and may increase flatulence (intestinal gas) and constipation. Digestion is also affected by a general decrease in enzyme and gastric juice production.

5. *Respiratory system changes*

Lungs show a decline in elasticity, which causes underexpansion. As a result, older adults are more at risk for pulmonary disease. Secretions are cleared from the lungs less effectively because ciliary action decreases, and the strength of the cough is decreased through muscle weakness.

6. *Nervous system changes*

Loss of neurons causes diminished tactile (touch) sensation and decreased ability to distinguish odors and tastes. A general slowing of neural response and reaction time occurs. Slower reaction time and diminished sight or hearing contribute to accidents in the elderly.

7. *Genitourinary system changes*

Decrease in renal function is caused by changes in both kidney structure and blood circulation to the kidneys. The bladder muscles weaken, and the ureteral and urethral muscles lose muscle tone. These changes contribute to the problems of urinary incontinence.

8. *Endocrine system changes*

Atrophy of the thyroid gland contributes to general metabolic slowdown. This means that all physical and chemical activity within the body declines. Hormone activity decreases as all glands decrease in function; for example, the ovaries (female reproductive glands) and testes (male reproductive glands) become smaller and less productive.

Changes of aging and their implications for nursing care are discussed in Part 2 of this book. It is important to remember that *each person ages on his or her own time schedule.* Persons of the same chronological age may differ greatly in physical changes and functioning.

Nurses in both acute and long-term care facilities need to realize that adjustments must be made in the care of elderly patients based on the loss and decline in physiological functioning. Adaptations required by geriatric (care of the elderly) nursing also occur on the psychologic level. As the aging process slows responses, the older adult is acutely aware of the many changes his or her body is undergoing. Loss of physical strength and peak function is often compounded by other losses: family members, spouse, identity in the work force, financial independence. Nurses can help by allowing for the slower pace and reaction time of the elderly person and recognizing their need for independence and respect.

□ *The Family and Home Care*

A surprisingly large percentage of older adults live near an adult child. It is the family that supplies 80 per cent of health-related and/or personal care to the elderly parent. The family prevents or postpones the need for institutionalization. Many families view institutionalization as a last resort when all resources fail.

Care of older adults with medical problems does not take place only in the hospital or nursing home. Soaring medical costs and changes in reimbursement for medical costs have created a tremendous expansion in home health care. Home care is a viable alternative for many elders and their families. Remember that less than 5 per cent of older adults are in institutional care, even though a high percentage of the elderly have multiple health problems.

The benefits of home care are many:
- maintenance of dignity, individuality, and control
- absence of rules, institutional policies, and depersonalization
- familiar surroundings and people
- enhanced healing, more responsibility for self care
- maintenance of independence
- lower costs for health care

There can be drawbacks. Home care may not be the answer if
- tension and pressure on family members cause severe family friction
- the home is small or crowded

- the responsible family member is unable to safely provide care
- the nature of the illness requires skilled, 24-hour care and complex medical treatment
- the patient does not want to be home

Home care is the right choice if the decision includes the patient, family, and supervising physician and if there is access to adequate home health services.

☐ THE HOME ENVIRONMENT

The following are suggestions for simple ways a home can be made safer and more suitable for home care of the older adult:

1. Eliminate or decrease the need for the older adult to use stairs. Using a room on the first floor that is close to a bathroom is ideal.
2. If the person is confined to bed, a radio, television, and telephone should be in easy reach. Clocks and calendars should be in view to help the person maintain orientation.
3. Grab-bars or hand rails can be installed in halls and in bathrooms next to toilet and shower.
4. Floor covering should be adapted to the needs of the elderly. Falls can be caused by scatter rugs, slippery floors, and shag rugs. Lighting is especially important; bedrooms, bathrooms and hallways all may need increased lighting to compensate for the reduced vision of the older adult.
5. If the person is hearing impaired, an amplifier can be installed on the telephone.
6. Adhesive strips or other nonslip surfaces can be placed in the bathtub. A bench in the bathtub can contribute to safety and comfort in bathing.
7. If utensils are hard to handle because of weakness or arthritis, handles may be enlarged with foam rubber, Velcro, and cloth.
8. Door handles also may be changed to a lever type for ease in handling.
9. Provision must be made for quick and easy evacuation in case of fire, depending on the level of mobility of the person. Smoke detectors are essential in the home for early warning.

Equipment can be purchased or rented to make caring for a confined, homebound older adult easier. Some examples are the following:

1. An electric bed to help the patient sit up or get in and out of bed.
2. Water bed, air mattress, or egg crate mattress to reduce the chance of pressure sores.
3. A trapeze to be installed above a bed to facilitate movement by the patient.
4. A commode to be kept next to the bed for ease in toileting.

☐ HOME HEALTH SERVICES

Local hospitals have discharge planning departments and social service workers to coordinate the transition from hospital to home. Physicians and community health agencies are appropriate resources for families whose elderly relative is not hospitalized, yet needs help.

Every state has a state agency on aging. These agencies are able to provide multiple services for older adults at home. The Area Agency on Aging is the only funded network for home care assistance for elders. For further information on the Area Agency for Aging in your state, write to the National Association of Area Agencies on Aging, 600 Maryland Avenue S.W., Suite 208, Washington, D.C. 20024. Their telephone number is (202) 484-7520.

There are other community services that provide in-home professionals for home health care. Professionals who make home visits include public health nurses and registered dieticians and speech, physical, occupational, and respiratory therapists.

There are *proprietary* (for profit) agencies that supply professional nursing services as well as supplemental care in the form of attendants, homemakers, home health aides, and companions, depending on the level of assistance the older adult needs.

☐ SUPPORT FOR FAMILIES

Families responsible for the care of the elderly at home have a formidable responsibility. There should be a physician available to supervise the medical aspects of care. Friends and relatives should be encouraged to assist with some of the aspects of care to prevent the situation from becoming burdensome.

Some ways in which the family and close friends may help would be with the following:
- any aspect of personal hygiene, i.e., bathing, shaving, grooming hair
- assisting the person in and out of bed
- helping to feed and to ambulate the person
- cooking
- housecleaning
- laundry
- yard maintenance
- errands
- filling out forms and contacting government agencies on behalf of the person

Local Red Cross chapters, home health agency nurses, or health department visiting nurses offer health training instruction for families and friends who feel they would benefit from this instruction.

In addition to the many physical services agencies can provide in home care, family caregivers may need help with the emotional strain of caring for an older adult. Community mental health centers and social services departments of local hospitals are able to direct people to appropriate self-help or support groups.

Support groups for family members provide a place for sharing the experience of caring for an elderly person with others in the same situation. The following sources can help in locating self-help groups in your area:

- Help: A Working Guide to Self Help Groups by Alan Gartner and Frank Riessman, c/o New Viewpoints, Dept. E-J, 730 Fifth Avenue, New York, N.Y., 10019 ($9.95).
- National Self Help Clearinghouse, Graduate School and University Center of the City University of New York, W. 42nd Street, Room 1227, New York, N.Y., 10036; telephone (212) 840-7606.

☐ RESPITE CARE

Caregivers (usually family members) need a change of pace and scene 20 minutes to 1 hour daily and weekly for part of a day once or twice a week. Many nursing, convalescent, and retirement homes offer what is called *respite care*. For a day or weekend, or longer, they will temporarily admit the client and assume full responsibility for his or her care. This enables the usual caregiver (family) to maintain well being and to return to the situation refreshed, restored, and better able to cope. (In some areas, hospitals also provide this service.)

☐ *Myths and Facts About Aging*

There are many myths about older adults. Read the following examples and see if you have ever confused a myth with a fact.

Myth: Old people are sickly and most of them are hospitalized.

Fact: Less than 5 per cent of the elderly are confined to institutions. Although more than 80 per cent of them have some type of chronic health problem, ranging from arthritis to vascular disease, better than 80 per cent are up and taking care of themselves. The myth that most older people are sickly may have grown from the fact that between two thirds and three fourths of hospital admissions are over the age of 65.

Myth: The poor can tolerate the impact of aging better than the affluent because the poor have never had anything anyway.

Fact: As the poor become older, their problems intensify. Many live in substandard housing. The necessities of life, i.e., food, shelter, and medical expenses, become discouragingly expensive to poor people. This has given rise to the next myth.

Myth: Elderly people don't need to spend much money for clothing, recreation, transportation, and so on.

Fact: They would like very much to spend money on these things, but the poor among them just can't afford to. The director of a Golden Age center made this revealing comment: "Today, there's barely a dress code anywhere. You may go where you wish and dress as you please. Anything goes. But these people (indicating the members) were raised in a generation where you *dressed* to go out. Not having what they consider 'suitable' clothes or enough changes of clothes often keeps many of our members from participating here."

Myth: The blue collar worker has a difficult adjustment to retirement.

Fact: No doubt some blue collar workers view retirement with concern, but many have good pensions and retirement benefits. In addition, they have worked regular hours for many years and have had time to find outside interests and hobbies. This is in marked contrast to the professional man who has committed all his time and attention to his career and faces retirement with nothing to take its place.

Myth: Old people are senile.

Fact: This is unkind stereotyping of the elderly when they exhibit forgetfulness, memory lapses, confusion, or slow reactions. Unfortunately, the term "senility" is used by lay persons and professionals alike and this indiscriminate labeling often postpones or clouds the diagnosis of treatable conditions. When any one of the just-mentioned conditions happens to younger people, it is treated lightly. If it persists, we become concerned and seek treatment. But when the person is 65 or older, it is easier to use the catchall term "senility."

☐ CHECKING WHAT YOU KNOW

One way to begin the study of new material is to determine what you already know. Complete the following True-False quiz by circling T or F and then check your answers on page 345.

T F 1. Life expectancy has increased through modern medical advances.

T F 2. Elderly people need at least 8 hours of sleep each night.

T F 3. A small percentage (5 per cent or less) of the elderly are institutionalized.

T F 4. For the adult past 65, chronological age and biological age are the same.

T F 5. Depression is quickly diagnosed in adults over 65.

T F   6. Senile patients escape depression because they are not in touch with reality.
T F   7. If the blood supply to the brain is impaired, the resulting damage to the brain is always irreversible.
T F   8. There is a definite decrease in the short-term memory of adults over 65.
T F   9. Elderly people do not tolerate pain well.
T F 10. Normal elderly people have no interest in sexual activity.
T F 11. Reminiscing is helpful in adapting to the aging process.
T F 12. Listening to elderly people is an effective way to learn about geriatrics and gerontology.

Chapter 1 ☐ Review Questions

Matching

_____ 1. homeostasis

A. "springiness" of skin

_____ 2. reduced hormone secretion

B. reduced bone mass

_____ 3. osteoporosis

C. sensory deficit

_____ 4. respite care

D. a warning signal to the body

_____ 5. diet

E. environmental cause of aging

_____ 6. turgor

F. fee for service

_____ 7. Medicare

G. body's equilibrium

_____ 8. hearing loss

H. temporary nursing home admission

_____ 9. pain

I. organic change of aging process

_____ 10. proprietary agency

J. federal health insurance

Study Questions

1. Research your community resources and list the names of agencies in your area that provide assistance for older adults in the home. What kinds of services do they offer? Is there a charge for services? How do older adults learn about these resources?

2. What are some safety measures and simple adaptations you would recommend for someone responsible for the home care of a frail elderly person?

□ REFERENCES

Butler, R., and Lewis, M.: Aging and Mental Health. St. Louis, C.V. Mosby Company, 1977, p. 141.

Developments in Aging, 1981: U.S. Senate. A Report of the Special Committee on Aging. Report No. 92-46, U.S. Government Printing Office, Washington, DC, 1981.

National Institutes on Aging, 1980: Epidemiology of Aging (Bethesda, MD: U.S. Department of Health and Human Services).

Objectives	Vocabulary

After completing this chapter, the student should be able to

- [ ] list the indications for home care
- [ ] describe differences among geriatric facilities
- [ ] explain what is meant by levels of care
- [ ] define Medicare and Medicaid and explain their roles in institutionalization
- [ ] design a nursing care plan for a nursing home resident
- [ ] describe the function of an ombudsman

ethnicity
Medicaid
Medicare
ombudsman
Supplementary Security
   Income

CHAPTER 2

Care Facilities for the Elderly

Chapter Outline

☐ Noninstitutional Care

☐ HOME CARE

The need for a decision about the long-term care of an older adult often comes at the end of a period of hospitalization in an acute care hospital. Once the acute problem is resolved, the person or the family, or both, must decide whether he or she can return to the previous mode of living or find an alternative. One of the functions of the professional discharge planner in the hospital is to help the patient and family in making this decision. Placing elders in institutions when there are reasonable alternatives must be avoided. Two alternatives are home care and group living.

Home care assistance is available through a state Area Agency on Aging (See Chapter 1).

Some of the services offered are health screening, homemaking (light housekeeping and meal preparation), chore service (heavy duty household work), mental health, and legal services. Most of these services are free, others have a nominal fee set on a sliding scale.

☐ GROUP LIVING

Congregate Housing and Communal Living

Another alternative to premature and inappropriate nursing home placement is group living, either in congregate housing or in communal living quarters.

Congregate housing is sheltered housing for elderly and handicapped adults. A residential complex is modified to accommodate their needs by installing wide doorways, ramps, low cabinets, and so forth. There is a security guard, and often a physican or nurse is on call for health emergencies.

Communal living simply means a group of people live together and share expenses. Jon A. Larkin, executive director of the Wilmington (Delaware) Senior Center, described an experiment in communal living in *Perspective on Aging* (National Council on Aging, 1980). A family of nine unrelated elderly persons live in a large, three-bathroom duplex. Each resident pays a nominal rent, which entitles him or her to a private bedroom and shared kitchen, living room, sitting room, and bathroom. The rent also includes utilities, two meals a day at the house, and one meal a day at the senior center. The criteria for living in the complex state that an applicant must have an income of less than $7000 a year and that he or she must be committed to the experiment of sharing a home with other people. Mr. Larkin states:

"Those who have worked to develop Brandywine House believe there is great potential for the same or similar alternative living arrangements for older persons:

"Cities can use boarded-up housing for a useful purpose—while preserving an established community. The cost of each project is returned to local government through the required repayment of rehabilitation loans.

"The elderly will no longer be herded into high-rise housing projects that encourage loneliness and introversion. Instead, their independence and outgoing spirit will be encouraged.

"Senior centers, with their wide range of services, will become even more integrated into the lives of the community's older people.

"Brandywine House is ideal for older persons who want their independence at reasonable cost. It may well be the forerunner of similar housing alternatives for the elderly in many other U.S. communities."

There are countless situations in which people have discovered for themselves that two or more can live less expensively when resources are pooled. Congregate housing and communal living are examples of exciting and optimistic innovations for housing the nation's elderly.

Adult Day Care

Adult day care originated about 15 years ago as an offshoot of day care for mentally and emotionally impaired persons.

Elderly adults attend the day care center for part or all of the day. The program may be limited to crafts and social activities, with a hot meal in the

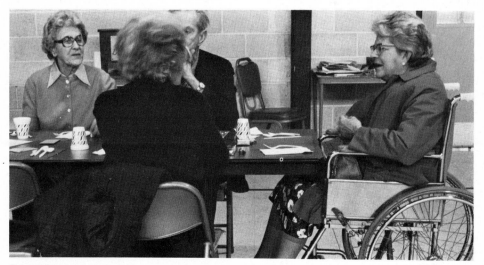

One of the most important contributions of a senior citizens center is that of adding variety to the lives of its participants. (From Dennis and Hassol, p. 267.)

middle of the day, or it may offer all-encompassing care of aged adults. Some centers offer breakfast, personal care (showers and shampoos for those who need this help), and even financial counseling. All of this is done to keep people in their own homes and functioning independently.

Day care centers are found in nursing homes, hospitals, and separate buildings. The residents of nursing homes do not use a day care center even though it may be located in their facility. However, many people who use a nursing home center have a more comfortable transition to the nursing home when this move becomes necessary because they are familiar with the building and the staff.

Admission to a day care center generally must be approved by a physician.

In the next chapter, you will find interviews with a director of an adult day care center and a day care supervisor who runs a program within a nursing home.

☐ Institutional Care

☐ GERIATRIC FACILITIES

Although the general public uses the term "nursing home" to describe any institution that offers health services for older adults, health care professionals are aware that the specific services in nursing homes are not available in all other geriatric facilities. Table 2–1 describes several different geriatric facilities.

Table 2–1 ☐ Defining the Geriatric Facility

Name	Definition
Domiciliary Housing	Units for independent living, social services, occupational/recreational therapy, and group dining provided
Health-Related Facility (HRF)	A recent development in geriatric care for elderly patients who have been rehabilitated in nursing homes, HRF serves those who require some health care services but not 24-hour supervision. Most clients come from domiciliary housing or private homes.
Skilled Nursing Home	The generic nursing home provides 24-hour nursing care, physical/social services, and related programs
Extended Care Facility	Developed through Medicare legislation/funding, it accepts patients discharged from acute care hospital. Skilled nursing and intensive rehabilitation are available.
Geriatric Center	This organization operates under long-term contract to provide housing, social services, and health care. It offers skilled nursing home, health-related accommodation, and domiciliary housing.

□ TYPES OF NURSING HOME CARE

All legitimate nursing homes are licensed and regulated by the state in which they are located. State regulations vary greatly. Nursing homes offer three types of service:

1. Nursing care utilizing the professional skills of nurses as well as physical therapy, diet therapy, and dental services.
2. Personal care, which means assistance with the activities of daily living.
3. Residential care, i.e., giving supervision for self-care residents. Level 4 homes (see box) are often called rest homes. To be eligible for acceptance into a rest home, the applicant must be well and able to take care of himself or herself. Some rest homes are committed to life care of residents. This means that if a resident becomes ill, he or she will be cared for in the home's infirmary, but there are no extraordinary measures—no IVs or respirators, for example. Infirmaries such as these give supportive care—even oxygen—but if more skilled nursing care is needed, the resident must go to a hospital.

All rest home residents are eligible for Medicare. Patients are all private-paying persons. Most rest homes have sliding scales, however, and when social security and pensions don't cover the regular charges, adjustments are made by the home.

There are four levels of nursing home care (see box). Some homes offer only one level and others offer more than one.

Level I. Intensive nursing and rehabilitation care facilities: these facilities provide skilled continuous care and an organized program of restorative services in addition to the minimum basic care and services.

Level II. Skilled nursing care facilities: these facilities provide continuous skilled nursing care and meaningful availability of restorative services and other therapeutic services in addition to the minimum basic care and services. They care for patients who show potential for improvement or restoration to a stabilized condition or who have a deteriorating condition that requires skilled care.

Level III. Supportive nursing care facilities: these facilities provide routine nursing services and periodic availability of skilled nursing, restorative, and other therapeutic services, in addition to the minimum basic care and services. They are for patients whose condition is stabilized to the point that they need only supportive nursing care, supervision, and observation.

Level IV. Resident care facilities: these facilities provide protective supervision in addition to minimum basic care for residents who do not routinely require nursing or other medically related services.

Levels of Care: Basis for the Classification of Long Term Care Facilities

Facilities may provide more than one type of care and are referred to as multi-level. All four levels must provide minimum basic care and services required by the Department of Public Health. Each level must provide social services and organized recreational and activities programs as an integral part of the total health care plan. In addition, each level is expected to utilize public and voluntary agencies in order to promote long-range social and health planning.

Many components enter into the determination, but reduced to simplest terms, the classifications are based on the personnel, the kind of care required (nursing or residential) and the physical plant of the facility.

☐ THE ROLE OF MEDICARE AND MEDICAID

Medicare is a broad program of national health insurance for persons 65 years of age or over that is administered by Social Security. There is a widespread belief that it covers all hospital and nursing expenses for elders, but this is by no means the case. The essential requirements are that a person must be admitted to a Medicare Certified Facility within 14 days of discharge from a hospital where he or she has been a patient for at least 3 days and must require *skilled nursing and rehabilitative care* for the same condition for which he or she was treated in the hospital. The program is subject to legislative and administrative changes, and although substantial help may be given in meeting expenses, eligibility and the extent of entitlement should be carefully checked with the Social Security Office.

Medicaid is a joint federal and state program administered through the Public Welfare Department. Medicaid is available in Level I, II, and III facilities. To qualify, it is not necessary to be receiving other Public Assistance as it is recognized that although some people may not need aid for basic living expenses, they may require financial assistance to meet the heavy cost of medical and nursing care. As in the case of Medicare, the program is subject to legislative and administrative changes, and any questions regarding eligibility should be cleared with public welfare for determination.

☐ PUBLIC ASSISTANCE AND LEVEL IV FACILITIES

Since Level IV facilities provide residential rather than medically related care, the board and room charges may be paid through the Social Security Administration under a federal program known as Supplementary Security Income (SSI). Applications for this benefit are made through the local Social Security office, not the public welfare department. Persons receiving the SSI benefit are automatically eligible for medical assistance. Because the health care provider is often asked about assistance programs by patients and families, it is necessary to be familiar with changing legislation. For specific, accurate information, however, the person should be referred to the appropriate governmental office.

Many facilities are making an encouraging move toward reducing the isolation of those within their confines and bringing them closer to the mainstream of community life. For example, Adult Day Care Centers offer supportive services to participants; arts and crafts, Family Group Therapy, and Meals on Wheels are some instances of programs for nonresidents (Levels of Care Facilities in Massachusetts, 1982).

□ *The Nursing Home Resident*

A profile of a typical nursing home resident would be a female (because 70 per cent of nursing home residents are women), probably afflicted with heart disease, cancer, or chronic brain disorder, or a combination of all three (Aiken, 1978). This woman has become a nursing home resident because she

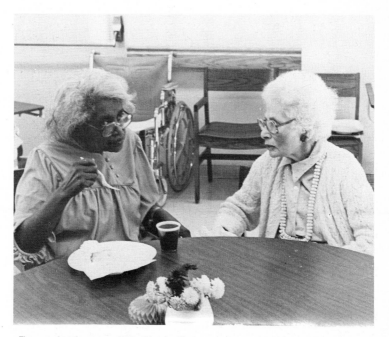

The nursing home resident typically has one or more chronic health problems that make it impossible for her or him to remain at home. Frequently, through good nursing care the person can return home.

requires continual supervision and extensive nursing care. Perhaps she has become confused, disoriented. She may also be incontinent. She no longer is able to live independently, and family members are not able to assume the responsibility of her care.

Often, the nursing home resident improves because of quality care, attention to nutrition, bowel and bladder training, and the distinct social advantage of being able to interact with other people.

☐ Choosing the Right Facility

Before making the arrangements for institutional care in either a nursing or rest home, other choices should be weighed, such as homemaker or home health aide assistance, Meals on Wheels, shopping and chore service, adult day care, and congregate or shared housing. There is a network of supportive services available to elders that may make it possible for a person to continue to live independently.

If, after weighing each alternative, nursing home care appears to be the appropriate solution, the physician or hospital must determine the level of care needed. Once this basic medical determination has been made, there are other factors to be carefully evaluated, not only physical needs but also personal, social, and emotional needs of the individual. There are wide variations in the quality of the facilities within a given level, and one facility may provide a better answer to these needs than another.

It is essential that there is personal and family involvement in the final selection. If, however, a person is not able to act on his or her own behalf or if no relative is available, the physician, hospital, or local social agency may be able to give the assistance needed.

After medical and personal decisions have been made, the location of the facility and the flexibility of the visiting hours are important factors in an individual's adjustment to institutional living. Is it near enough for family or friends to visit frequently? Those who are ambulatory will want to know if the facility is close to transportation, church, library, and other cultural and recreational resources and if it is close to shopping.

Geriatric facilities, just like people, have their own characteristics. A small, quiet home with an informal atmosphere may appeal to one person, whereas a larger facility where more activity is going on may be better suited to another person.

For a person who speaks or understands little or no English, it is a great morale lifter if someone on the staff can speak or understand his or her native language. In selecting a facility, it is necessary to know what is available. Many facilities should be visited before making a final choice. This is the most reliable way to find out which one is most likely to meet one's personal needs and interests.

□ EVALUATING THE NURSING HOME

Features to check include the following:
1. a current state nursing home license?
2. a current administrator's license?
3. special services (hairdresser, barber, podiatrist)?
4. financial assistance program?
5. location
   a. near a hospital?
   b. convenient for family?
6. hazards
   a. lighting—is it adequate?
   b. safety rails—are they located in bathrooms and corridors?
   c. federal and state fire safety codes—are they enforced?
7. bedrooms
   a. are there four or fewer residents to a room?
   b. are call bells, fresh drinking water, reading lights by all beds?
   c. individual clothes closets and drawers?
8. cleanliness and lack of unpleasant odors
9. kitchens—are there separate areas for food preparation, dishwashing, and garbage disposal?
10. activity rooms?
11. examination rooms?
12. general atmosphere
   a. convenient visiting hours?
   b. does staff call patients by name?
13. services
   a. is a physician available in an emergency?
   b. is physical therapy available?
   c. is a speech therapist available?
14. activities (group and individual)
   a. do patients go on outside trips?
   b. are there volunteers in the home?

□ FINANCIAL AGREEMENTS

All financial agreements must be in writing. There are several ways to meet financial requirements: social security payments, personal assets, welfare assistance, health insurance, and Medicare/Medicaid.

□ FAMILY REACTIONS TO NURSING HOME PLACEMENT

There are several principles that guide nursing practice in long-term-care facilities. Knowledge of the aging process, effects of illness and institutional-

HERITAGE HALL NURSING HOME NURSING HISTORY AND ASSESSMENT

PATIENT'S NAME: _____ FILE NO.: _____

DATE OF ADMISSION: _____ LEVEL OF CARE: _____

HEALTH HISTORY: From Referral and Physician

Current Diagnosis: _____

Past Diagnosis: _____

Pertinent Lab. Findings: _____ Medications: _____

_____   _____

Allergies: _____   _____

SENSORY AND COMMUNICATION:

| Hearing Loss: | YES | NO | Vision: | YES | NO |

Hearing Loss: YES | NO   Vision: YES | NO

    Left Ear: _____ | _____   Glasses: _____ | _____

    Rt. Ear: _____ | For Reading: _____ |

    Both: _____ | All Day: _____ |

    Hear/Aid: _____ | Special Eye Care: _____ |

        Type: _____   Specify: _____

    Provision for Batteries: _____   Last Eye Exam: _____

    Communication: Speech: _____   Able to Read: YES _____   NO _____

        Able to Write: YES _____   NO _____   RT. _____   LT. _____   HAND

        Attention and Memory Span: _____

_____

        Judgment: _____

NUTRITIONAL STATUS: Admitting Wt.: _____ Approx. Height: _____

    Overweight: _____ Underweight: _____ Losing Wt. _____ Gaining Wt. _____

CARDIOVASCULAR STATUS:	**RESPIRATORY STATUS:**	**SKIN CONDITION:**
Pulse Rate: _____	Rate of Resp.: _____	Appearance: _____
Blood Pressure: _____	Shortness of Breath: _____	Edema Present: _____
Postural Hypotension:_____	Cyanosis: _____	Ulcer: _____
Angina: _____	Cough: _____	Rash: _____
Other: _____	Other: _____	Wound: _____
		Other: _____
_____	Does Pt. Smoke: _____	_____

JOINT RANGE OF MOTION: Limited or Normal RA__ LA__ RL__ LL__ Paralysis__ Contractures__

BLADDER AND BOWEL FUNCTIONS:

    Bowel: Continent ____ Incontinent ____ Colostomy ____ Comments: _____

        Laxatives (specify) _____ Enemas _____ Frequency _____

    Bladder: Continent: ____ Incontinent: __ __ Foley: ____ Other: _____

SAFETY NEEDS: Siderails _____ Restraints (type): _____

DO NOT REMOVE FROM CHART

Figure 2–1 ☐ Nursing home nursing history and assessment. (Courtesy of Heritage Hall Nursing Home.)

Illustration continued on opposite page

LEVEL OF FUNCTIONAL INDEPENDENCE

A. HYGIENE   YES | NO   COMMENTS   **BATHING**   YES | NO

Brushes teeth _____|_____   _____   Upper Body _____|_____

Oral Care _____|_____   _____   Lower Body _____|_____

Applies Cosmetics _____|_____   _____   Back _____|_____

Shaves _____|_____   _____   Comments: _____

Hair Grooming _____|_____   _____   _____

Toilet Hygiene _____|_____   _____   _____

Other _____|_____   _____   _____

DRESSING   YES | NO   COMMENTS   **EATING**   YES | NO

Shoes _____|_____   _____   Diet-Special Needs _____|_____

Stockings _____|_____   _____   Feed self _____|_____

Underclothes _____|_____   _____   Dentures _____|_____

Pants/Slacks _____|_____   _____   Comments: _____

Shirt/blouse _____|_____   _____   _____

Other _____|_____   _____   _____

B. MOBILITY—LOCOMOTION

Bed Mobility YES | NO   **Transfer** YES | NO   **Ambulation** YES | NO

Turns self _____|_____   Dangle _____|_____   Self _____|_____

Comes to sitting   Pivot _____|_____   Device _____|_____

position _____|_____   Stand _____|_____   Assist Persons(s) _____|_____

Comments: _____

_____

_____

EMOTIONAL—SOCIAL—RECREATIONAL

1. A. Feeling about present situation: nursing home/hospital; illness _____

_____

B. Family relationships: _____

_____

2. A. Orientation and Understanding: _____

_____

B. Social Attitude: _____

_____

C. Type of activity (bed-group-limited): _____

_____

D. Problem List: (carry over to Plan of Care) _____

_____

_____

DATE: _____   SIGNED: _____ R.N.

Figure 2–1 *Continued*

ization on the aged patient, and adaptation of textbook procedures and nursing routines to meet individual needs are some of the obvious ones. The skilled geriatric nurse is also aware that many families responsible for the supervision of frail or ill older adults recoil when nursing home placement is suggested. They dread the idea of putting their spouse or parent in what they fear may be a cheerless institution with indifferent personnel. Patience, reassurance, and counseling are additional nursing responsibilities.

☐ Admission to the Nursing Home

☐ NURSING HISTORY

When a patient is admitted to a long-term-care facility, a thorough assessment of the patient's physical condition and level of functioning is made. Depending on the specific facility, the assessment of the patient is conducted by staff members from several disciplines, including a physical therapist, occupational therapist, social services representative, and physician. Usually an interdisciplinary meeting is held to discuss the patient's needs and to plan a comprehensive program. As part of the holistic assessment of the patient, a nursing history is taken and, from this, a nursing care plan is developed.

The nursing history collects data in a structured, organized way. It should be flexible and should be designed to illustrate the needs of the patient and to fit the requirements of the particular health care agency that admits the patient. It is helpful if the family can also be interviewed. If the patient is brain damaged or comatose and no family cooperation can be obtained, no history is taken.

It isn't always easy to gather information for a nursing history from an elderly person. It requires sensitivity, and good communication skills on the part of the interviewer, especially if the patient cannot hear well. About 25 per cent of persons over 65 have some hearing impairment. In such cases, the interviewer should position herself so that the person being questioned can see her or his lips and eyes. If the patient is profoundly deaf, it may be necessary to resort to writing.

The interviewer should be aware that a patient's vocabulary may not be the same as his or her own. If the interviewer asks, "How often do you void?" the patient may look blank. "How often do you urinate or pass water?" may be language more suitable for some individuals.

When asking about medications, be sure that the patient understands that these include over-the-counter drugs as well as prescriptions.

Gathering data is an important first step in developing effective plans of care, but some questions may be interpreted as being intrusive. Avoid making the patient feel uncomfortable. Allow enough time to gain the patient's confidence. After all, the quesions can be postponed for a while and can even be asked informally while assisting the patient with the activities of daily living.

☐ NURSING CARE PLANS

Most hospitals and long-term-care facilities have nursing care plans. These are designs for the patient's care based on a summary of the patient's problems, suggested approaches to the problems, and an evaluation of the action to be taken. The nursing team, the patient's family, and sometimes various resource persons (dietitians, physical therapists, and so on) contribute to the care plan. The physician is chiefly concerned with the patient's medical diagnosis and treatment, although often he or she is an important resource person.

Nursing care plans should be dynamic and constantly changing to meet the changing needs of the patient. Although every health care agency has a different method of maintaining care plans (kardexes and looseleaf books are often used), they all share one common problem: keeping the plans up to date. This can be done daily or at the end of each shift. In some states, interdisciplinary meetings are required regularly to revise and update plans of care.

☐ *Patient's Rights*

Human rights is a sensitive issue. Wars have been fought to defend dignity; people have died defending their integrity. In the past 25 years awareness of individual rights has been highlighted by the civil rights movement, the women's movement, and consumer action groups. Passionate belief in individual rights has at times resulted in protests, political action, and even violence.

☐ WHAT IS A RIGHT?

By "right" we mean something enforceable in a court of law. Where there is a right there is a corresponding duty that can be legally enforced.

When patients are admitted to a hospital or nursing home, they forfeit certain freedoms. For example, they lose the freedom of mobility because they may not wander in and out of hospital rooms or from floor to floor. A hospital gown is substituted for their own clothing. Unfortunately, sometimes a room number is even substituted for their name. (Have you ever heard a nurse say, "X-ray just called for 320B"?) Meals are served at the convenience of the hospital and even bedtimes seem to be scheduled. Obviously, there must be structure and regulation in patient care or chaos would result. However, patients have the right to determine how they are to be treated.

In 1972, the Division of Nursing of the American Hospital Association presented, for the first time anywhere, a Patients' Bill of Rights. The preamble states "These rights will be supported by the hospital on behalf of its patients as an integral part of the healing process. It is recognized that a personal rela-

HERITAGE HALL NURSING HOME PLAN OF CARE

PATIENT'S NAME: _____ FILE NO.: _____

INTERDISCIPLINARY MEETING HELD—DATE: _____

PRESENT AT MEETING—SIGNATURE: _____

_____

_____

_____

_____

OVERALL PLAN OF CARE AND GOALS: _____

_____

_____

_____

_____

DATE	PROBLEM	GOAL	APPROACH	DISCIPLINE RESPONSIBLE	DATE RESOLVED

DO NOT REMOVE FROM CHART

Figure 2–2 ☐ Nursing home plan of care. (Courtesy of Heritage Hall Nursing Home.)

HERITAGE HALL NURSING HOME—NURSING CARE FLOW SHEET

	MONTH/YEAR DATE:	SUN			MON			TUES			WED			THURS			FRI			SAT		
	SHIFT:	N	D	E	N	D	E	N	D	E	N	D	E	N	D	E	N	D	E	N	D	E
HYGIENE	BATH: B-BED T-TUB S-SHOWER																					
	C-COMP A-ASST S-SELF																					
	SPECIAL SKIN CARE																					
	MOUTH CARE																					
	SHAVE (A-AIDE OR P-PT)																					
	SHAMPOO																					
	PERI CARE																					
	MANICURE																					
DRESS	DRESS: C-COMP A-ASST S-SELF																					
	UNDRESS: C-COMP A-ASST S-SELF																					
AMBULATE	AMBULATES: DISTANCE																					
	S-SELF A-ASST W-WALKER																					
	WHEELCHAIR																					
	BED TO CHAIR																					
	BED REST																					
REST	SLEPT: ALL SHIFT																					
	AT INTERVALS																					
	NOT AT ALL																					
SAFETY	RESTRAINT: W-WAIST O-OTHER																					
	GERI-CHAIR																					
	RELEASED EVERY 2 HRS																					
	SIDERAILS UP																					
MENTAL STATUS	ORIENTED (TIME, PLACE, PERSON)																					
	DISORIENTED																					
RESTORATIVE BY N.A.	BOWEL & BLADDER TRAINING																					
	ROM ACTIVE																					
	ROM PASSIVE																					
	ADL TRAINING																					
ACTIVITY	VISITORS																					
	ATTENDED ACTIVITIES																					
	OUT FOR DAY / OVERNIGHT																					
	PHYSICAL THERAPY																					
	HAIRDRESSER / BARBER																					
ELIMINATION	CONTINENT: BLADDER																					
	BOWEL																					
	INCONTINENT: BLADDER																					
	BOWEL																					
	FOLEY CATHETER (YES / NO)																					
	COLOSTOMY (FOR BM)																					
		B	D	S	B	D	S	B	D	S	B	D	S	B	D	S	B	D	S	B	D	S
NUTRITION	ATE: ROOM																					
	FEEDING GROUP																					
	DINING ROOM																					
	WITHOUT ASSIST																					
	ASSIST																					
	FED																					
	ATE SOLIDS: INDICATE A / ALL; P / PARTIAL; N/NONE																					
	DRANK LIQUIDS: INDICATE A / ALL; P / PARTIAL; N / NONE																					
	BETWEEN MEAL LIQUIDS*																					
	BETWEEN MEAL FEEDINGS*																					
	COMMENT ON NURSE'S PROGRESS NOTE																					
	*"R" IF REFUSED																					

FURTHER COMMENTS TO BE MADE ON NURSE'S PROGRESS NOTE

PATIENT'S NAME: _____ RM.: _____ DR. _____ FILE NO.: _____

Figure 2–3 □ Nursing care flow sheet. (Courtesy of Heritage Hall Nursing Home.)

tionship between the physician and the patient is essential for the provision of proper medical care." Patients' rights rest on these basic premises.

☐ GUARDING PRIVACY

There are still daily violations. For example, one of the rights listed in the Patients' Bill of Rights reads: "The patient has the right to every consideration of his privacy concerning his own medical care program. Case discussion . . . [is] confidential and should be conducted discreetly." Yet, Mrs. Y, a 65-year-old arthritic, was on her way to the X-ray Department in a large, modern medical center. She asked the young man wheeling her to stop at the nurses' station so she could ask for something for pain. Her physician was at the desk and overheard the request. He walked over to the patient and said, "Look, you have had enough medicine for the time being. I think you're making a mountain out of a molehill! You're not going to have anything more at this time." The patient was humiliated and even the orderly transporting the patient was embarrassed.

Another right reads: "The patient has a right to considerate and respectful care." However, in one 400-bed chronic care facility, patients who can stand are bathed standing at a sink in their rooms. Those awaiting tub baths are stripped naked and placed in a wheelchair, clutching a skimpy bath blanket to cover themselves. They wait in line in a drafty corridor until it is their turn to be bathed. Nurses are responsible for the actions of ancillary personnel. Affronts to dignity and lack of respect are direct violations of patients' rights. The supervising nurse can be held liable.

"The patient has a right to obtain from his physician complete and current information concerning his diagnosis, treatment and prognosis in terms he can be reasonably expected to understand." Yet, often a patient's query about his diagnosis or treatment is met with cliches such as, "Let me do the worrying," or "It's nothing for you to be concerned with," or with bewildering medical jargon.

☐ RIGHTING THE WRONGS

"Too little time," "not enough help," and "too many patients" have long been offered as excuses for the indignities and discomforts inflicted on patients. Since the Bill of Rights was first issued in 1972, hospitals and nursing homes all over the country have either adopted it or designed their own versions.

But there are still problems, and enforcement is difficult. Some states set fines for violations, but violations are not always easy to prove. Elsewhere, ombudsmen (officials empowered to investigate complaints about injustices or abuses) are the voices who speak for patients.

No document will ensure careful, considerate treatment for patients. Only people can do that. Health care professionals must work together to recognize the dignity of the individual.

☐ NURSING HOME OMBUDSMAN

In the early 1970s, the Department of Health, Education and Welfare introduced the concept of advocacy groups for nursing home residents. Each state has a Department of Elder Affairs and nursing home ombudsmen whose purpose is to investigate and resolve the complaints of nursing home residents.

This is where state uniformity ends, however. The state office may have ties on a municipal level with a Council of Churches, a Council on Aging, or a Home Care Corporation that, in turn, uses salaried or volunteer persons to fulfill advocacy goals.

A nursing home ombudsman is a person who visits one or more nursing homes at least once a week for the purposes of getting to know the patients and staff, assessing the nursing home environment, and identifying problems in patient care. In talking to nursing home residents, the ombudsman is available to receive complaints. Problems are discussed with the nursing home administrator, the director of nursing, or both. Problems that cannot be resolved by the nursing home staff are submitted to a coordinator of ombudsmen. Complaints received and the actions taken to resolve them are recorded on standardized forms.

Ombudsmen are given a training course during which some basic differences between nursing homes and hospitals are stressed. One difference is that the nursing home resident has a much longer stay than a hospital patient with a resulting greater social isolation that causes a need for emotional attachment to persons other than staff and fellow residents.

Ombudsmen are counseled to keep relationships friendly but professional and to respect the confidentiality of the patients and their diagnosis and treatments. They avoid criticism of the home, its personnel, and its policies, and they offer support and loyalty in a dignified, cordial, and business-like manner.

☐ *Geriatric Care Abroad*

A look at long-term care in other countries can be useful to those of us interested in the aged. Europe has faced many of the same problems that affect geriatric care in this country. Lack of security in the big cities, the breakdown of the extended family, and economic instability are all factors that have influenced the rapid development of health care in the last few decades.

Great Britain, Denmark, and Sweden are countries that have implemented alternative noninstitutional living arrangements that have helped to solve many geriatric problems.

Before it instituted the National Health Service in 1949, England had a dismal record of caring for the elderly ill. They simply admitted old people to hospitals, kept them confined to beds, and, in most cases, did not treat them. Eventually these people died from either the primary illness or secondary problems.

Sweden had most of their elderly confined to poorhouses or nursing homes until the 1950's, when they developed alternative living arrangements for the aged. These include

- Loans to help modify an elderly person's home to accommodate disabilities.
- Housing allowances to permit elderly persons to select housing best suited to their needs.
- Pensioner hotels, some with supervision.
- Homes with continuous supervision and nursing service.

Denmark had a centuries' old tradition of taking care of their sick and aged relations at home. It was considered disgraceful to receive aid. That changed with various governmental policies in the early 1900's, and in the 1960's more sophisticated geriatric care was developed, for example, day care.

Two innovative European ideas are floating beds and rotating beds. Floating beds are beds that are held in a hospital for a limited period of time so that those who are caring for an elderly or infirm person can receive much-needed relief. Rotating beds are beds reserved in a hospital also. The family shares care with the hospital by having the patient at home for 6 weeks, then in the hospital for 6 weeks, then back in the home for another 6 weeks, and so on. When the system of rotating beds is used, efforts are extended to the family to encourage home care, i.e., certain remodeling (perhaps widening doorways to receive wheelchairs and installation of special plumbing) is paid for.

Many European countries recognize that geriatrics is a demanding speciality and, to attract competent and sufficient personnel in this discipline, a salary differential is offered.

Chapter 2 ☐ Review Questions

DISCUSSION QUESTIONS

1. Many families experience severe guilt when they have made the decision to institutionalize an elderly relative. How can the nurse help the family deal constructively with this problem?
2. Mrs. X, 79, lived alone and independently until she fell at home and fractured her hip. She is now recovering from surgery in a hospital from which

she will soon be discharged to a nursing home. Circumstances are such that nursing home placement will most likely be permanent.

What physical and emotional problems can the nurse anticipate?

What discharge planning can help ease the transfer from the hospital to the nursing home?

3. As a clinical component of Chapter 2, select an elderly medical/surgical patient to follow through discharge from the hospital. Research the discharge planning. Will your patient go home? Are support services needed? List and explain.

a. If your patient is going to a nursing home, why? What are the advantages? Disadvantages?

b. As a variation of this project, you might select a nursing home resident and investigate the circumstances that led to placement. Do you see alternatives? If so, why were they not used?

TRUE/FALSE

_____ 1. Medicare is a national health insurance that is administered by the Department of Public Welfare.

_____ 2. Adults over 65 automatically qualify for Medicaid.

_____ 3. A Level IV facility may be correctly termed residential.

_____ 4. Guilt is the most common reaction of families when they place a family member in a nursing home.

_____ 5. Alternative living arrangements for elders who need care are severely limited.

_____ 6. Nursing care plans are seldom used in long-term-care facilities.

_____ 7. An ombudsman investigates and resolves complaints of nursing home residents while maintaining strict confidentiality.

_____ 8. Leaving a patient uncovered while giving him or her a bath is an invasion of privacy and therefore a violation of his or her rights.

_____ 9. Patient's rights is a recent issue with no past history.

_____ 10. Communication skills are an important part of obtaining a nursing history.

☐ REFERENCES

Aiken, L.: Later Life. Philadelphia, W.B. Saunders Company, 1978, p. 154.

Levels of Care Facilities in Massachusetts, 1982. A social services publication of the Women's Educational and Industrial Union.

Perspectives on Aging, 1980. National Council on the Aging, Inc.

Objectives	Vocabulary

After completing this chapter, the student should be able to

- ☐ identify therapeutic goals in long-term-care settings
- ☐ list stereotypes of older adults
- ☐ define ageism
- ☐ describe reasons for the loss of interpersonal skills by elders
- ☐ discuss the principles of communication and relate them to the special needs of the older person
- ☐ list members of the rehabilitation team and describe the purpose of the team
- ☐ identify goals of rehabilitation for the elderly

Vocabulary

articulation
aural
heterogeneous
homogeneous
incontinence
psychologic
physiatrist
physiologic
rehabilitation

CHAPTER *3*

Relationships Between Elders and Caregivers

□ *Elders and Illness*

Nursing care of the aged implies care of the chronically ill and long-term treatment. The goals are not the same as those for nursing care of acutely ill patients in the general hospital setting. Only a small percentage of the chronically ill will get well enough to live independently of any supportive services.

Health problems are far more common among the elderly than among younger adults. Chronic disabling conditions occur more frequently and are likely to persist for longer periods of time than among those who are younger. In 1980, nearly half (45 per cent) of all noninstitutionalized persons aged 65 and over were reported to have a chronic health condition that limited their activities (Burnside, 1984). In contrast, less than a quarter (24 per cent) of those ranging in age from 45 to 64 and only 1 in 16 (7 per cent) of those younger than 45 were so limited.

Acute conditions, defined as those conditions lasting less than 3 months and involving medical attention or activity restriction, occurred less frequently but were responsible for more days of disability among the elderly than among those under age 65. In 1980, persons 65 years of age or older averaged 1.1 episodes of disability from acute conditions, compared with 8.8 days of restricted activity and 3.6 days of bed confinement for those in the 45 to 64 age range, and 10 days of restricted activity and 4.5 days of bed confinement among those under 45 years of age. For each episode of illness, those who were 65 years of age or older averaged 9.3 days of restricted activity (Burnside, 1984).

□ *Attitudes of Caregivers*

There is a relationship between attitudes of caregivers and characteristics of the elderly. These attitudes surface in acute care settings as well as in long-term care.

Therapeutic goals in long-term-care settings often are limited to preventing or retarding further physiologic or mental deterioration, or both. Aggressive rehabilitation and dramatic responses are infrequent. The responsiveness of many elderly patients needing intermediate or skilled care often is so minimal that even the most persevering caregiver may become frustrated and discouraged.

Fewer than 20 per cent of the people employed primarily or solely in programs that are specific for the care of elders have had formal training. The number of health care professionals who are knowledgeable about the aging process and who have the special skills of caring for the elderly is sadly inadequate. (Burnside, 1984).

Caregivers in nursing homes often indicate that older adults are slow, hard to deal with. They become annoyed with elders' complaining, incontinence, lack of self feeding, and lack of appreciation. These attitudes often reflect social stereotyping. Some of these stereotypes are that aged persons are slow (mentally), generally ill, tired, unproductive, and defensive (Heller and Walsh, 1976).

The unfavorable regard of older adults extends into acute care settings. There is a view of elders as a homogeneous group of invalids sitting out their days as spectators in life. This type of thinking leads toward custodial care, in which the caregiver values being nice to the patient rather than aggressively using all available resources necessary to restore the patient to optimal health and functioning.

The fact is that older adult populations are heterogeneous. They include biologically superior individuals who will enjoy a middle age that extends into their nineties. Other older people will have many health problems; most of them will make adaptations in their lifestyles and environments that will allow them to lead independent lives. Still other older adults will have relatively minor health or social problems but great deficits in functional skills. Health professionals must remember that a 75-year-old person has an average life expectancy of 10.4 years. Consequently they can aim to maintain or improve functional ability during those 10 years (Paniccuci, 1983).

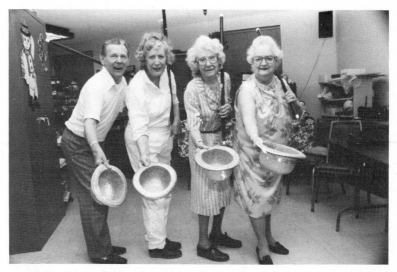

The nursing home can provide companionship and activities for the elderly. (Courtesy of Ring Nursing Homes.)

☐ Ageism

By ageism we mean negative attitudes and practices that discriminate against the aged (Lilliard, 1982). If society values youth over age, there is both a social and an economic emphasis on youth-oriented goals. This emphasis is communicated through special interest groups to legislators who control federal funding, and educational institutions seeking federal monies design curricula and programs to satisfy the legislative charge. Thus, new nurses can be influenced by society's values.

New nursing school graduates are seen to choose areas of nursing that are perceived as having higher status, such as intensive care units and emergency rooms. Caring, in the sense of providing on-going support to elderly patients who have no chance of cure, is given low priority (Paniccuci, 1983).

The medical profession also has been reluctant to devote study and energy on behalf of the geriatric patient. There is a dearth of material on geriatrics in medical school curricula, and geriatrics is the least preferred medical specialty.

The irony is that the older adult owes increased life expectancy to the very health professions who hold aging in low esteem.

☐ Loss of Interpersonal Skills

Many ill elderly persons are demanding, self centered, and unappreciative. They show little interest in those around them: nurses, family, and other patients. There are a number of physiologic and psychologic reasons why interpersonal skills deteriorate in the ill elderly.

Sensory deficits, declining strength, and loss of spouse and friends all contribute toward an ill older adult's negative feelings and responses. An understanding of these reasons may decrease the relationship between the patient's ability or willingness to respond in a friendly, cooperative, appreciative manner and the caregiver's feelings about providing nursing care. Education about aging and pathology combined with articulation of attitudes toward individual patients could lead to awareness of the possible relationship between attitudes and care given. It could also lead to more sensitive and compassionate nursing (Elliot and Hybertson, 1982).

☐ Communication

Sensory losses in general are major impediments in nurse-patient communication. Communicating effectively is basic to understanding the elderly. A review of the communication process follows.

There are four basic elements in the process of communication:
1. the sender
2. the message
3. the channel
4. the receiver

By applying the principles of communication with an understanding of the special needs of the elderly, the nurse can ensure better communication.

The sender may communicate through speech, writing, gestures, posture, and facial expressions. Whatever channel the sender is using, the message must be clear. If the message is not clear—either because of noise, interference, distraction, or language barrier—the communication process will break down.

The channel selected (verbal, written, or nonverbal) must be appropriate to the message. For example, a long list of instructions to an elderly patient would best be communicated in writing, with the most important ones reinforced verbally. If there is interference with the receiver, the communication process will again be ineffective. A person's emotional state, physical discomfort, level of consciousness, and age-related changes must be taken into consideration to ensure effective communication.

When working with the aged, allow for visual or aural deficits, or both, diminished pace, and a slowed reaction time in order to communicate appropriately. Be sure the person has his or her eyeglasses on and that they are clean. Hearing aids should be kept in the same safe place (with extra batteries) so that they are accessible. Allow the elderly person time to process the message and to respond.

Sensory deficits, language barriers, haste, and misunderstanding contribute to poor communication. Moreover, facial expressions, gestures, and body movements speak volumes. Nonverbal signs of communication strongly influence the ability to convey warmth and understanding qualities caregivers must have.

☐ *Rehabilitation*

Rehabilitation begins when the patient enters the hospital. The goal of caregivers is to encourage independence. Today, the patient who enters the acute care setting is likely to be an older adult, often over 75, with multisystem physiologic and, possibly, social problems (Panicucci, 1983). There are some health professionals who feel that these elders do not have the rehabilitative opportunities readily available to younger patients. This age discrimination is said to result from the attitude held by some caregivers that elders have less important reasons for being rehabilitated or maintained at their present functioning level.

More and more, health care professionals are recognizing the potential for rehabilitating elders. Ideally, the rehabilitation team is headed by physiatrist, a doctor whose specialty is rehabilitation and who is therefore prepared in physical, emotional, social, and economic aspects of rehabilitation. Other members of the team are physical/occupational/speech/recreational therapists, audiologist, social worker, psychiatrist, rehabilitation nurse and vocational rehabilitation counselor.

In developing a plan of care, the team gathers data about the patient's health status and functional ability before hospitalization or institutionalization. Data are also gathered about lifestyle goals, daily living activities, desired levels of independence, relationships with others, and the effects of environmental factors. The family is an integral part of the plan because most older adults value family ties and have come to depend on family members for assistance in long-term care.

Developing an acceptable level of activity is challenging when the patient will not be able to maintain the previous level of functioning. Attention should be placed on adapting the environment to meet the patient's needs: changing the location of the patient in the home, for example. Perhaps a dining room could be made to serve as a bedroom if the patient is not able to climb stairs. In this instance, the patient would be offered an opportunity for optimal independence in accordance with the level of function.

☐ Elders, Geriatric Nursing, and the Future

Despite the fact that the elderly population is steadily increasing, nursing's interest in geriatrics remains low. This is of particular concern, considering that 85 per cent of the elderly have at least one chronic illness and that 70 per cent of all acute care hospital beds are occupied by elderly persons (Tollett and Adamson, 1982). This population has grown faster during the 20th century than any other segment of the population and can be expected to do so until the first third of the next century!

Although there has been research exploring the need for geriatric/gerontologic content in curricula, there has been little research indicating how the content should be implemented. Some educators think that gerontology content should be placed in specific courses and others feel that integration throughout the curriculum is best.

Fortunately, virtually all agree that a background in geriatrics is necessary for nurses. Positive attitude, absence of stereotyping, and innovative teaching methods will benefit the vast numbers of aged patients who seek health care.

Working with elders can be frustrating, but it is also potentially very rewarding. Many elders are weak, deteriorating in body and spirit. They experience feelings of rejection, depression, and bitterness. The geriatric nurse needs skill and energy to help elders ventilate their feelings in order to respond to their complex needs.

Older adults have different backgrounds and disabilities, but they all share some common needs: understanding, acceptance, and the knowledge that someone cares. By improving the understanding of long-term-care patients and upgrading the care of the ill elderly we ensure our own care in the future.

☐ *Personal Points of View*

The following are interviews with health care professionals whose specialty is geriatric nursing.

☐ INTERVIEW WITH A NURSING HOME ADMINISTRATOR

"There are four main reasons why people are admitted to nursing homes: either the patient is living in an undesirable situation, which can mean he is

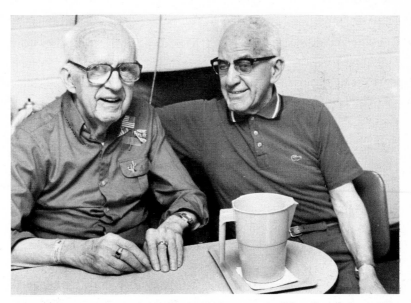

Close friendships often develop in long-term-care facilities. They truly can be "homes" to many residents. (Courtesy of Crescent Hill Nursing Center, Springfield, Massachusetts.)

living with a married son or daughter who doesn't want him, or he is living in a rundown apartment, or simply that he is unable to manage at home. *Or*, the patient is placed here by a son or daughter (maybe with great reluctance). Now the reaction from the person who comes from an undesirable situation is positive. This place [indicates his nursing home] looks like heaven after what he's been living with. But the patient who is *placed* here has a definite negative reaction. That patient feels he's been committed.

"We recognize that placement is difficult for both parents and children (and in some cases, spouses). We try to ease the transition from hospital or private home to nursing home as much as possible. The prospective resident is visited in the hospital by a social worker and a registered nurse. They objectively assess the elderly person. Then we have an orientation for patient and family. We also have monthly meetings with the families of our residents in groups; at these meetings we attempt to raise and examine any problems that the families may be facing.

"It's important to recognize that most families have great ambivalence about placement. They are almost invariably torn between feelings of relief and guilt when the placement is made.

"We have a supportive staff here. They realize that families as well as residents need encouragement. You know, the days are gone where a nurse was lowering herself to work in a nursing home. We consider geriatrics a dynamic specialty. Every once in a while we have a nurse or attendant leave because they are unsuited to this type of nursing. It's not dramatic work and our patients don't get better. Rarely is anyone discharged. The plain fact is that our patients *die*. Most of them die—unlike those in a hospital who recover and are discharged."

The administrator was asked how he handled the situation of having a resident admitted to an acute care facility for care.

"This is a problem and about the only way to deal with it is the way our resident physician does. We get them into the hospital, have the problem taken care of, and get them back to the home as fast as possible. If we don't, we see confusion where there previously was no confusion. We see instant senility. It's very destructive. We have to face the fact that nursing home patients don't do well in hospitals if they have to stay there too long."

☐ INTERVIEW WITH A WOMAN WHO PLACED HER MOTHER IN A NURSING HOME

This interesting story is about a woman with arteriosclerosis and how her disease progressed from occasional forgetfulness to dangerously inappropriate behavior. Reading this should provide insight into some of the stress, frustration, and anxiety endured by family members as they observe the inevitable deterioration of an aged parent.

"To look at my mother you couldn't imagine a thing wrong with her. Outwardly she was a beautiful woman. But she had arteriosclerosis from the time she was just 62 years of age. I guess you could say it killed off her brain cells. She became forgetful. Very forgetful. As long as my father was alive he used to cover up for her, so we didn't notice it too much. At least not to the point where we did anything but joke about it.

"I used to bring all my clothes to her to be altered. One day I saw that she had unaccountably sheared off about three inches from a very expensive dress. That was my first indication that there was something really wrong with my mother. It was horrendous, both for me and for my father. You see, there was a 15-year age difference between them and my father always hovered over mother. When she became 'ill,' he took care of her like you would a retarded child . . . with tenderness, love, and protection. But then he died very suddenly. So, what was to become of mother? They had lived together for over 40 years in the home we were raised in. A big 12-room house. That house was their 'roots' and it seemed cruel to change things. But my brother and I had to face the fact that there was a serious problem. At this time we were both against the idea of a nursing home. In fact, it was unthinkable. We were busy enough selling the home and all the furnishings and accumulation of 40 years.

"Well, I decided that I could take care of her. I was working at the time but I decided to cut down to four days a week. I would take mother from Thursday to Monday and then my brother and his wife would take over the rest of the time.

"My sister-in-law had a job, too, and one day she came home to find that mother had taken all the drapes down and had hidden them. Then she'd forget that she'd eaten and would go to the refrigerator and eat enormous quantities. She'd eat seven meals a day and slowly she got enormously heavy. She was always accusing them of not giving her anything to eat.

"Another time she hid my husband's wallet. We had a terrible time trying to find it. Then she had a temper tantrum when I suggested she wear a hat to some function we had to attend. She actually threw the hat out of the window. All this was thoroughly uncharacteristic behavior for my mother. After all, my mother had been an impeccably dressed woman—every hair in place, weekly manicures. My mother never had a crooked seam or anything less than immaculately white gloves. Now it didn't bother her to wear the same dress five days in a row—food stains, ripped hems, torn stockings. It was very upsetting to all of us. It became such an emotional issue that we were forced to consider alternatives. We decided she wasn't bad enough for a regular nursing home, so we put her in a rest home. It was a mistake, but we didn't realize that until later.

"The home looked cozy enough and Mother had a nice room with a radio, TV, and attractive furnishings. But she'd wear the same dress every day until I came to change it. Of course I'd go four or five times a week to do her laundry, change her clothing, and kind of supervise. But it wasn't working out. There were 12 women residents and one attendant. It was perfectly fine for people who had their wits about them (they had room and board) but for my mother, well, she needed closer watching. If I didn't give her a bath she wouldn't have one. If I didn't dress her she'd wear the same thing all the time. Things came to a head when one day I took her shopping and got the shock of my life when she undressed. Her slip was dirty and everything she had on seemed to be soiled. It was embarrassing.

"Now you probably are wondering why we didn't do something right away. Well, when it's your mother, you come to those decisions slowly. At last my brother and I had her transferred to a place where she would be supervised in all her activities.

"If I could make one point I would say *become involved*. Don't just tuck a person away and forget about him. Ask questions. Don't be brushed off. And above all, be there. See what's happening. They'll respect you for it and you'll know you did the right thing."

☐ INTERVIEW WITH A GERIATRIC NURSE

"This is a private-pay, Level II and III nursing home. At a glance, you would have to say it looks great here—the decor, the lounges for the residents, the activities available. Our dietitian sees all the residents daily and tries very hard to accommodate everybody.

"I've been working here 7 years and I truly love it. I work hard, but there is not the pressure of hospitals. We do have some problems, however. For one, we have no full-time nurses. Oh, I tried it, but I just couldn't keep it up. We have no orderly, so we are responsible for all our lifting and moving. I have wonderful nurses to work with, but we have a problem with our assistants. The aides. We hire them right off the streets. Now, that means that for every ten you train (on-the-job training), you have maybe one that stays with you. The others, well, some we have to let go. They aren't rude to the residents, but they just have no feeling for this type of work. Others have an extremely high absentee rate.

"To get back to the nurses; the reason we have no full timers is that everyone feels as I do. The sameness of geriatrics becomes a pressure when you don't have enough help. Pay definitely has to be upgraded here. If we could attract a better quality, *trained* aide, that would make a tremendous difference. I think education is the only way to solve the problem of geriatric nursing today. Here we feel that the hospital RN or LPN looks down on those of

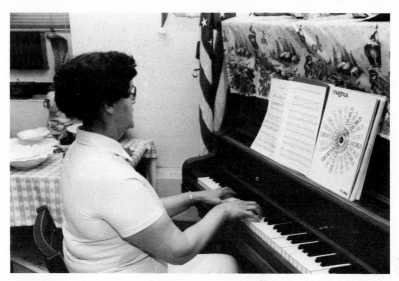

Health care providers in long-term care often join into activities. Here a licensed practical nurse leads a sing-along for residents. (Courtesy of Crescent Hill Nursing Center, Springfield, Massachusetts.)

us who prefer working in a nursing home. I've heard it said that many think we couldn't get work anywhere else. Well, that's not true. Every nurse here, to the best of my knowledge, is here because she loves geriatric patients. We take time to listen to our residents. It becomes frustrating, though, when you find yourself working shorthanded. When that happens I always say to the residents, "I'll be back," and I make every effort to get back to them. But it can bother you. All of the residents have their own needs. Some are lonesome, some are depressed. You can't just hand out a pill and forget about them.

"We don't have the dramatic recoveries here that take place in hospitals. But we do see changes that make this work very rewarding. We have a woman here who came in to us a year ago bedridden and unresponsive. She was like a vegetable. We got her as a transfer from another nursing home. Well, it turned out that at one time she had had seizures so she was put on Dilantin. They examined her Dilantin levels and found that they were excessive. After she was off the Dilantin she slowly showed improvement until now she can walk a few steps with assistance and she is lucid. She had been practically comatose.

"The only way I see the future of geriatric nursing improving is to attract younger nurses. The only way that will be done is if students have more emphasis on geriatrics in their education. It is *not* second-rate nursing. It's challenging, a fertile field for innovative techniques, and extremely satisfying. The future of geriatrics lies in the nursing schools."

☐ INTERVIEW WITH A DIRECTOR OF AN ADULT DAY CARE CENTER

"This center is just like a nursing home except that our clients go home at 4 PM. When they come in in the morning (a van brings them to the center), they have juice, coffee, and toast. We also offer complete grooming services if they need it. We have a shower room and attendants who assist with showers, hair care, and oral hygiene if necessary. We serve a hot meal at noon, also. We offer all kinds of crafts along with day trips, and even weekend trips in some instances. We encourage, but don't force, involvement.

"We get our referrals from VNA, Homemakers, and physicians. I guess our only restrictions are incontinency and confusion that would be disturbing to others. We aren't equipped to handle either of those situations. I'm not saying that we don't have anyone who isn't confused—we do. But it is not disruptive.

"People seek this center for several reasons. We have many here who need to socialize. They live alone and it is good for them to be with other people. We have some who are retarded. There is one elderly woman who lives with her younger sister. Day care gives the sister some relief.

"Day care may be used as a transition. Some go from the nursing home to day care and then to their own home. Day care is also useful for people who come from a hospital situation (say, after having had a stroke) because they can have all their therapies here. We have physical therapy, speech therapy, diet therapy, and, most important of all, we have good peer socialization.

"In order to be accepted into day care, patients must be approved by a physician. This is a medically approved program. Then, if they are medically approved, they may also have to be approved by the Medicaid office. (Most of these participants are Medicaid patients.) It just isn't enough to say they are lonely and need other people around them. It's not a drop-in center; we have a structured program, you see. People come for reasons of their infirmities or disabilities or advanced depression. Not just because they are a little lonely.

"I find that now we are taking on a much sicker clientele. We had one lady last year who had four heart attacks before she had her fifth one right here. It wasn't as upsetting as you might think. Oh, we did feel sad but, remember, this is a group who is very realistic about death. One man said, 'Well, Edna always said her biggest fear was that she would die alone. And look! She died among all her friends.'

"Any nursing home that wished to develop a day care center would have to contact the Department of Public Welfare. They in turn send criteria that have to be satisfied before anything further can be done. Then you are either approved or not approved.

"A rate-setting commission sets fees. People who qualify for Medicaid are completely paid for by the state. Their program and their transportation are both paid. But they must meet the criteria of being Medicaid approved. The others are private paying. Some are on fixed incomes that are just slightly above what the state allows for Medicaid and I have a problem with that.

"Now, for people who hold private insurance policies with an insurance company or Blue Cross Extended Care, 80 per cent is paid for. We are getting more people interested in and paying for day care.

"Our aim for day care here is to get the patients to function independently. We want them to live on the outside for as long as possible. We have discharged people from this program, people who are better.

"An innovation in day care, as I mentioned before, is to get the patient out of the nursing home and back into the community. This is a comfortable transition. It also works the other way around. When a person who is coming to day care reaches the point when nursing home admission is necessary, the move into our nursing home is not as traumatic. For one thing, a new admission already knows most of our staff and, best of all, there are friends here. My day care group knows many, many residents. I guess you could say we bridge the gap between dependence and independence in more ways than one."

Chapter 3 ☐ Review Questions

MATCHING

_____ 1. homogeneous   A. rehabilitation specialist

_____ 2. ageism   B. aural impairment

_____ 3. sensory deficit   C. nonverbal communication

_____ 4. interpersonal skills   D. discrimination against aged

_____ 5. touch   E. similar

_____ 6. physiatrist   F. effective

_____ 7. functional   G. relationships with people

TRUE/FALSE

_____ 1. Nearly half of all noninstitutionalized persons over 65 have chronic health conditions that limit activity.
_____ 2. Fewer than 20 per cent of persons employed in programs for older persons have formal training.
_____ 3. A social stereotype of an aged person is one who is appreciative.
_____ 4. The average life expectancy of a 75-year-old is about 2 years.
_____ 5. An important sensory loss in the elderly is a decline in hormone production.
_____ 6. Facial expressions are a negligible means of communication.
_____ 7. Rehabilitation should begin shortly before a patient is discharged from the hospital.
_____ 8. Seventy per cent of all acute care hospital beds are occupied by elderly persons.
_____ 9. Hospital admission of a nursing home patient can cause confusion where there was no pre-existing confusion.
_____ 10. Adult day care offers respite to families of frail, dependent elders.

DISCUSSION QUESTIONS

1. How does stereotyping reinforce ageism? Describe two examples of ageism in modern day living.
2. Mr. Wallace lives in a nursing home. He needs to be hospitalized for surgery. What are some problems the nurse should anticipate when he is admitted? Supply a solution for each problem listed.
3. Mrs. Riordan is 85. She is about to move into a nursing home. What are some barriers to communication that nursing home personnel can help to overcome?

☐ **REFERENCES**

Burnside, I.: Working With the Elderly: Group Processes and Techniques. Monterey, CA, Wadsworth Health Sciences Division, 1984. p. 92, 95.
Elliot, B. and Hybertson, D.: What is there about the elderly that elicits a negative response? J. Gerontol. Nurs. 8(10): 568–571, October, 1982.
Heller, B., and Walsh, F.: Changing student's attitudes toward the aged. J. Nurs. Educ. 15:11, January, 1976.

Lilliard, J.: A double edged sword: Ageism and sexism. J. Gerontol. Nurs. 8(11): 630–634, November, 1982.

Panicucci, C.: Functional assessment of the older adult in the acute care setting. Nurs. Clin. North Am. 18(2): 355–362, June, 1983.

Tollett, S., and Adamson, C.: The need for gerontologic content within nursing curricula. J. Gerontol. Nurs. 8(10): 576–580, October, 1982.

Objectives	Vocabulary

After completing this chapter, the student should be able to

☐ define dementia
☐ list examples of dementias
☐ explain the difference between dementia and pseudodementia
☐ identify causes and symptoms of depression
☐ identify characteristics of Alzheimer's disease and list nursing implications
☐ explain the differences between multi-infarct dementias and transient ischemic attacks
☐ describe the therapeutic approaches to mental disorders of older adults
☐ give examples of cognitive processes

cognition
insidious
labile
noncompliance
pejorative
pernicious anemia
psychomotor
somatic
succumb
toxicity

CHAPTER 4

Psychologic Aspects of Aging

☐ *Dementia*

The types of mental disorder that an elderly person may have and the severity are critical in determining the treatment he or she will receive. Dementia is characterized by a decrease in intellectual ability, memory loss, disorientation, and impaired judgment. In older adults, it is critical to exclude depression when assessing what appears to be intellectual deterioration since depression may mimic dementia in many respects. When depression is present, vigorous therapy with antidepressive drugs should be instituted (Covington and Walker, 1984).

Ten to fifteen per cent of patients with dementia have reversible illnesses; thyroid disease, drug toxicity, hepatic disease, and pernicious anemia are but a few of the disorders that respond to treatment (Covington and Walker, 1984).

Dementia is the most important geriatric psychiatry problem and affects at least 5 per cent of the elderly. It leads to confusion in appropriate diagnosis because this country, unlike European countries, has not studied and researched geriatric and gerontologic problems for very long. Dementia is often confused with depression (pseudodementia), and indeed, the patient may have both disorders at the same time.

Initial symptoms of dementia often present as lack of interest in personal appearance, poor judgment, apathy, or irritability. The physician who knows his or her patient may detect subtle personality changes early on and thus be able to treat a reversible condition before any permanent change occurs.

Older adults usually have several medical conditions for which a broad array of medications has been ordered. These drugs can cause symptoms of dementia. Examples of drugs that can trigger such symptoms are antihistamines, antihypertensives, sedative-hypnotics, and alcohol. In addition, malnutrition (due to financial problems, poor dentition, isolation, or anorexia) is common in elders and also can produce the same symptoms. All situations must be carefully evaluated in order to treat the disorder dementia.

With time, certain classic symptoms of dementia appear. They are
1. recent memory impairment
2. impaired intellectual function
3. poor judgment
4. fluctuating mood (labile affect)
5. disorientation
6. psychotic symptoms: (a) illusions; (b) delusions; (c) hallucinations

Any symptoms of dementia must prompt a family member or health care professional to seek treatment for the patient. At no time should such signs be disregarded as simply normal aging.

The word senile merely means old. Therefore, senility does not describe a disease, and, furthermore, the term is felt by many to be pejorative.

Chronic organic brain syndrome and acute or reversible organic brain syndrome are terms used by some to refer to those dementias that could not be treated (chronic) and to deliriums (mental disturbances of relatively short duration) that respond to treatment (acute), respectively (Mace and Rabins, 1981). These terms are inaccurate and nonspecific; therefore, they are now inappropriate to use.

☐ *Depression*

Depression is common and often very serious in the older adult. White males in their eighties are at highest risk. Other risk factors include bereavement, illness, isolation, alcoholism, and dementia.

Depressed elders also have somatic complaints: loss of appetite, weight loss, fatigue, sleep disturbances, and low energy level.

The multiple losses elders experience—family, friends, strength, job, and so on—predispose them to depressive illness. Moreover, the drugs used for the common medical conditions experienced by older adults also produce depression. For example, reserpine used for hypertension and beta-blockers used for angina may produce a dose-related depression in 15 per cent of the patients taking them (Schrier, 1982). Older adults are also candidates for reactive depression via psychologic losses, i.e., the marked changes in self image caused by loss or thinning of hair, enlarged nose and ears, loss of teeth, wrinkles, and stooped posture.

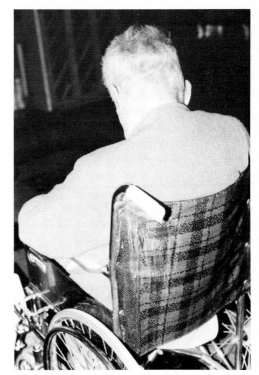

White men in their eighties are at great risk for suicide. It is believed that they suffer most from feelings of lost power and control.

A slowing of perceptual or psychomotor functioning may be falsely attributed to "old age" due to cultural stereotyping of the elderly. It is important for the nurse to remember that depression is a treatable cause of dementia. In a study of patients seen at the Johns Hopkins Hospital, about 25 per cent of those who had symptoms of dementia were depressed (Mace and Rabins, 1981); 82 per cent of these patients recovered after being treated for the depression. No health care professional should ever dismiss depression.

☐ Hypochondriasis

Many elders develop exaggerated concern about illnesses, both real and imaginary. There are several reasons for this: decline in vigor, awareness of limitations and disabilities, and, particularly, awareness of approaching death.

Older adults who have excessive contact with their physicians may be doing so for many reasons: reassurance and security, attention getting, and fear. Fear may occur if the person identifies a symptom in himself or herself that is a symptom in someone else who actually has been diagnosed as ill.

Unfortunately, if the person has been *labeled* as a hypochondriac, it is possible to overlook a new illness.

☐ Alzheimer's Disease

Alzheimer's disease is named after the German physician Alois Alzheimer, who identified the condition in 1907. Recent studies show that nearly 20 per cent of the population now living will develop some type of severe dementia before death and that 50 to 65 per cent of these people will have the neuropathologic changes that characterize Alzheimer's disease. It is estimated that Alzheimer's disease affects 3 to 4 million Americans at the present time (Steffl, 1984).

The cause of Alzheimer's disease is still unknown, although there are clues that implicate viruses, a reduced number of neurotransmitters, and possibly aluminum. Vasodilators and antipsychotic drugs (neuroleptics) sometimes help in the management of the patient.

A cure is as yet undiscovered, but supportive care can prolong the early stages before the more helpless and terminal stages begin. Supportive care can help the patient exist on a satisfactory, productive level and is often given within the loving, compassionate family setting. Those who allow the patient to live life at his or her own pace, reduce the patient's stress, and relieve him or her of the functions he or she is no longer able to perform offer realistic options. The person who must be institutionalized is the one without family or who presents safety hazards and is an unmanageable burden to the family. The course of the disease is divided into four stages: early, advanced, later, and terminal (Wolanin and Phillips, 1980).

□ EARLY STAGE

The patient in the early stage of Alzheimer's disease gradually loses interest in the environment and in personal affairs. There may be a lack of social courtesies and a vagueness and uncertainty in initiating action. The patient will be unable to remember nouns (he or she will recognize them but be unable to recall them). In this stage, he or she will be able to live at home with supportive care from the family if responsibilities are decreased. Attention to health care with the reduction of environmental change and stress can prolong this stage. If the patient lives alone, he or she will need the assistance of a social agency to help keep his or her affairs in order. For example, the patient will need help in paying bills and managing income. He or she must not be allowed to drive.

□ ADVANCED STAGE

The advanced stage of Alzheimer's disease is marked by a decline in the ability to care for personal needs or affairs. Memory deficits are obvious, both in recall and in retention. The patient may be disoriented as to day and night. He or she will forget appointments and important dates, lose belongings, hide things, and be unable to follow simple directions. Health and hygiene will be ignored.

The family can remain the primary caregiver provided they have some outside support. Institutionalization will be required if there is no supportive family reinforcement.

□ LATER STAGE

Aimless wandering and disorientation to time and place characterize the later stage of Alzheimer's disease. The patient will not be able to identify his or her caregiver. Fine motor skills decline. There will be deterioration in the basic activities of daily living. The patient will be incoherent and will compulsively touch and examine objects with hands and mouth. Institutionalization is usually needed at this time unless there is a strong supportive family structure. When the patient is institutionalized, the change is extremely stressful. Care is custodial, but there are still activities that the patient can enjoy; walking, music, and certain group efforts are some examples. Sleep is impaired, and anxiety and confusion are present on awakening.

☐ TERMINAL STAGE

This last stage of the disease can be compared with the terminally ill patient who is receiving total care. The patient does not respond to communication and does not recognize family, friends, or familiar objects. He needs help with all basic physiologic processes. Death is caused by infection, pneumonia, renal failure, or decubitus ulcers.

☐ NURSING IMPLICATIONS

The following are nursing measures for the Alzheimer's patient:
- Use time cues such as calendars, clocks, newspapers, trips out of doors, written lists, and reminders to maintain reality orientation.
- Physical activity combined with proper nutrition can stimulate a sluggish appetite, prevent loss of muscle tone, minimize fractures, and encourage sleep.
- Maintain structure and routine; there should be no abrupt changes in residence, life-style, food, or medication.
- Avoid sensory overload. Restrict conversation to one topic at a time, limit visitors to one or two at a time; limit choices. Too many decisions cause anxiety and confusion.
- Maintain communication and affectional ties. Use frequent identification by name.
- Use positive reinforcement and praise to help maintain physical and social skills.
- See that dental and foot care are not neglected.
- When there is a deterioration in toileting, be consistent with bowel and bladder routines.
- Inform families about the Alzheimer's Disease and Related Disorders Association, Inc., 360 N. Michigan Ave., Chicago, IL 60601.
- Suggest families contact their local Visiting Nurses Association and Public Health Nurses for information about support groups for families of Alzheimer's victims.

☐ POINTS TO REMEMBER

- Alzheimer's is characterized by gradual behavior and personality changes that may be barely noticed at first.
- Many dementias cause problems that are similar to Alzheimer's disease but that might be reversible. For example, trauma, infections, drug toxicity, metabolic disorders, and circulatory disturbances are often to blame for symptoms of the disease.
- A comprehensive physical assessment including a general medical workup in addition to extensive neurologic and psychologic tests is essential for ruling out other dementias.

- Environmental adjustments can reduce stress and frustration.
- Research is being done on experimental, memory-enhancing drugs, but they are unapproved and unavailable as yet for the general public.

□ Grief Reactions

By the time an older adult has reached the age of 70, it is inevitable that he or she has experienced the death of a significant other: spouse, friend, colleague, or adult child. The loss of a spouse can be particularly destructive; *the risk of mortality for the survivor is increased by 600 per cent in the year that follows.* Professional treatment may be required.

□ Multi-Infarct Dementia

Repeated small strokes that destroy small areas of the brain cause *multi-infarct dementia (MID).* These injuries affect memory, coordination, and speech.

The main difference between Alzheimer's disease and multi-infarct dementia is the progression of the disease. Alzheimer's has an insidious onset. Families cannot recall a specific time when the patient developed memory loss because the changes came about so gradually. However, in MID they do recall a time when the patient did not exhibit symptoms of a brain disorder. Alzheimer's progresses steadily; MID does not. In fact, sometimes the patient seems to get a little better.

Present treatment of MID includes maintaining adequate cardiac function and controlling hypertension. Some cases of MID are halted by the prevention of further strokes. In others, the disease advances.

□ Transient Ischemic Attacks

Intermittent episodes of cerebrovascular insufficiency are called TIA's, or *transient ischemic attacks.* The poor supply of blood to the brain causes such symptoms as weakness, nausea, dizziness, and even, in some cases, paralysis. The episodes may last only a few minutes or several hours, often disappearing without residual effects.

It is important to report TIA's to the physician immediately; they are a meaningful warning signal of instances of cerebrovascular disease. Their recognition provides an opportunity to institute preventive measures in hopes of warding off a stroke.

☐ *Suicide*

Suicide, one of the ten leading causes of death in the United States, is considered to be the result of an emotional disorder. Although suicide rates are on the rise among young males (especially adolescents), the elderly white male (over age 85) is also at high risk. Until 1983, 11 per cent of the population (the elderly) accounted for 25 per cent of the suicides.

Risk factors for suicide include loss of spouse, living alone, recent physical illness or physical change, and low socioeconomic status.

Bereavement is a significant factor. Despair and depression, which usually contribute to distortion of intellectual abilities and outlook on life, prevent the person from exploring acceptable solutions to his or her problems.

Appropriate treatment of bereavement is support. Also, many patients respond to counseling, attention to physical problems, and frequent telephone contact. The elderly depressed patient may also require antidepressants. In some cases, a short inpatient stay may be necessary.

☐ *Alcohol Misuse and Abuse*

Alcohol consumption is on the increase. The elderly are particularly at risk to the effects of alcohol misuse and abuse. Excessive or prolonged use of alcohol by older adults can lead to somatic, psychologic, social, and other serious consequences. Alcohol misuse also can interfere with the successful management of some chronic diseases and heighten the risk of drug interactions and their effects.

The elderly are at a heightened risk of succumbing to alcohol abuse after retirement from meaningful work. Loss of status, power, and income trigger abuse, as do loss of spouse, family members, and friends. The stress of relocation should not be overlooked.

Some clues to alcoholism include insomnia, rapid onset of mental confusion, uncontrollable hypertension, frequent falls, and self-neglect (Lamy, 1984).

Alcoholism in the elderly is often overlooked because so many older problem drinkers are retired and therefore "hidden" at home. Symptoms of alcoholism occur frequently in the older adult who is *not* a problem drinker: gastritis, insomnia, anemia, and depression.

☐ *Psychotropic Drugs*

The body's mechanisms for distributing, detoxifying, and eliminating drugs may be impaired in older adults. Side effects are more common in older people than in younger adults. To help to avoid potential side effects from drugs, smaller dosages of the drug are usually administered.

Nurses are responsible for knowing the drugs their patients are taking and the relationship between the drugs and the symptoms presented. Psychotropic drugs are frequently used by elders, and a major part of Chapter 5 is devoted to discussing them.

□ *Therapeutic Interaction*

Psychotherapy, medication, and a range of other methods help geriatric patients with mental disorders. Good management depends on "what can be treated" and "what works." Currently, not much can be done for the damaged thought centers of the brain, but the patient's mood and behavior can be improved.

Disorders associated with mild to moderate brain damage and depression, alcoholism, and drug addiction may improve with individual psychotherapy. Group therapy has been found to be useful in increasing the patient's self esteem. These techniques, however, have limited value when the patient has dementia (chronic organic brain syndrome).

Ways to encourage the mental health of the elderly include the following:
- Encourage independent living and activity through the Visiting Nurses Association and other community agencies.
- Assess noncompliance. Does the person take prescribed drugs appropriately? How well does he or she follow directions?
- Nursing home care: visit, telephone, write!
- Compensate for memory deficits with reminders, appointment books, calendars, and daily newspapers.
- Provide environmental stimulation for patients with dementia: continuity of care, night lights, family photos, an open window to orient to sounds of outside.
- Show respect for the elderly; address each patient by his or her surname unless otherwise requested. Sit near the patient; touch.
- Provide counseling. Allow for conversation with the physician or nurse during regularly scheduled appointments; help the patient to adjust, do not try to "cure"; be supportive during grieving process; and give reassurance (Schrier, 1982).

□ PETS

Pets have positive effects on the health of elderly people. In many cases pets may provide the main source of socialization for the isolated older adult.

Pets meet many needs: they are someone to talk to, someone to care for. They amply satisfy the need for touch. Pets, especially dogs and cats, enable an older person to deal with anxiety, loneliness, and depression caused by the many losses in old age.

Activities directors in long-term-care facilities can provide many instances in which pets have directly contributed to the support of the mental well-being of residents. Pets, like children, stimulate childhood memories so useful in reminiscence groups (reminiscence in this context meaning the normal life review that gives meaning and significance to one's life). Pets have also been used successfully in remotivation groups, a technique designed to stimulate communication skills and environmental interest.

☐ REMOTIVATION TECHNIQUES

Older adults with the diagnosis of confusion caused by chronic brain syndrome, senile brain disease, or cerebral arteriosclerosis have benefited by the use of remotivation techniques to help bring them back to reality.

The leader is a member of the nursing home staff who conducts a patient-group interaction program with six to eight patients (residents). There are basically three steps planned to renew the client's interest in everyday life and

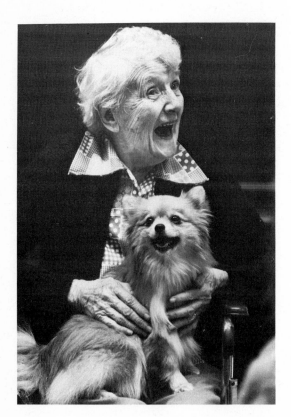

Research has shown that pets provide beneficial interactions for older adults. Some facilities have pets in residence; in others, volunteer groups bring pets to the patients on a regular basis. (Courtesy of Ring Nursing Homes.)

in social surroundings. Initially, the leader greets and welcomes each individual to establish a "climate of acceptance." Then the leader forms "bridges of reality" by showing pictures and talking about the world in which we live and the kinds of work people do. Topics are "basic": gardening, pet care, cooking, and so on, capitalizing on the client's interest. Lastly, the leader thanks the group for their participation in the 45-minute session and extends to them an invitation to attend the next meeting.

Although this procedure does not ensure success in all cases, the social benefits are important. In many cases, there is a return of appropriate behavior that allows for maximum independent functioning.

□ REALITY ORIENTATION

In a broad sense, reality orientation means continually orienting the confused patient to his or her identity, location, and time and encouraging him or her to interact with others. The first reality orientation program was organized in the late 1950's in a Kansas Veterans Administration Hospital by James C. Folsom. It was suggested that most of the work be done by attendants, since they spend more time with patients than anyone else. However, it should be used by everyone who comes in contact with confused geriatric patients, especially those who have been institutionalized a long time or who have moderate to severe organic brain impairment.

Folsom organized classes that consisted of no more than four patients to an instructor, who was usually an attendant. The original facts taught were

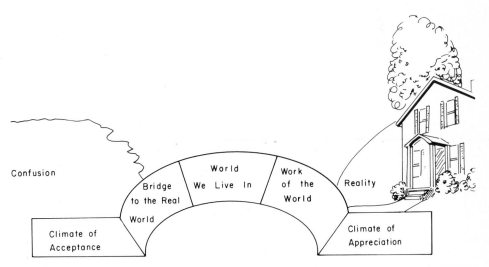

Figure 4–1 □ Remotivation therapy is one method to build bridges, leading to a greater recognition of reality for persons who are confused or who have some degree of brain failure. (From Rambo, p. 77.)

the patient's name and location and the date. New facts (age, home town, former occupation) were not introduced until the patient relearned the three basic facts. However, the Do's and Don't's listed here should be followed all the time by staff personnel. Set routines, consistency, and sincere, friendly interest provide the best foundation for effective reality orientation.

Do's and don't's of reality orientation*

Do's

1. Do set a routine and stay with it.
2. Do call the patient by his correct name and title (Mr. Smith) unless he specifically asks you to use his first name.
3. Do look at the person you are speaking to; make eye contact.
4. Do reinforce orientation through the use of clocks, calendars, and written reminders (writing in color helps because it is attention grabbing).
5. Do carry on conversations about familiar subjects.
6. Do initiate simple activities, such as brushing teeth or combing hair, that require purposeful movement.
7. Be consistent.
8. Be honest. (Two elderly ladies were sitting side by side in the lounge of a large nursing home. One had had a stroke and was paralyzed. However, she understood what was going on around her and, with difficulty, could speak. The other lady, who had organic brain syndrome, sat rocking in her chair and crying for her mother. No matter how the attendants tried to pacify her, she would not stop crying. With a great effort, the stroke patient said to her, "I think your mother passed away and I'm sure she's in heaven. Don't you think she's in heaven?" To everyone's surprise, the crying stopped. Confused people have shown remarkable ability to cope with the truth.)

Don't's

1. Don't rush. (Especially, don't push wheelchairs fast—it makes patients dizzy.)
2. Don't give patients involved tasks to do.
3. Don't give complicated instructions.
4. Don't become impatient or discouraged. Allow patients time to answer your questions or to do what you ask.
5. Don't fail to repeat, over and over if necessary, instructions or basic information.
6. Don't agree with a confused person's incorrect statements. Gently correct them.
7. Don't forget to encourage independence in whatever small way you can.
8. Don't underestimate the importance of touch. It's the most positive means of communication we have and sometimes it's the only means.

---

*Adapted from the reality orientation program at the Veterans' Administration Hospital, Tuscaloosa, Alabama.

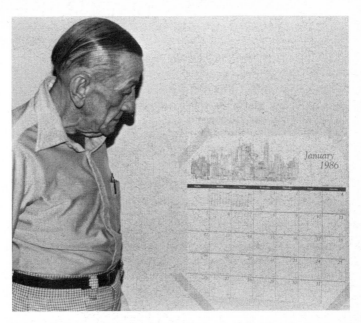

A calendar is useful for keeping patients oriented. For some patients, simpler means are needed, such as being near a window so that they can distinguish night from day.

Acknowledging the fact that reality orientation is based on the principles of client involvement and dealing with the "here" and the "now," health care workers must be prepared to devote 24 hours a day and 7 days a week to the job. Caregivers should be sure that the patient is in a room with windows so he or she can distinguish day from night and describe weather and seasons. The therapy is more successful when the patient has photographs of the family, his or her own clothing to wear, and, if possible, his or her own bed linens. All of these factors help to reinforce reality and help them maintain their identity. Whatever structured activity and social interaction of formal reality therapy classes the patient is exposed to will be welcome side benefits.

Not all patients will be successful despite the most sincere efforts of a dedicated staff. There will always be those who respond only when allowed to hold a doll or if the nurse acknowledges some fantasy that the patient is experiencing. That, too, is reality.

□ REMINISCENCE

In 1974, Butler and Lewis wrote: "The life review is characterized by the progressive return to consciousness of past experiences and particularly the resurgence of unresolved conflicts." Reminiscence, an adaptive mechanism of aging, is a universal occurrence in older people. Although it is agreed that everyone reminisces, whether young or old, the act of remembering one's past is more intense in the elderly.

Reminiscence is a part of the life review. Emotions that surface during this process may vary. Pain, discomfort, and depression often accompany reminiscence as unresolved conflicts and life's disappointments are remembered. However, reminiscence that ranges from mild storytelling to nostalgia also encourages serenity, wisdom, and frankness in old age that can bring about an acceptance of one's life as being meaningful and having had purpose.

Although it may be difficult for family and caregivers to listen to the same stories repeated frequently, reminiscence is a natural adaptation to aging. A group approach offers the advantage of helping more people as well as providing the opportunity for increased interaction and socialization.

Reminiscence groups may easily be established informally wherever interested older adults gather. Leaders do not have to be trained professionals if the goal of the group is simply social. Formal groups, either in institutions or in independent living situations, that have a therapeutic purpose should be facilitated by trained professionals.

□ COGNITIVE PROCESSES

Since nurses may see only sick older people, it is easy to fall into the habit of generalizing that "all old people become sick." Informed health professionals know that less than 5 per cent of elders are institutionalized and that most older adults have several chronic problems that interfere with optimal health. Nevertheless, most elders function very well. It is unfortunate for nurses to embrace the popular opinion that cognitive processes decline with age. Research indicates that this is not true.

Cognitive processes, the way we manipulate information, include the following:
1. *interpretation*
2. *storage and retrieval from memory*
3. *evaluation*
4. *reasoning*

□ IMPLICATIONS FOR NURSING

- Rigidity. Older adults are labeled "rigid." This does not mean that they cannot learn. What is difficult and sometimes interferes with learning new skills is the *unlearning* of the old ones. The degree of rigidity seems to be determined by culture and experience.
- Caution. Caution increases with aging. The decline in so many abilities of the older adult promotes feelings of uncertainty and fear of failure.

- Memory. Memory involves several stages: registration—the entrance by a stimulus into the memory system—retention, and recall. Older adults quite naturally will have difficulty with recall; their brains have been admitting stimuli for many years. To lose memory is neither natural nor inevitable as one grows older.
- Pace. Elderly people have slower reaction times. When they are hurried, they feel reluctant, frustrated, or anxious. A calm, unhurried manner on the part of the nurse or aide will generate trust and cooperation. Coax and encourage elders and allow them enough time to respond appropriately to your requests.
- Change. Elderly people became elderly by coping successfully with change. Wars, depressions, births, and deaths were changes they survived. Now that they are elderly, however, they may not react well to change. There is security in structure and routine, whether one lives in one's own home or in a long-term-care facility. For example, bedtime rituals are common: saying prayers, using certain covers or pillows, and raising or lowering the window.

  Sometimes a change that seems right and good can cause serious emotional harm. A prime example is a move. When an elderly parent is widowed, often the children feel that it is wise for him or her to sell the family home and move into something small that is easier to care for. On the surface, the idea seems to have merit. Maintenance is costly and tiring. The property will bring a good price, and so on. But beware. Selling the family home can cause depression and anxiety in the parent and guilt in the child who suggested it. It is not a foolproof solution.
- Need for self-esteem. Many times health care personnel talk over, around, and about their patients rather than to them. Conversation does not have to be lengthy. A cheerful greeting, a remark about the weather, a smile, or a friendly touch on the arm all communicate interest. Saying, "Good morning, Mr. Ryan," with eye contact, will raise his feeling of self worth several degrees.

  Treating older adults as children fosters childish behavior and regression, not progression. A mark of good nursing care is to promote independence in patients.

□ POINTS TO REMEMBER

- Encourage independence and activity. Investigate social agencies that support independent living, such as Visiting Nurses Association, Meals on Wheels, and home health care agencies.
- Measure the degree of noncompliance. Sensory deficits or memory impairment often cause the geriatric patient to omit medications or to take them inappropriately.

- Nursing home placement. If long-term care is the answer, recommend a facility with activities and rehabilitation policies designed to improve the client's level of independence.
- Memory deficits. Use an ID bracelet or necklace with the client's name and telephone number; set regular, simple schedules for activities of daily living (ADL); keep the environment simple and uncluttered (leave the furniture in the same place); avoid overstimulation and pressure; label closets and drawers; use pictures of family and friends; maintain physical activity and independence appropriately and give choices when feasible.
- Environmental stimuli. For clients in long-term care who have some dementia, room placement is important. They should have a room within sight of the nurse's station with the door open and a night light on. Personal orienting items such as pictures, collectibles, and so on are also helpful. The restless patient might be allowed to go to an activity room, where he or she might read or watch TV until tired enough to sleep.
- Respect for clients. Tone of voice when addressing nursing home residents indicates respect. Method of address (Mr., Mrs., or first name if the resident agrees) is important. Do not use "baby" names: "Dearie," "Honey," and so on. Speaking to the client at eye level and touching the hand or arm while talking are also gestures of respect.
- Listening. A sympathetic ear and gentle reassurance are often the most effective of therapies.

Chapter 4 ☐ Review Questions

MATCHING

_____ 1. depression

_____ 2. psychotic symptoms

_____ 3. dementia

_____ 4. delirium

_____ 5. somatic complaint

_____ 6. Alzheimer's disease

A. acute mental disorder

B. bring patient back to reality

C. life review

D. the way we manipulate information

E. pseudodementia

F. intermittent episodes of cardiovascular insufficiency

_____	7. transient ischemic attacks	G.	sleep disturbance
_____	8. remotivation techniques	H.	hallucinations
_____	9. reminiscence	I.	chronic mental disorders
_____	10. cognitive processes	J.	slow, insidious, imperceptible memory and personality changes

DISCUSSION QUESTIONS

1. What are some characteristics that older adults exhibit that lead to their erroneously being labeled "senile"? What would be the correct assessment of their actions?
2. Name some causes of depression in elderly persons and discuss ways of maintaining their mental health.
3. How do the losses elderly persons endure contribute toward hypochondriasis?
4. What are some ways nurses can increase the self esteem of some of their elderly patients?

□ REFERENCES

Bromber, S., and Cassel, C.: Suicide in the elderly. J Am Geriatr Soc, _30_(11):698–703, 1983.
Covington, T., and Walker, J.: Current Geriatric Therapy. Philadelphia, W.B. Saunders, 1984.
Lamy, P.: Alcohol misuse and abuse among the elderly. Drug Intell Clin Pharm, _18_:649, 1984.
Mace, N., and Rabins, P.: The 36 Hour Day. Baltimore, Johns Hopkins University Press, 1981.
Schrier, R.: Clinical Internal Medicine in the Aged. Philadelphia, W.B. Saunders, 1982.
Steffl, B.M.: Handbook of Gerontological Nursing. New York, Van Nostrand Reinhold, 1984, pp. 124–126.
Wolanin, M.O., and Phillips, L.: Confusion: Prevention and Care. St. Louis, C.V. Mosby, 1981.

Objectives

After completing this chapter, the student should be able to

- [ ] list reasons why elders are at risk when taking medications
- [ ] relate the pharmacologic implications of physical changes in aging body systems
- [ ] describe reasons for noncompliance in elders and suggest remedies
- [ ] explain the origin and use of psychotropic drugs
- [ ] identify drugs associated with cognitive dysfunction
- [ ] suggest ways to deal with insomnia in older adults
- [ ] explain why medication withdrawal in elders can cause problems

Vocabulary

cognitive
dementia
dyscrasia
extrapyramidal
hypochondriasis
labile
tardive dyskinesia
vermiform

CHAPTER 5

Pharmacologic Aspects of Care of the Older Adult

☐ *Factors That Place the Elderly at Risk from Problems with Medications*

One quarter of all prescription drugs sold in the United States are taken by persons over 65. One half of all adverse drug reactions are experienced by older adults. Why are there so many serious problems with the older adult and medications? Some factors are readily apparent. *Changes in body composition in the elderly* (increased percentage of fat and decreased percentage of water) *change the intensity and duration of action* of some drugs. Although not enough research has been done on the absorption and metabolism of drugs in the elderly to be certain about drug actions, it is generally believed that medications are metabolized at different rates in older people than in younger people. Therefore, either the drug may not be effective or *toxic effects may occur because the drug accumulates in the body* due to reduced excretion.

A second cause of problems is that *older people take many more drugs simultaneously, frequently mixing prescribed and nonprescribed drugs.* (Nonprescribed drugs are called over-the-counter, or OTC, drugs.) The more drugs

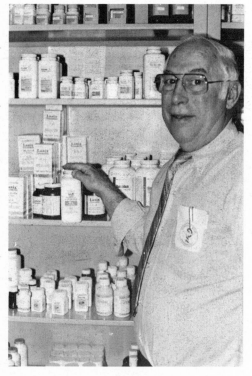

The older adult frequently is taking several prescription and nonprescription drugs. In the hospital pharmacy pictured here, the pharmacist is the best source of information about drug interactions. Most nursing homes do not have a pharmacy on site. Since a physician is also infrequently on the premises, an additional responsibility is placed on the nurse for monitoring potential drug interactions.

a person is taking, the more chances exist for drug interaction. Prescribers of drugs have become keenly aware of the possibilities of drug interactions. Sometimes, however, the elderly person forgets to tell the prescriber about all other medications he or she is taking. The nurse is a key person in monitoring drug actions and side effects in the community, the hospital, and the nursing home. She or he needs to be aware of the actions of all the drugs a patient is using, to monitor the drugs a patient is taking, to help teach the patient to monitor himself or herself, and to alert the physician about the appearance of side effects. Table 5–1 summarizes problems associated with age that have an impact on drug use.

Older adults develop illnesses at a time when they are experiencing a decline in organ function and general reserve capacities. *Changes in the body's systems due to aging affect the way drugs work in the body.*

Integumentary System. There is a reduction in the secretion of drugs through the skin. Phenothiazides can produce photosensitivity because the drugs bind with melanin.

Cardiovascular and Urinary Systems. Decreased effectiveness of the heart as a pump decreases effective circulation. One result is that less blood is supplied to the kidneys. The kidneys' ability to perform filtration functions is decreased. There is a general decrease in the excretion of any water-soluble drug.

Neurologic System. Conduction velocity of peripheral nerves declines, and there is known to be increased central nervous system (CNS) sensitivity to many drugs ingested by the elderly.

Special Senses. The inability to read fine print on medication labels and to distinguish color differences among shades of blue, green, and purple may result in the elderly person making mistakes when taking drugs. Because the sensation of taste is diminished, his or her ability to distinguish between drugs is impaired.

Table 5–1 □ Problems of the Elderly Having Impact on Drug Use

Increased use of drugs because of more chronic diseases.
Adverse drug effects potentiated by physiologic changes of aging.
Increased risk of drug interactions owing to increased numbers of drugs being ingested.
Erratic or dangerous drug-taking behavior because of vision and memory changes.
Lack of money to purchase needed drugs.
Similarity of drug side effects to manifestations of normal aging.
Failure to adequately monitor the responses to drug and drug-taking practices.
Use of over-the-counter drugs in addition to prescriptions without informing doctor or nurse.
Failure to reevaluate ongoing need for the drug, or drug dosage.
Seeing more than one physician and purchasing drugs at more than one pharmacy so no one has an accurate drug profile.
Discontinuance of drug by the patient without consultation.
Using medications shared by other persons who had similar conditions.

(From Carnevali, D.L., and Patrick, M.: Nursing Management of the Elderly. Philadelphia, Lippincott, 1979, p. 169.)

Endocrine System. A decrease in hormone levels may cause behavioral changes. These changes contribute to inappropriate medication or overmedication of the elderly patient.

Digestive System. Most drugs are absorbed through the intestinal mucosa. A few are absorbed through the stomach. Two factors that interfere with drug absorption in the elderly are that (1) there are fewer secreting cells in the mucous membrane and (2) the elderly produce less gastric acid.

Indirect components of impaired drug absorption are reduced blood flow secondary to cardiovascular changes and decreased intestinal motility. Also, decreased liver size can cause patients to lose a significant amount of desired drug effect, and the liver becomes smaller with advancing age.

Genitourinary System. The normal changes in renal function can cause inefficient and slowed drug excretion in elderly persons. There is general diminution in excreting any water-soluble drug. Moreover, many older adults have such disorders as dehydration, pneumonia, congestive heart failure, and urinary tract infections that add more stress to the aging genitourinary system.

Musculoskeletal System. In older adults, the ratio between lean body mass and fat changes. There is a reduction in the proportion of lean body mass to total body weight. With the increase in fatty tissue, the volume of distribution of fat-soluble drugs increases and there is the chance of longer drug action.

Older adults often misuse drugs. They may share drugs liberally with friends and acquaintances. ("Too expensive to throw them out" and "It worked just fine for me" are two of the reasons given for this dangerous practice.) They often neglect to reliably inform their physicians about current prescription and OTC drugs they may be taking. In addition, because they may be seeing several different doctors for various problems, no one physician may have a total understanding of the patient's medication history. The elderly usually fail to make use of one of their best resources for information— their pharmacist.

Elderly patients are more apt to display noncompliance than any other age group. Although noncompliance may not be directly related to age, older people exhibit noncompliance more because they have more incidences of multiple chronic diseases that require greater numbers of medications for a longer period of time. Noncompliance is also a method of maintaining control and independence for some elderly people.

Other reasons a patient may not comply with a prescribed drug regimen include inability to pay for the drug, inability to get to a pharmacy, physical inability to prepare the medication or open the package, and lack of understanding of the drug's purpose.

There are compliance aids. A medication calendar, personal patient profiles (kept by the pharmacist), and unique packaging devices that help the person remember when and which drugs to take have been developed to encourage compliance. The problem of noncompliance offers an opportunity for

an interdisciplinary effort among professionals in medicine, nursing, and pharmacology to coordinate and reinforce measures to improve the quality of patient care.

☐ Nursing Considerations to Prevent Drug Misuse

Drug misuse among the elderly can be a significant medical problem that
can go unrecognized. The following measures can improve safety:
- Provide color-coded charts and special pill boxes that can help the elderly person remember when to take specific drugs.
- Obtain drug histories from patients and provide drug information in
  language the patient can understand. Never assume that because the
  patient does not ask questions, he or she understands directions.
- Encourage the elderly patient to write out a list of questions for the
  pharmacist or physician, so that he or she does not forget. Some questions that should be asked about every drug include the name of the
  drug, the condition it treats, the main effect it will have, any possible
  side effects to watch for, the relationship of the drug to food and to
  other drugs.
- Explain to patients that they should tell the physician about all drugs
  presently and recently taken, including OTC drugs, and to mention any
  history of adverse reactions and any allergies.
- Stress that no one of any age should share medications with anyone.

☐ Psychotropic Drugs

An estimated one third of the population of the United States is at some
time given a prescription for psychotropic medication; a major emphasis in
this chapter is on this group of drugs. In recent years, there has been criticism
about psychotropic drugs being overprescribed for institutionalized patients.
In long-term care, for example, the level of a patient's anxiety and the use of
tranquilizers may not correlate. In one study exploring the relationship between the use of tranquilizers and the characteristics of nursing home residents, several factors surfaced: Being female, having a "low mental status,"
and being termed uncooperative or unfriendly toward staff all increased the
likelihood of a person being prescribed tranquilizers.

Psychotropic drugs first appeared in the early 1950's. At that time, the
word "neuroleptics" was employed to refer to the group of drugs originally
called major tranquilizers and now termed antipsychotic drugs. These are
mood-altering drugs that change behavior yet do not oversedate the patient

when appropriate dosages are used. The desired effect is that the patient interact in a normal fashion in his or her environment. Tables 5–2 and 5–3 describe the major indications for psychotropic drugs.

Psychiatric disorders commonly associated with the elderly are defined here.

- *Depression.* A profound sadness, common in the elderly as a reaction to their many losses, depression may also have physical causes (e.g., it may be drug induced, as in reserpine prescribed for hypertension). It may be a result of alterations in the concentrations of chemicals in the brain called neurotransmitters. Monoamine oxidase (MAO) levels increase and norepinephrine levels decline with aging.
- *Anxiety.* Anxiety is an intense feeling of discomfort associated with fears and threats that have no basis in fact.
- *Hypochondriasis.* Exaggerated concerns about illnesses real or imagined may result from a person's awareness of gradual physical decline.
- *Grief reaction.* A mourning reaction due to loss of spouses, friends, and other family members, grief reaction may be almost continuous in some elders.
- *Dementia.* Dementia is a chronic organic brain syndrome. Symptoms may vary from mild memory impairment to disorientation accompanied by psychotic symptoms.
- *Neurosis.* The emotional maladjustment of a person who uses poor judgment but who does not lose touch with reality is called neurosis.
- *Paranoia.* Paranoia is a mental disorder in which the patient describes with logic and conviction impressions of being persecuted.

Table 5–2 ☐ Indications for Psychotropic Drugs

Symptoms	Drugs
Psychotic behavior	*Antipsychotic drugs*
1. severe agitation	1. phenothiazines
2. delusions	2. haloperidol
3. hallucinations	
Anxiety	*Minor tranquilizers*
1. somatic symptoms	1. diazepam
2. hypochondria	2. mebrobamate
3. demanding, frightened behavior	3. chlordiazepoxide
Depression	*Antidepressants*
1. apathy	1. amphetamines
2. unbearable sadness	2. methylphenidate
3. hopelessness	3. tricyclics
4. somatic symptoms	4. MAO inhibitors
Insomnia	*Sedative/hypnotics*
1. difficulty falling asleep	1. barbiturates
2. early awakening	2. chloral hydrate
3. awakening feeling exhausted	3. nonbarbiturates
4. frequent awakening during the night	

- *Psychosis.* A severe mental disorder, psychosis is characterized by personality disorganization. Stress and biochemical factors contribute to the cause.
- *Mania.* Mania is a type of psychosis in which the patient is hyperactive and excited, has flight of ideas, and is emotionally unstable.
- *Manic-depression.* The psychiatric disorder with an emotionally labile patient exhibiting mood swings from mania to depression is termed manic-depression or bipolar disease.
- *Extrapyramidal symptoms.* These symptoms originate in the descending nerves out the pyramids of the medulla. They include *tardive dyskinesia,* abnormal movements of the face (grimacing, vermiform tongue movements, puffing of cheeks, chewing, licking of lips). Other symptoms are akathisia (severe restlessness), tremors, muscular rigidity, and weakness. Symptoms usually are irreversible and are always dangerous to the frail elderly because of the possibility of falls or other injuries. These symptoms are also referred to as parkinsonism.

☐ Disturbed Behavior

Agitated and disturbed behavior may result in a prescription for a psychotropic drug, but good nursing care may be able to identify the reason for

Table 5–3 ☐ Drugs Used in Mental Disorders

Disorder	Category	Example	Side Effects
Schizophrenia Schizophrenic affective disorders Mania (acute) Psychosis in the elderly	Antipsychotic	phenothiazines (e.g., Thorazine, Sparine) butyrophenones (e.g., haloperidol, [Haldol])	Tardive dyskinesia, blood dyscrasia, change in menstrual pattern, abrupt onset of milk flow, rashes, jaundice, extrapyramidal effects
Manic depression	Manic episode control	lithium (Lithane)	Drowsiness, tremors, thirst, nausea and vomiting, polyuria
Depression	Tricyclic antidepressants	imipramine (Tofranil) amitriptyline (Elavil) doxepin (Sinequan)	Extrapyramidal effects, dry mouth, drowsiness, blood dyscrasias
	MAO inhibitors	phenelzine sulfate (Nardil) isocarboxazid (Marplan) tranylcypromine sulfate (Parnate)	Hypotension, restlessness, anorexia, insomnia, dry mouth, overstimulation

NOTE: Certain foods are contraindicated when the patient is on *monoamine oxidase (MAO) inhibitors.* For example, aged cheeses, bananas, beer, red wines, and chocolate should not be ingested. Also, narcotics, which are used for deep-seated pain, particularly meperidine, must be used with great caution if the patient is receiving MAO inhibitors—either antidepressives or some antineoplastics—since the combination may precipitate respiratory depression, hypotension, and coma. (Covington and Walker, 1984.)

the behavior and eliminate the need for the drug. Agitated and disturbed behavior can be caused by social problems such as losing a spouse or moving into a nursing home. Some psychologic problems experienced by the elderly (physical losses, decline in self esteem) cause stress that increases in frequency and severity.

When the geriatric patient presents a behavioral problem, staff should try to find out why he or she is acting unacceptably. Appropriate action is determined by assessing individual behavioral problems. Take time to allow for hearing and visual problems. The geriatric patient needs to be allowed to make choices regarding his or her life and behavior. The attitude of the caregiver strongly influences patient behavior. Appropriate interventions may be social or environmental changes, counseling, medication, or behavior modification.

Gentle persistence and persuasion are often effective in overcoming agitation and getting the patient to act appropriately. Eliminating the fear of retaliation or punishment frequently reduces the behavior. Always make a sincerely interested attempt to find out what is causing the behavior problem.

Health care providers agree that medicines can never replace human interactions and attentive attitudes. We acknowledge that drugs can and do cause undesirable side effects—even more so in the elderly.

Homeostasis, that automatic regulator that maintains our physiologic response, is impaired in the elderly. This is why caregivers must anticipate undesirable drug effects in the elderly. Remember that physiologic changes in absorption, circulation, and metabolism affect drug actions in the aged person.

☐ MENTAL IMPAIRMENT OR CONFUSION

Drugs that may cause confusion include digoxin, antiparkinsonian drugs, antidepressants, and hypotensive agents. Nurses who have the responsibility of administering drugs to geriatric patients should review the following important points:

- When taking a drug history, inquire specifically about OTC drugs. These seemingly innocuous medicines may produce exaggerated drug interactions. (Examples include aspirin and certain antihypertensives.)
- The lowest dosage that is effective should be used. (Think "low and slow.")
- Geriatric stereotyped behavior such as forgetfulness and confusion can be drug related. *Severe memory loss is never a normal part of the aging process.*

☐ COGNITIVE DYSFUNCTION

All drugs, OTC or prescribed, can cause cognitive dysfunction. Those most frequently encountered by health care personnel are psychotropic drugs, alcohol, antihypertensives, cardiovascular medications, cimetidine, and hormones. Properly used, medications benefit the elderly; psychotropic drugs are useful for treating specific problems such as psychotic symptoms or depression. The nurse must learn to recognize which drugs may be causing behavioral changes, rather than labeling an older person "senile," which often prevents accurate assessment of their problem.

Some common examples of psychotropic drugs include:

Antipsychotic drugs	Antidepressant drugs
Thorazine	Tofranil
Sparine	Serentil
Vesprin	Norpramin
Mellaril	Elavil
Serentil	Aventyl
Compazine	Sinequan
Stelazine	Marplan
Trilafon	Parnate
Navane	Nardil
Haldol	
Moban	

☐ ANXIETY

Anxiety is fairly common in older adults. The feeling may be intense or vague. It is described as feeling threatened—but for no apparent reason. Often people who are anxious regress by becoming more dependent; therefore, the caregiver must understand the cause of the anxiety or try to determine the cause.

Not all anxiety is bad. The mentally healthy person develops mechanisms to cope with anxiety and institutes changes that foster mental health. Note that the major symptom of anxiety is fatigue. If the anxious patient does not improve on benzodiazepines, he or she may have an underlying depression.

Patients will display physiologic, behavioral, and emotional signs of anxiety.

Table 5–4 ☐ Examples of Disorders That Cause Acute and Chronic Confusion

Acute Confusion	Chronic Confusion
TIA's	cerebral arteriosclerosis
cardiac failure	senile psychosis
metabolic problems (diabetes, hyperthyroidism)	Alzheimer's disease
alcoholism	multi-infarct disease
hepatic failure	
renal failure	
anemia	
fecal impaction	
dehydration and electrolyte imbalance	
drugs	

- Physiologic. The patient will complain of shortness of breath, dizziness, headaches, and heart pounding. Tension, fatigue, and diaphoresis are additional possibilities.
- Behavioral. The anxious person will feel panicky and may act in an obsessive compulsive manner. He or she will be easily distracted and poorly motivated and may lose problem-solving ability.
- Emotional. The patient's complaints will include nervousness, apprehension, and worry. However, when asked why he or she is worried, the patient will probably not be able to explain.

In an acute situation, the nurse would try to change the patient's environment. The idea is to relieve immediate stress. Relaxation exercises and breathing techniques designed for relaxation for 15 to 20 minutes are helpful. Walking about with the patient or giving him or her specific *simple* tasks to do helps to channel the excess energy. The patient requires the feeling of being needed at this time. Medications should be limited to 1 to 2 weeks, and drug therapy should be used only as an adjunct to psychotherapy.

As effective as psychotropic drugs are, and as fortunate as we are today to have them, no drug *cures* disturbed behavior. Frequently nonpharmacologic intervention is as effective as medication. Being a good listener and showing interest and concern for the individual are positive factors for the caregiver to remember.

☐ DEPRESSION

Signs of depression are observed emotionally, physiologically, and intellectually. The patient will appear extremely sad. He or she describes feelings of hopelessness and worthlessness. The patient probably has withdrawn from most social experiences and has an uncharacteristic lack of interest in his or her usual activities. Simply put, he or she cannot enjoy anything and feels very sorry for himself or herself. The patient may express suicidal thoughts ("I don't see much point to going on. No one would miss me.") Family and friends may be impatient and tell him or her to "cheer up" and pull himself or herself together. This is futile.

Depression is frequently accompanied by insomnia. The patient will mention vague bodily complaints such as headaches, backaches, and a feeling of weakness. There will be irregularities of appetite and a consequent reduction in energy. There is little if any interest in sex. In a true depression the patient will be unable to think clearly or concentrate. There will be memory lapses.

Depression can be masked in the confused older adult. It requires painstaking diagnosis. Since depression usually responds to treatment, it is important to recognize the symptoms of depression rather than just assuming they are part of the aging process. Depression is the most frequent psychologic disturbance in the elderly.

□ INSOMNIA

Insomnia may be described as sleeplessness during the normal sleeping period. It is a problem shared among 30 million people, between 12 and 15 per cent of the United States population. About five million Americans take some form of sleeping pill and 5 per cent of this number are over the age of 60. Insomnia is discussed in this chapter because it frequently becomes part of a chemical cycle. Pharmacologic agents contribute to the development of insomnia; drugs are taken to solve the problem; they in turn may cause problems, including further insomnia (Covington and Walker, 1984).

Many elders assume they have insomnia because their sleep pattern is not what it was when they were younger. Actually, normal aging is associated with an increase in the number of awakenings at night, a decrease in deep sleep, and a decrease in REM (rapid eye movement) sleep. REM sleep is one of the cycles of sleep, during which the eyes move rapidly and dreaming takes place. The need for REM sleep depends on the amount of stress and anxiety one is experiencing. Sleep scientists have concluded that it is a time when the body adapts emotionally, and therefore it is important for psychologic restoration.

The most common reason the older adult wakens during the night is to go to the bathroom. Other reasons for sleep disturbance in the older adult are overstimulation, depression, nocturnal myoclonus, and chemicals.

The most common drugs that cause interference with sleep are

1. appetite suppressants
2. OTC remedies such as diet aids and cold medicines that contain phenyl-propanolamine
3. caffeine
4. alcohol (acts paradoxically in most elderly)
5. narcotics (act paradoxically in most elderly)
6. psychotherapeutic agents
7. steroids
8. reserpine
9. Inderal

There are other factors that contribute to insomnia besides drugs. The nurse will want to evaluate for

1. hypoxia
2. pulmonary congestion
3. hypoglycemia (and other endocrine disorders)
4. pain
5. having to defecate or void
6. depression
7. anxiety or stress

Given the fact that the elderly as a group take a large number of medications, health professionals agree that the best approach to sleep disturbances is a nonpharmacologic one. The following should be tried first:

1. regular daily routine including some form of exercise
2. no food at bedtime
3. warm bath (followed by back massage, if possible)
4. small glass of warm milk (tryptophan is a natural sedating substance in milk that is activated by warming it)
5. quiet room—or wear ear plugs (the kind that mold to the ear)
6. avoid daytime naps
7. share worries and anxieties with an interested listener
8. avoid *any* beverage with caffeine
9. set a certain hour for sleep in a room that is used for sleep only
10. keep the bedroom cool
11. use mild pain relievers such as aspirin (the discomfort of arthritis and poor circulation is common in older people)

Drugs used for sleep disorder management are flurazepam (Dalmane), temazepam (Restoril), and triazolam (Halcion). However, these drugs can have side effects when combined with other medications the elderly client may be ingesting.

Antihistamines have been used but they can cause acute toxic delusions. Chloral hydrate has sedative effects but has been known to cause gastric distress. Hypnotics and barbiturates are contraindicated as long-term sleep aids since they can cause confusion and can depress cardiac and respiratory function.

Weaning from sedative-hypnotics must be done gradually to avoid agitation, nightmares, and rebound effects.

Often just informing the older adult of the expected sleep quantity and quality helps adjust the wrong perception of his or her sleep requirements.

☐ Discontinuing Medications

Bearing in mind that the older adult is extremely sensitive to drugs, caregivers must withdraw drugs slowly. Several factors affect discontinuing medications: the drugs, the reason they were administered, the dosages, and the length of time given. Certain drugs, psychotropics for example, can precipitate dangerous withdrawal problems. Cardiovascular drugs and anti-inflammatory drugs can cause rebound symptoms when withdrawn too abruptly. Patients should understand their medication regimen as well as caregivers do, and both groups should be aware that there are problems resulting from sudden drug withdrawal.

☐ Drug Misuse and the Elderly

Although it is almost always unintentional, drug misuse by the elderly is a problem of growing concern. What happens is this: Older adults usually have several health problems for which they are being treated. Unfortunately, these people rarely question the two best sources of drug information: their physician and their pharmacist. Noncompliance is a contributing factor to drug abuse. Either the patient does not take the prescribed drug or he or she takes it incorrectly. Most often the patient neglects to inform his or her physician about the medications, OTC or otherwise, that he or she is presently taking.

Another reason elderly persons misuse drugs is that they visit several physicians. Records are incomplete and drug histories are almost impossible to elicit.

Older adults who live independently must accept responsibility for learning more about all their medications and for using their pharmacists and physicians—not their friends—as their resources. They need to be reminded to ask questions about possible side effects. Above all, they should be encouraged to have more respect for OTC drugs, many of which used to be obtained by prescription only.

The elderly are susceptible to adverse drug reaction and are more prone to drug-induced disease states (e.g., tardive dyskinesia). Drug responsiveness is altered in older people because of changes in the process of drug handling: absorption has decreased, the liver's ability to metabolize has diminished, and renal function has deteriorated. Moreover, lifestyle and nutrition strongly affect drug activity.

As the number of drugs used rises, so do the chances of errors and drug reaction. In light of all this, consider that many diseases the elderly have do not need any drugs. Nonpharmacologic approaches to the health problems of the geriatric client should be explored.

Chapter 5 □ Review Questions

MULTIPLE CHOICE

_____ 1. The increase in fat composition and the decrease in muscle mass of the older adult means that
  A. the older adult needs more protein in the diet
  B. the older adult excretes drugs at a different rate
  C. the older adult needs a vigorous exercise program
  D. most older adults are seriously obese

_____ 2. Lithium is a useful medication for the treatment of
  A. digitalis intoxication
  B. angina
  C. narcotic overdose
  D. manic-depressive behavior

_____ 3. Elderly persons are prime candidates for drug problems because
  A. they see too many physicians
  B. they fail to follow directions correctly
  C. they have multiple chronic diseases
  D. they do not have easy access to pharmacists

_____ 4. An elderly person who experiences anxiety will be helped if the nurse
  A. obtains an order for a tranquilizer
  B. tells the family to visit more frequently
  C. tries to determine the cause of the anxiety
  D. encourages the patient to rest

_____ 5. The best approach to sleep disturbances in the elderly would be
  A. a quiet room
  B. avoiding daytime naps
  C. a regular daily routine that included some form of exercise
  D. all of the above

_____ 6. Which of the following is _not_ a symptom of depression?
  A. hopelessness
  B. self pity
  C. selfishness
  D. social withdrawal

_____ 7. When withdrawing drugs from the older adult, the nurse must remember
  A. that documentation is the most important factor
  B. that the elderly are extremely sensitive to drugs, so withdraw slowly
  C. to discontinue the most frequently taken drug before any others
  D. that diuretics are seldom withdrawn

_____ 8. The following drugs are antidepressants except
  A. imipramine
  B. haloperidol
  C. Marplan
  D. Parnate

_____ 9. The symptoms of Parkinson's disease include:
  A. tremor
  B. loss of muscle tone
  C. dry mouth
  D. all of the above

_____ 10. When the geriatric patient presents a behavioral problem, the nurse should
  A. restrain the patient
  B. determine why the patient is acting unacceptably
  C. consider medicating the patient
  D. change the patient's environment

TRUE/FALSE

_____ 1. Food plus drug interaction is as important as drug plus drug interaction.

_____ 2. The aging process has an insignificant effect on drug excretion.

_____ 3. One reason that drug "holidays" are given to elderly patients is that drugs are stored longer in their body fat.

_____ 4. Nearly half of all drugs can cause cognitive dysfunction.

_____ 5. One of the goals in nursing the geriatric patient is relief of all the patient's anxieties.

_____ 6. Normal aging is associated with an increase in the number of awakenings at night.

_____ 7. Impaired liver function prevents proper metabolism of drugs.

_____ 8. Cardiovascular drugs that are abruptly withdrawn can cause rebound symptoms in the older adult.

_____ 9. A side effect of tricyclic antidepressants is exhibition of extrapyramidal effects.

_____ 10. Cardiac failure can be a cause of chronic confusion.

□ REFERENCES

Burnside, I.M.: Nursing and the Aged. New York, McGraw-Hill, 1976.

Covington, T.R., and Walker, J.I.: Current Geriatric Therapy. Philadelphia, W.B. Saunders, 1984.

Dement, W.L.: Normal sleep and sleep disorders. In Usdin, G., and Lewis, J.M.: Psychiatry in General Practice. New York, McGraw-Hill, 1979.

Eisdorfer, C., and Fann, W. (ed.): Psychopharmacology and Aging. New York, Putnam Press, 1973.

Fielo, S., and Rizzolo, M.A.: The effects of age on pharmacokinetics. Geratr Nurs, 1985, p. 328.

Judd, E.: Nursing Care of the Adult. Philadelphia, F.A. Davis, 1983.

Levenson, A.J.: Neuropsychiatric Side Effects of Drugs in the Elderly. New York, Raven Press, 1979.

Libow, L.S.: Pseudosenility: Acute and reversible organic brain syndrome. Geriatr Soc, 21:112–120, 1973.

Milliren, J.W.: Some contingencies affecting the utilization of tranquilizers in long-term care of the elderly. J Health Soc, 18:206, 1977.

Rambo, B.J.: Adaptation Nursing: Assessment and Intervention. Philadelphia, W.B. Saunders, 1984.

Ray, O.S.: Drugs, Society and Human Behavior. St. Louis, C.V. Mosby, 1972.

The Relevance of Sleep Research to the Nursing Profession: A Review of 25 years of Intensive Sleep Research. Roffwarg, H., and Hartman, M. (eds.). Roche Products, 1980.

Scherer, J.C.: Introductory Clinical Pharmacology. Philadelphia, J.B. Lippincott, 1975.

Schrier, R.W.: Clinical Internal Medicine in the Aged. Philadelphia, W.B. Saunders, 1982.

Soloman, K., and Vickers, R.: Stereotyping the Elderly: Changing the Attitudes of Clinicians. Presented at the 33rd Annual Meeting of the Gerontological Society of America, San Diego, CA, November 25, 1980.

Todd, B.: Drugs and the elderly: Why are some drugs withdrawn slowly? Geriatr Nurs., 4:321, 1983.

Objectives

After completing this chapter, the student should be able to

☐ define aphasia
☐ list causes of aphasia
☐ describe anatomically and physiologically the aphasic zone
☐ compare expressive with reactive aphasia
☐ list nursing considerations of the aphasic patient
☐ describe treatment of the aphasic patient
☐ develop a guide for families of aphasic patients

Vocabulary

dilemma
gyrus
motor
posterior
sensory
superior

Imagine the extreme frustration of aphasic stroke patients. Their intellect is usually normal, but they are unable to communicate their most basic thoughts. Is it any wonder that these patients may become irritable, excited,

CHAPTER **6**

The Aphasic Patient

and even aggressive when they find that, although they think clearly, they have no way of communicating their thoughts and needs?

☐ Definition and Causes

Aphasia is a neurologic disorder that affects any and all factors in the comprehension of language. This disorder can involve speaking, reading, writing, and understanding spoken language.

Aphasia may be sensory (receptive aphasia) or motor (expressive or executive) aphasia. Most aphasias are mixed, a combination of both sensory and receptive. Global aphasia is the term given to total aphasia, in which no language ability is retained.

Trauma, cerebral vascular disease, lesions, or infection may cause the disorder. Commonly the problem is caused by left hemisphere damage due to vascular disease. Nearly 99 per cent of right-handed people and 60 per cent of left-handed people who have aphasia experienced a left-hemisphere injury.

The principal speech center in the brain is called Broca's area. In the aphasia zone, that section of the brain where varieties of aphasia are associated, Broca's area is located in a convolution (gyrus) adjoining the middle cerebral artery. The many combinations of muscular movements needed to speak each word are stored there as codes. Each word requires a combination or a sequence of combinations of muscular contractions for its expression. These combinations of muscular contractions are stored in the cells of Broca's convolution, and they govern the cells of the motor area responsible for the muscular contractions. Damage to Broca's convolution results in motor aphasia.

Sensory aphasia results when there is damage to Wernicke's area of the brain—the posterior part of the superior and middle temporal gyri. The normal function of Wernicke's area is the recognition of spoken language. The patient has normal hearing but cannot understand spoken language.

Expressive Aphasia
1. speech slow, labored
2. good understanding of writing and talking
3. can repeat single words with difficulty

4. object naming poor
5. patient aware; usually frustrated, depressed

Receptive Aphasia
1. speech fluent, words incorrect
2. words and sounds incorrect
3. unable to understand writing, talking; repetition is poor
4. object naming poor
5. may not be aware; in acute stage, often not depressed

☐ Nursing Considerations

Communication involves sending and receiving messages. Speech is our fundamental method of communication. Whether fully or partially impaired, the aphasic patient experiences profound frustration at its loss.

There are powerful changes in social relationships, economic status, and body image and esteem that the aphasic patient faces. He or she feels isolated because of the burden of communication restraint. Therefore, speech rehabilitation should begin as soon as the patient is medically stable.

The nurse can help reduce the frustration and isolation of impaired speech by the following:
1. anticipate patient needs to reduce frustration, worry, and concern
2. reinforce vocabulary with nonverbal communication: pictures, gestures, body language
3. speak in a normal tone
4. avoid baby talk or a patronizing tone; continually reassure to allay anxiety
5. remember pace; allow time for response
6. respect the patient's intellectual status; it is the same as before he or she became aphasic
7. explain the patient's environment to him or her; encourage responses

With professional speech therapy and the cooperation of all who come in contact with the patient, many aphasics regain most of their ability to communicate. Because the nurse should know what the speech therapy consists of so that she can reinforce it in her contacts with aphasic patients, a brief summary of it is presented here.

☐ Treatment*

Patterns of disability vary widely from case to case. Generally, concentration on the functions *least* impaired is recommended so as to inspire hope in the aphasic. Let him see progress. The general language disability is recognized and improvement aimed for in all areas. The therapist begins and ends each session with things the patient can do. Attempts are made very early in the illness to teach basic communication skills, e.g., how to call for the nurse, how to ask for water, and how to say hello, goodbye, yes, and no.

Parallel Talking. All who speak to the patient should speak clearly and simply. The use of gestures and written and pictured materials at times is very helpful. Therapists practice parallel talking; that is, they tell the patient what he is doing, feeling, or perceiving in simple short sentences or phrases. Often

---

*For the sake of clarity, in this section only, the patient will be referred to as "he" and the therapist will be referred to as "she."

the patient will join in and say a word the therapist is "fumbling" for. It's a basic part of therapy, but it has to be done well. The therapist must know when to hesitate, and it has to be at *exactly* the right moment that the patient is experiencing the thought that the therapist "fumbles" to express. It's also important not to overreact when the patient says the correct word. Just agree and then repeat what the patient has said in the context of the entire statement.

Stimulation. The aphasic lives in a confusing world. Depending on which function is affected, the newspaper seems to be pages of obscure hieroglyphics; he recognizes a clock, but can't tell time. His wife may be talking to him, but he doesn't understand her. He asks her for a glass of water, but she hears only unintelligible jargon.

The speech therapist must first identify what the patient *can* do. For example, can he copy the letters of the alphabet? If not, can he trace over them? Together they will begin at some level at which he or she can function and practice it until the skill is comfortable for the patient. The therapist will try other stimulation. She may have him repeat a sound, a word, or a gesture. Together they may each butter a piece of bread. She will take his hand and touch his ear, knee, and the table with it saying the names as she does this. The therapist might have the patient lipread "four" as she places four pennies on the table and then have him count to four aloud.

In each session the therapist will review the stimulation, praise success, and treat failure matter-of-factly. Success comes as the aphasic's confusion decreases and the lost functions begin to return.

Inhibition. Brain injuries make it difficult to curb emotional outbursts. Laughing, crying, and even tantrums are often observed. The patient may persevere too long. For example, he may start a sentence with "I want" and then, like a broken record, repeat it over and over, being unable to actually tell what it is he wants. The patient needs to be trained to inhibit himself; to stop what he is doing, first at the direction of the therapist and ultimately on his own. The aphasic should practice silently, or with a mirror, or learn to pantomime what he wants.

A therapist will even use "inhibition cards" for patients who can read. The message might be "**WAIT**," or "**STOP LAUGHING**," or "**WHISPER FIRST!**"

Translation. This means training the aphasic to change from one type of symbolism to another. For instance, he will listen to the sound of a cat meowing on a tape recorder. Then the therapist will ask him to identify and spell the name of the animal he heard and then to write (or print) the name of the animal. The object is to give the patient experience in shifting from one set of symbolic meanings to another.

Memorization. Aphasics may be asked to memorize a sequence of movement. This may be an exercise or picking out several objects in a definite order. For example, the therapist may give the patient a catalog and ask him to pick out three items in the order in which they are written on a blackboard. Or the patient's name will be spelled out in block letters on a table and then scrambled so that he has to rearrange them to spell the name correctly. Finally, the patient will be required to memorize prose and poetry. This helps to reinforce word associations and also reviews the basic structure of language.

Scanning and Concentrating. An aphasic may be compared to someone who accidentally lands on another planet. Sights and sounds are foreign, even overwhelmingly so. Basic tools and implements used by the natives are mysterious. He must observe and scan for meanings, but he needs the therapist's help. Together they will bring order out of confusion. For example, she may give him a magazine and have him point out all the hats. She will then ask him to stop her every time she says a word beginning with "h." She will have him connect the hat pictures with his own hat. They are selecting and classifying skills most of us take for granted but that have to be relearned by the aphasic.

Organization. The words "scramble," "jumbled," "confused," and "chaotic" have been used liberally to describe the world of the aphasic. He needs routines, schedules, and structure. The therapist begins with very basic pattern training. The patient may be asked to stack a series of boxes in graduated sizes. Maybe he has to be taught how to set the table or turn the pages of a book from right to left. Together, therapist and patient may sing old, familiar songs. All the planned activities require concentration and scanning by the patient and parallel talking by the therapist.

Formulation. Often the aphasic cannot find the words he needs and is overwhelmed with such depression that he stops right there. He needs direction and encouragement to try a new and different way that makes sense. Parallel talk and self talk can help him find verbal symbols that elude him. The following excerpt from a speech therapy session shows how this is done*:

> *Therapist:* All right, John. Let's begin. Talk to yourself. Say what you do. Like this. [She opens her purse, takes out a pencil, and writes his name. As she does so, she speaks in unison with her activity. "Open purse . . . here pencil . . . write name." The therapist hands him the purse and signals him to repeat her behavior.]
> *John:* [Opens purse] 'Oen puss . . . no . . . poos . . no . . . oh dear, oh my . . . ' [gives up].
> *Therapist:* OK. You got mixed up on purse . . . purrse . . . Never mind. Say the whole thing. [She repeats action]
> *John:* Open puss . . .
> *Therapist:* And here pencil . . .
> *John:* Pencil . . . and now I write mame . . . no . . . mama . . . no
> *Therapist:* Write name . . . name . . . like this. [Demonstrates]
> *John:* Write name like . . . [writes "John"] . . . John . . . John . . . write no good.

---

*Excerpt from speech therapy session taken from *Speech Correction Principles and Methods*, by Charles VanRiper, Prentice-Hall Inc., Englewood Cliffs, N. J., 1963, p. 453.

Therapist: Fine! You did it! Now, let's do it again. Talk to yourself. Say what you're doing.

Nurses and family members can describe the activities of daily living in this way and soon the patient will parallel talk as he observes the behavior of others. But this is only the beginning. He has to learn to make change, do mental problems, or, if that's not possible, do simple problems on paper. The aphasic will also be asked to write simple sentences and to write what he is about to say before he says it.

Body Image Integration. If the patient feels as if he has landed on another planet when he is confused by the strange sounds and sights caused by aphasia, he also wonders if his skin has been invaded by an alien. He is not now who he used to be. The family and health care professionals often reinforce this by treating him as if he were a child. An understanding of the situation can prevent this from happening.

What must it be like to find out that overnight one has an arm or a leg or a tongue that will not obey commands? The patient has to be reintroduced to his body all over again. While giving range of motion, the nurse can name the parts of the body she's working with. When teaching lip and tongue movement, it's helpful to use a mirror. A numb hand can be stimulated by massaging it with raw rice. A good therapist and good nursing care can accelerate body image integration.

Psychotherapy. The catastrophic effect of stroke cannot be underestimated. The anxieties about money, jobs, and family responsibilities can be overwhelming and certainly can be legitimate reasons for psychotherapy. Many therapists feel that a well-adjusted person who becomes aphasic has a better chance of ultimate adjustment than a neurotic individual who becomes aphasic. They caution about the problem of psychotherapy with a person who cannot communicate. It is extremely difficult to treat someone who cannot tell you what he understands or does not understand. Often a trial period of therapy is the only way to approach the situation.

☐ *Aphasia and the Family*

By examining some of the widespread changes in family life, it is easy to see how depression in the aphasic patient is precipitated. There is a loss of role, of status. Deprivation of responsibilities and enforced dependence erase identity.

Many aphasics are older adults, often with sons and daughters who have families of their own. It is not uncommon for these people to face the dilemma of dividing their attention between their children and their parent. Much of the time families make heroic efforts to be helpful and many aphasics owe their recoveries to the warmth, understanding, and encouragement of that invaluable support system.

Caregivers agree that stimulating and understanding companionship fosters motivation. But families need direction.

The first priority is open and thorough communication with the physician. There should be a clear understanding about the patient's physical and medical needs. These needs are rarely static and contact should be ongoing for assessment and re-evaluation. Even the aphasic who is healthy and under the supervision of a speech therapist will have other needs. For example, there may need to be a referral to a vocational rehabilitation agency. Caregivers will usually offer guidance by means of suggestions rather than rigid instructions. The family can adapt them.

An important suggestion is to observe when the patient is most responsive to visitors. When energy levels are high and the patient is rested, he or she will be able to respond to and benefit from company. At first, there will be difficulty in following multiple conversations, and the number of visitors should be limited.

Families often know instinctively how to keep the aphasic patient involved and stimulated in what is going on. Past interests and hobbies can give valuable clues. Pets can provide pleasure as well as interest. The family will also have to make adjustments when the patient does not respond. If people are relaxed and allow enough time for action and responses the patient will have less anxiety and more small successes.

Feelings of anger and resentment are common, and loved ones are often shocked and guilty to find that they are experiencing them. They may try to deny them. Sometimes an objective third party, a clergyman, physician, or therapist, may help the family to understand that they are experiencing natural emotions, legitimate reactions. Families get tired too.

Suggestions for families of aphasic patients follow:

1. *Seek good professional assistance.* The regular advice of a physician is best. The aphasic may need diagnostic tests, medications, nutritional advice, and prescribed exercises. Trained social workers, psychologists, and psychiatrists are helpful when there are emotional problems. Remind the family, however, that others besides the skilled team can help the patient recover. Most aphasics improve because of their affectionate support systems, i.e., the family.

2. *Discover how well the patient can communicate.* Although diagnostic studies will be used to determine the aphasic's ability, the family should observe the patient's language, or lack of it, also. How does the aphasic communicate? Can he or she gesture? Can he or she express thoughts,

ideas? Efforts to study this will help a person understand what the therapist is doing and ultimately will benefit the patient.

3. *Take a good look at your own feelings.* Aphasia affects the family profoundly. Reactions vary from anxiety and being too helpful to being discouraged and resentful. All these feelings are natural, but they must be recognized. Sometimes an objective, uninvolved third party such as a physician, a clergyman, or a psychologist can be helpful.

4. *Spend time with the patient when he or she is most responsive.* Aphasics feel isolated because of the severity of their communication problem. Most family members encourage visits with old friends, but it's important to realize that the patient tires easily. During the recovery period, gradually increasing the length of visits is a sensible approach to including the patient in social interaction. The patient's motivation and response will be at a high level *only* when rested, so company will be welcome at appropriate times during the patient's daily schedule.

5. *Make a check list of his or her special interests and use material from it when you spend time with him or her.* The patient's special interests are as distinctive as each patient is. Sports, hobbies, favorite foods—any and all activities form a basis for stimulating the patient. The aphasic's reactions and attitudes have to be closely watched, and endeavoring to interest him or her can be a hit or miss affair. If the response is unfavorable, discard the idea and try something else. Change the subject or just leave the patient alone if he or she seems upset or restless.

6. *Accept the patient as he or she is at the moment.* Outbursts of temper are common. A relaxed, matter of fact attitude is important here because the patient has less control over his or her emotions than before the illness. Be encouraging but avoid false optimism and cliches.

7. *Use every opportunity to increase his or her independence.* The patient can actually be held back if people do too much for him or her. The family should aim for daily *small* successes in feeding, dressing, and other activities. They should encourage gains and minimize losses.

8. *Include the patient in family affairs.* It's irritating to be talked about as if you are not even present. Worse, it's demeaning. Provide for the participation of the patient in conversations, decisions, and activities as much as possible and within reason.

9. *Be alert for signs of depression.* It is common in aphasic patients. It is especially noticeable in those who do not have severe auditory verbal agnosia (lack of understanding of spoken language) and who are painfully aware of their own errors. Suicide is a possibility in the untreated depressed patient. Caregivers should take seriously any self-destructive threats. Sometimes the attempts are not overt. For example, "forgetting" to take medications, other forms of noncompliance, and refusing therapy or meals are indications of passive suicide.

Booklets for the Family (Darley, 1982)

American Heart Association: Aphasia and the Family. New York, American Heart Association, 1965.

Boone, D.: An Adult Has Aphasia. Danville, IL, Interstate Printers and Publishers, 1965.

Cohen, L. K.: Communication Problems After a Stroke. Minneapolis, Kenny Rehabilitation Institute, 1971.

Crickmay, M. C.: Help the Stroke Patient to Talk. Springfield, IL, Charles C Thomas, 1977.

Sarno, J. E., and Sarno, M. T.: Stroke: The Condition and the Patient. New York, McGraw-Hill, 1969.

☐ Conclusion

Most aphasics have been impaired by stroke. Rehabilitation consists of an interdisciplinary effort among physical, occupational, recreational, corrective, and manual arts therapies.

Behavioral changes often occur because of brain damage. There may be mood swings, irritability, inappropriate laughter, and tears. Continuity of care and supportive services are essential. Caregivers accept emotional lability pragmatically and without embarrassment, attempting to reduce the level of frustration and to encourage more effective communication.

Chapter 6 ☐ Review Questions

MULTIPLE CHOICE

1. The principal speech center in the brain is called
   A. Broca's area
   B. Wernicke's area
   C. gyrus
   D. convolution
2. An example of receptive aphasia is
   A. slow and labored speech
   B. fluent speech
   C. parallel talking
   D. perseveration
3. Depression in the aphasic can be precipitated by
   A. fatigue
   B. poor nutrition

C. lack of intensive psychotherapy
D. enforced dependence
4. Family members can help the aphasic by
   A. spending time with him or her when he or she is most responsive
   B. seeking good professional assistance
   C. encouraging independence
   D. all of the above
5. Commonly, aphasia is caused by
   A. right-hemisphere damage
   B. left-hemisphere damage
   C. damage to the organ of Corti
   D. aging process

TRUE/FALSE

_____ 1. Global aphasia is the term given to total aphasia; no language ability is retained.
_____ 2. Expressive aphasia is characterized by slow speech.
_____ 3. Brain injuries make it difficult to curb emotional outbursts.
_____ 4. A competent speech therapist can fulfill most of the aphasic's needs.
_____ 5. Past interests and hobbies of the aphasic patient will serve no useful purpose and, in fact, will cause depression.

DISCUSSION QUESTIONS

1. What are the causes of aphasia other than strokes?
2. Give examples of nonverbal communication as related to the activities of daily living.
3. What are some ways the nurse can help the family of the aphasic patient?
4. What are some ways the nurse can help the aphasic patient?

□ **REFERENCES**

Agranowitz, A., and McKeown, M.: Aphasia Handbook for Adults and Children. Springfield, IL, Charles C Thomas, 1975.
American Heart Association: Aphasia and the Family. New York, American Heart Association, 1979.
Blanco, K.: The Aphasic Patient. J Neurosurg Nurs, 14 (1):34–37, 1982.
Burnside, I. M.: Working with the Elderly: Group Processes and Techniques. Belmont, CA, Wadsworth Health Sciences, 1984.
Coleman, J. C.: Abnormal Psychology and Modern Life. Glenview, IL, Scott Foresman, 1976.
Darley, F. L.: Aphasia. Philadelphia, W. B. Saunders, 1982.
Judd, E. W.: Nursing Care of the Adult. Philadelphia, F. A. Davis, 1983.

Luckmann, J., and Sorensen, K.: Medical Surgical Nursing: A Psychophysiologic Approach. Philadelphia, W. B. Saunders, 1980.

Rambo, B. J.: Adaptation Nursing: Assessment and Intervention. Philadelphia, W. B. Saunders, 1984.

Schuell, H., et al.: Aphasia Theory and Therapy. Baltimore, University Park Press, 1974.

VanRiper, C.: Speech Correction Principles and Methods. Englewood Cliffs, N.J., Prentice-Hall, 1963.

Objectives	Vocabulary
After completing this chapter the student should be able to	augment emphysema incest
☐ list the normal physiologic processes that cause changes in the sexual organs of older adults	neuter sociogenic testosterone
☐ explain why there are negative attitudes toward elders who express their sexuality	
☐ describe how negative attitudes of others affect sexual behavior in older adults	
☐ list reasons why adult children oppose or discourage sexual activity between their elderly parents	
☐ describe the nurse's role in acknowledging the right of elders to sexual expression	

CHAPTER *7*

Sexual Aspects of Aging

Chapter Outline

RESEARCH FINDINGS
CULTURAL ATTITUDES AND STEREOTYPES
AGE-RELATED CHANGES
    Changes in Women
    Changes in Men
BARRIERS TO SEXUAL EXPRESSION
    Misinformation
    Chronic Illness
    Fear of Heart Attack
    Medications
    Excesses in Food and Alcohol
    Lack of Partner or Opportunity
    Loss of Self Esteem; Masculinity
      and Femininity
    Depression

NURSING ACTIONS
    Acknowledge Elders as
      Sexual
    Examine Personal
      Attitudes
    Reinforce Sexual
      Identity
    Encourage Good
      Health Habits
    Respect Privacy
    Meet Social Needs
    Refer for Medical Help
    Provide Teaching
REVIEW QUESTIONS
REFERENCES

☐ *Research Findings*

Masters and Johnson's classic work, *Human Sexual Response*, gave us our first knowledge about the changes in anatomy and physiology of the sexual organs and our first insights into how aging affects sexual response patterns. Although there are circumstantial and emotional factors that may cause an aging person to refrain from sexual intercourse, there are no inherent physical changes in the aging process of the healthy person that negate sexual behavior or satisfaction.

Since then, other studies have augmented this original work. One of the more thought provoking is the Starr-Weiner Report on *Sex and Sexuality in the Mature Years*. This study is especially useful because it does not emphasize changes, either physiologic or behavioral, in terms of *losses*. Instead, it teaches us that there is a strong need to accept a range and variability of sexual expression. The elders surveyed concentrated less on goal-oriented sexual expression and more on a diffuse and widespread means of expressing sexuality. For example, they noted that touching, pleasuring, and cuddling are expressions of sexual experience that offer satisfaction. This indicates that the quantity of sexual expression is less important than the significance or quality. The greatest barrier remains one of attitude by society in general and by the elderly themselves. Older people, unfortunately, believe the stereotypes of sociogenic aging.

☐ *Cultural Attitudes and Stereotypes*

Older men and women are strongly influenced by the current attitudes of society towards sex. Most people will admit that sexuality is one of the most interesting of all human subjects. Curious, then, is the fact that until quite recently the sexual aspects of aging received little attention from researchers or health professionals. Our culture still rejects, to a great extent, the idea that sex is normal and healthy in the later years. It is possible that we have avoided studying this important aspect of aging because professionals also believed that sexual feelings and behaviors did not exist for most of the aging.

In a recent discussion, a group of health professionals was asked to associate words for characterizing sexually active older adults. They selected words and phrases such as hard to imagine, nonexistent, impossible, slow, and infrequent. It seems hard to acknowledge that aged persons participate in active sex because of the assumption in our society by both young and older adults that elderly persons do not have sexual desires, are physically (therefore, sexually) unattractive, and are too fragile physically to engage in sexual activities.

Elderly men who display sexual interest are labeled "dirty old men," but elderly women do not merit even that kind of attention. They may be called "old bags" or "crocks," thus being successfully neutered and encouraged to slide rapidly into sexual oblivion. The media, the families, and society in general view the elderly as asexual and therefore, as deviant if they express sexual needs, desires, or behavior. Adult children discount the possibility that their aging parents are, or even could be, sexually active.

During the age of sexual revolution and amid tolerant attitudes toward any sexual practice, it seems paradoxical that there exists a puritanical approach to gerontic sexuality. There are several reasons. The persistence of the Oedipus complex and incest taboos, the extolling of a youth-oriented culture, and the association of aging with illness (thereby focusing attention on the minority of elders who are sick rather than on the majority who are healthy and active) are all issues contributing to negative attitudes. Another interesting reason for inhibiting sex among the elderly by adult children is the fact that it protects inheritances, it eliminates older adults from competing sexually with younger adults, and nonsexual elderly are easier to control. (The older person who has a sexual partner has an ally, and therefore, strength.)

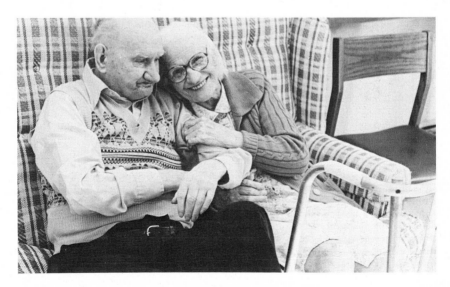

The expression of affection and sexual feelings is legitimate behavior among older adults. (Courtesy of Ring Nursing Homes.)

☐ Age-Related Changes

☐ CHANGES IN WOMEN

Changes in a woman's sexual organs seem to be related primarily to the loss of estrogen production after menopause. Lower estrogen levels cause a loss of elasticity and a thinning of the mucous membranes of the vagina. Consequently, the older woman experiences slower lubrication during sexual excitement than the premenopausal woman. Masters and Johnson found that women who were participating in regular sexual activity, regardless of age, maintained their ability to lubricate better than those who chose not to engage in sex. Also, women who take replacement hormones will experience a more gradual change in vaginal mucosa. Those women who find their lack of lubrication makes penetration uncomfortable can be advised to use a water soluble gel to compensate for nature's lack.

Whereas vaginal changes are to be expected, the clitoris, the major organ of sexual excitation, retains its high degree of sensitivity throughout life. Other characteristic physiologic responses to sexual stimulation may diminish (breast changes, skin flushing, and uterine contractions) as a woman ages but not enough to interfere with pleasure. Many of the changes of aging go unnoticed by the woman whose sexual life remains vigorous and satisfying.

Although women of any age may develop a urinary tract infection if bacteria pass into the paraurethral glands or to the bladder after sexual intercourse, older women especially are encouraged to void at this time. Voiding will flush out organisms that inhabit the lower urinary tract.

☐ CHANGES IN MEN

A man also experiences changes as he ages, but he, too, can rest assured that the changes are of degree, not kind. Testosterone levels gradually decrease with age, causing characteristic physical changes and changes in the timing of sexual response. The older man usually finds that erection takes longer to achieve, but he is able to maintain it longer. This aspect of aging is particularly welcomed by the couple disturbed during their younger years by premature ejaculation. The older man also experiences less urgency about ejaculation than his younger counterparts—in fact he often enjoys intercourse without the need to ejaculate. Lower levels of sex hormones diminish the response of the man's nipples, scrotum, and testes to sexual excitement and orgasm. Men experience longer periods of time between erections as they age and some have difficulty re-attaining a "lost" erection during an act of intercourse. The man who is unfamiliar with these expected changes may fear he has become impotent and put aside his sexual life prematurely and unnecessarily.

For both man and woman, then, the physical changes caused by the decline of sex hormone production do not seem to change the capacity for sexual response significantly. It has been reported, however, that the number of sexual encounters lessens as one ages in America. What might account for this if physical changes are not the cause?

□ *Barriers to Sexual Expression*

Several factors have been discussed in research literature and cited by older persons themselves as influencing their decrease in sexual activity. Some of these are misinformation, chronic illness, fear of heart attack, medications, overindulgence in food or alcohol, fatigue, loss through death or separation, lack of new partners, loss of self-esteem, and depression. Some of these factors are personal, some circumstantial, some social. A few are beyond the control of either the nurse or the client; others can be prevented or modified. We will consider them individually to see if we as nurses can have a positive role in changing these inhibiting factors.

□ MISINFORMATION

How and if an older person continues to express sexual needs is often related to cultural beliefs and previously learned expectations. Most of our present older generation grew up in an era of sexual silence, an era in which great gaps in sexual knowledge existed. When gaps in knowledge exist, humans tend to invent answers. With time and repetition, such "answers" become accepted as truth. Some of the "truths" about sexuality prevalent in the early 1900's that still affect the attitudes of older persons are that "nice" women do not experience sexual excitement, sexual interest beyond a certain age (for either sex) is perverse at worst and abnormal at best, masturbation causes physical and mental illness, and it is "bad" to think or fantasize about sex.

Persons who continue to hold these ideas may have had feelings of guilt about sex throughout much of their lives. They may actually welcome the changes of aging as a reason to stop psychologically uncomfortable sexual behaviors altogether. We need to accept such a choice with respect while not avoiding our professional responsibility to present better information about normal sexuality to them. Others, however, do not share these attitudes and beliefs, and it is these older persons who can most benefit from information-sharing and counseling with health professionals. It is this group who may need some sexual information in order to fully enjoy all their capacities as they age.

☐ CHRONIC ILLNESS

Chronic illnesses, such as arthritis, emphysema, and vascular disease, may inhibit some older couples from continuing their sexual activity. When properly treated with medication and physical therapy, however, a couple can often maintain their sexual relationship in spite of illness. Changes in love-making positions that may be less stressful for the affected partner could be of help. Side-lying postures for intercourse are often comfortable for both partners. Chronic diabetes is about the only disease that seems to cause impotence in the aging man. As with any type of serious sexual dysfunction, referral for a thorough evaluation of cause is in order before hope is lost.

☐ FEAR OF HEART ATTACK

Fear of heart attack during sexual activity is common among the older generation, particularly among those who have already had coronary difficulties or whose partner has heart disease. It has been shown through research that sexual activity, particularly in familiar surroundings with a familiar partner, is akin to any form of moderate exertion. Older persons need to be informed of this research and reassured that sexual activity and heart attack are not directly related to each other. Counseling about less stressful positions for intercourse may also help, although trying new positions seems to actually increase stress for some couples. The warning signs of increased stress should be taught to all cardiac patients, and they should consult with their physician if these signs occur during or shortly after sexual activity.

☐ MEDICATIONS

We know that certain drugs used in the therapy of hypertension, coronary disease, and chronic depression can cause a loss of sexual desire or drug-induced impotence, or both. The older person who must use such drugs should be familiar with their expected side effects and report to their doctor if changes in sexual functioning occur. Sometimes an equally therapeutic agent can be substituted for the one causing the problem.

☐ EXCESSES IN FOOD AND ALCOHOL

Overindulgence in food and alcohol can cause sexual problems for anyone but seems to be particularly troublesome to the older man. Encouraging everyone to enjoy food and drink wisely and to keep a good balance between rest and exercise is a nursing responsibility. The older person who is in good physical condition is more likely to enjoy *everything*, including sex!

☐ LACK OF PARTNER OR OPPORTUNITY

Loss of loved ones through death is a sad but common experience for older persons. Saddest of all during the later years may be the loss of one's love partner, for new sexual relationships are often very difficult to establish. Two cultural biases mitigate against the formation of new relationships—the idea that older persons should not be interested anyway and, secondly, the feeling that sex is for married persons only (at least if you're over 60!). Less effort is made by friends and relatives to introduce the older person to potential partners than would be the case for younger widows and widowers. Places where younger people go to meet new people are often unwelcoming and suspicious of older persons. Sons and daughters often have strong feelings against remarriage and extremely negative feelings about any other form of sexual relationship for their parents. Until recently, even some tax and Social Security laws made it financially unprofitable to remarry after 65. Chances are that persons who lose their sexual partner late in life will spend their remaining years alone.

Another form of separation can be equally devastating to an older, sexually active couple. Circumstances may necessitate the move of one of them from the home to a nursing home or other supervised living situation. Although the husband or wife (or lover) will be encouraged to visit, there is hardly ever enough privacy for the intimate relationship to be continued. Semi-private rooms, unlocked doors, and staff moving freely in and out are hardly conducive to loving! Even if both partners move to supervised living, they are often separated and given a roommate of their own sex.

More consideration must be given to the institutionalized elderly. "Petting rooms" have been suggested as an aid to privacy. This seems to be an artificial solution, however. More natural, and thus more appropriate, would be designated periods during the day when residents know they will not be disturbed in the comfort and security of their own rooms.

In the acute care setting, nurses can also help provide privacy and the opportunity for physical contact between a patient and his or her partner. Holding hands, hugging, kissing, fondling, and lying side by side are all actions that can provide great comfort to the patient. A great deal depends on the attitudes of the nursing staff; if they consider such contact inappropriate "sexual" behavior, they are depriving their patients of an important aid to recovery.

☐ LOSS OF SELF ESTEEM; MASCULINITY AND FEMININITY

Probably the greatest inhibitor of healthy sexual functioning in older age is loss of self-esteem and the development of a negative self-image. It is difficult to maintain one's positive self-image in a culture as devoted to youth worship as ours is. Loss of skin and muscle tone, graying hair, wrinkles, and "liver spots" are certainly not revered by Madison Avenue and Hollywood! The attitude that young is beautiful and sexy and that old is not pervades the thinking of many of us.

But being sexual and sexually attractive is more than one's physique; it involves those elusive qualities called masculinity and femininity and doing things that make one feel good about being a man or being a woman. When middle-aged persons were asked what makes them feel successful as a man or a woman, women tended to answer: dressing attractively; smelling good; being a good cook or homemaker; wearing make-up and jewelry; helping others; being a good wife, mother, or daughter; and receiving compliments. Men mentioned such things as being successful in their work; managing money well; participating in sports or other activities with men; discussing politics and world events knowledgeably; advising younger people; being attractive to women; and being a good lover. (These activities may seem stereotyped to the reader and, in one sense, they are. Many of our older citizens grew up in an era when "masculinity" and "femininity" were more rigidly defined than nowadays.)

When one feels good about oneself and one's self-confidence is high, something is communicated to others that translates into sexual attractiveness, regardless of age. Unfortunately, many of our older citizens live in environments that are not sensitive to the importance of helping them maintain a positive self image. Premature cessation of those activities that previously built self esteem, such as dressing attractively or participating in sports, sap the zest from life for them, as it would for us.

☐ DEPRESSION

Any of the factors discussed previously may lead to transient or chronic depression in our older clients. Frequently, several of the factors are operating simultaneously in their lives. The depressed person rarely has much energy for any of life's activities, including sexual activity.

☐ *Nursing Actions*

What can the nurse do in the face of all the possible inhibitors just discussed? The nurse can have a positive role in helping older persons continue to enjoy their sexual capabilities by following the suggestions listed:

Acknowledge Elders as Sexual. Caregivers need to give legitimacy to the normalcy of sexual needs among elders. The tendency to infantilize the elderly may have been one of our unconscious ways of avoiding our own discomfort about sexual expression at their age. Once we recognize and accept them as sexual persons, our relationships with them must change. That very change in our behavior can contribute much to the older person's positive self-image, which in turn will help him or her feel sexually attractive. Occasionally, a client's sexual needs and desires will be directed at the health care professional. Although we recognize flirtatious or seductive behavior as inappropriate to a professional relationship, we may find ourselves unable to cope with our own feelings in such situations. We may be tempted to simply avoid further interaction with the client. Gentle reminders about limits or, better yet, an open, frank discussion of their needs and feelings is more productive and caring than avoidance. If the professional feels unprepared to confront inappropriate behaviors alone, the assistance of a supervisor or coprofessional should be sought.

Examine Personal Attitudes. Recognize our own obstructive attitudes about sex among the elderly. It is almost impossible not to have learned some negative attitudes during our own growing-up years. Once we recognize our own attitudes, we can begin the process of re-education for ourselves as individual practitioners and for the profession as a whole. The new information being generated by research is not only important but also interesting.

Reinforce Sexual Identity. Help older persons continue those activities that contributed to feelings of masculinity and femininity in their younger years. Here is an opportunity to assess and individualize our nursing care for each client. Once we know what *they* choose for themselves, we can direct our efforts toward providing continuation of similar activities. We may need to provide transportation so that an older client can participate in community affairs or go to the beauty parlor or barber. We need to encourage women to continue cooking (or at least, to share recipes with the cook) and to encourage widowers to learn to cook for their own better nutrition. Providing activities that men can identify as "masculine" (woodworking, crafts, beer and poker parties, a pool table) in a long-term facility is also helpful. Opportunities for people to gather together to discuss politics or to watch sporting and other events can be provided in most settings. Other creative approaches will undoubtedly occur to health care professionals once they give priority to the maintenance of the older person's self image.

Encourage Good Health Habits. Encourage good physical habits through exercise, rest, and nutrition. Too often, we tacitly encourage older persons to spend most of their waking hours sitting around, which only compounds the natural loss of tone and circulation.

Respect Privacy. When a "couple" already exists, provide opportunities for privacy. In some supervised living situations, policies may have to be revised in order to provide an older couple with time alone together. We should beware, however, assuming that every older couple wants to continue being roommates! It should be their choice, supported by us and re-evaluated from time to time. If they do choose to share the same room, using their own bed in the new setting may encourage them to continue already established sexual patterns.

Meet Social Needs. Provide social outlets and encourage new friendships that may lead to intimate relationships. We are sometimes guilty of treating a newly forming couple as "cute" and joking about their relationship. Older persons, highly sensitive to criticism and poorly educated about sexuality in old age, will conform to what we are implying, thereby losing valuable opportunities to replace lost partners.

Refer for Medical Help. Refer clients to physicians for health check-ups (including pelvic exams) and re-evaluation of medications. Pain on intercourse, impotence unrelieved by changes in eating or drinking styles, and chronic depression need a specialist's intervention. The informed, interested doctor is our most valuable collaborator in re-educating our older clients toward healthier living and continued sexual expression. Using his or his or her authority judiciously, the physician can reinforce the nurse's teaching and counseling and provide reassurance.

Provide Teaching. Share new-found information on normal sexual functioning in older persons with clients, families, and professional peers. We cannot hope to accomplish much in a vacuum that continues to repress sexual

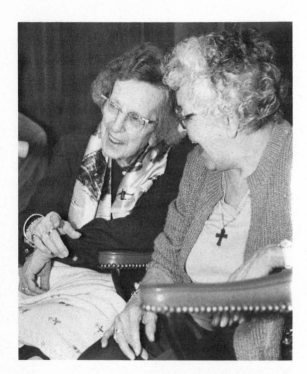

Attractive clothing, jewelry, and hair styling may be an important part of an older woman's self image. (Courtesy of Ring Nursing Homes.)

knowledge and to perpetrate sexual mythology. Fortunately, most persons are interested in knowing more about that ever-fascinating subject of human sexuality! Changing deep-seated attitudes is, of course, difficult and the nurse needs to accept this. It is our responsibility, however, to continue to try to influence persons of all ages towards healthier sexual attitudes and more informed decision-making about their sexuality.

A nurse and a psychologist who conducted a human sexuality course at a community senior center noted comments by participants on the significance of sex over the life span: "To me, sex is not solely sexual intercourse," stated an older woman. "I have clearly found that holding hands with a male I liked, being in the circle of his arms, or laying my cheek on his has been most reassuring, especially when I was unhappy, distressed or grieving."

An elderly male summed up his feelings about sex for him now: "Sex for most older adults is the same as our other appetites—it lessens, but sometimes it's special because we don't feed it as often." (Boyer and Boyer, 1982)

Although this knowledge will not make us qualified sexual therapists, it can add a new dimension to our nursing of older persons. What has been learned in recent years can help nurses assist the aging to continue to enjoy their sexuality, thus enhancing the quality of their lives.

Chapter 7 ☐ Review Questions

MULTIPLE CHOICE

1. Sexual behavior in older adults
   A. decreases because of age
   B. decreases because of poor health
   C. may be affected by circumstantial and emotional factors
   D. is normally absent
2. Elderly adults participate in sexual expression
   A. only when they are married to each other
   B. seldom, because they are frail and weak
   C. only if they are in good health
   D. in diffuse ways such as touching, pleasuring, and cuddling
3. Sexual aspects of aging
   A. are not well known by health professionals, the elderly, or society in general
   B. are well known by physicians, nurses, and psychologists
   C. are well known by older people
   D. are being carefully researched on a long-term basis

4. Families of the elderly often discourage sexual expression between elders because
   A. nonsexual older people are easier to control
   B. they are concerned about their parents overexerting themselves
   C. geriatric sexual expression is abnormal
   D. sexually active elders are prone to infections
5. The sexually active older woman
   A. will develop a urinary tract infection
   B. should always take replacement hormones
   C. may not even notice many of the changes of aging
   D. should strictly limit sexual activity

TRUE/FALSE

_____ 1. Sexual expression is often related to cultural beliefs.
_____ 2. Misinformation is no longer a barrier to sexual expression of older adults.
_____ 3. Chronic illness eliminates any sexual expression by elders.
_____ 4. Drug-induced impotence is always irreversible.
_____ 5. Persistence of the Oedipal complex into adulthood causes negative feelings in the children of elders.
_____ 6. Relaxed elderly partners can enjoy satisfactory sexual experiences.
_____ 7. The frequency of intercourse always decreases with aging.
_____ 8. Institutionalized elderly have no need of sexual expression.
_____ 9. Most elderly are well informed about sexuality in advancing years.
_____ 10. Professional persons have healthier attitudes toward sex than nonprofessionals.

DISCUSSION QUESTIONS

1. Suggest ways in which nursing home residents can be helped to form new relationships.
2. How can older adults who live independently be encouraged to form new relationships?
3. Are there some elderly who do not want to make new friends? Would you try to change their attitude? Why?

□ REFERENCES

Aiken, L.: Later Life. Philadelphia, W. B. Saunders, 1978.
Boyer, G., and Boyer, J.: Sexuality and aging. Nurs Clin North Am, 17(3):421–427, 1982.
Butler, R. N., and Lewis, M. I.: Aging and Mental Health. 2nd ed. St Louis, C. V. Mosby, 1983.
Byers, J. P.: Sexuality and the elderly. Geriatr Nurs, 4(5):293–297, 1983.

Comfort, A.: A Good Age. New York, Crown Publications, 1976.

Friedman, J. S.: Sexuality in older persons: Implications for nursing practice. Nurs Forum, 18(1):92–101, 1979.

Griggs, W.: Staying well while growing old . . . sex and the elderly. Am J Nurs 78(8):1352–1354, 1978.

Masters, W. H., and Johnson, V. E.: Human Sexual Response. Boston, Little, Brown, 1966.

Stanford, D.: All about sex . . . after middle age. Am J Nurs, 77(4):608–611, 1975.

Starr, B., and Weiner, M. B.: On Sex and Sexuality in the Mature Years. New York, Stein and Day, 1981.

Watts, R. J.: The physiological interrelationships between depression, drugs and sexuality. Nurs Forum, 17(2):168–183, 1978.

Objectives

After completing this chapter, the student should be able to

- [ ] list physical, economic, social, and psychologic issues associated with nutrition and the older adult
- [ ] list ways to improve nutrition in the elderly
- [ ] explain the basis of hospital-induced malnutrition
- [ ] state measures used to care for the nutritional needs of the acutely ill older adult
- [ ] suggest solutions to the problems of inadequate protein intake, dental deficiencies, anorexia, and other nutritional problems common in the elderly

Vocabulary

anorexia
cellulose
hemodialysis
malabsorption
malnutrition
osteoporosis

CHAPTER 8

Nutritional Factors

Chapter Outline

Almost all gerontologic researchers agree that nutrition is a factor in the aging process. As people age, the chances of developing a chronic illness are greater. It has become evident that an inadequate or improper diet contributes toward some of these illnesses. On the other hand, improved nutrition is therapeutic for many who have chronic diseases.

☐ Components of Nutritional Problems

Commonly, there are three overlapping components of nutritional problems: the physical, the economic, and the psychologic.

☐ PHYSICAL COMPONENT

Illnesses and Disorders

Improper nutrition can contribute to a number of problems, including heart disease, obesity, iron deficiency anemia, osteoporosis, dry skin and decreased mucus secretion, polyneuritis, and cancer. Research has shown some clear connections between certain eating patterns and disease, whereas other relationships are still being investigated. In particular, high fat content in the diet has been linked to disease.

Heart Disease. The leading cause of death in this country, heart disease strikes men and women in their peak productive years and continues through old age. Heart disease has been linked to high levels of saturated fats in the diet.

Obesity. Obesity is common, especially among postmenopausal women. As we age, our physical activity tends to decrease at the same time that our bodies' need for calories is decreasing due to a lower metabolic rate. If calories are not trimmed to accommodate this decrease, obesity is the inevitable result. It is not sufficient just to eat *less*. An obese elderly person presents a complex problem because if activity cannot be increased to help burn up the excess calories, the diet has to be adjusted to a lower calorie level while still allowing for sufficient amounts of calcium, protein, and iron.

Weight control in the elderly is a challenging objective. The rewards include less cardiovascular disability, less discomfort for the arthritic, and increased muscular strength.

Iron Deficiency Anemia. The most prevalent nutritional deficiency in the elderly is iron deficiency anemia, probably because the consumption of meat is limited because of high prices and restricted budgets. A lack of green and yellow vegetables in the diet also helps to cause this problem.

Osteoporosis. This condition is characterized by abnormal loss of bone mass, making the bones more fragile. It is encountered in persons after the age of 50 and is more common in women than in men by a ratio of about four to one. Inadequate calcium intake has been shown to contribute to the development of osteoporosis. Osteoporosis develops slowly, and it may be many years before a person becomes aware of overt changes. Thus it is important that the younger person be aware of the importance of calcium in the diet and establish good eating habits long before old age.

Dry Skin and Decreased Mucus Secretion. Common in older persons, these conditions may be partly caused by vitamin A deficiency.

Polyneuritis. This inflammation of many peripheral nerves at the same time can be due to a thiamine deficiency. (Thiamine is present in whole grain cereals and breads.)

Cancer. Links between diet and some kinds of cancer are being studied by researchers. It appears that there is a definite link between diets high in fat and low in fiber and the development of colon cancer. The National Cancer Institute has recommended that Americans decrease their consumption of animal fats and increase consumption of fruits, vegetables, and grains.

Physical Problems That Contribute to Nutritional Deficiencies

Dental Problems. Nearly two thirds of all Americans over age 65 have lost all of their natural teeth. By middle age, 25 million people are endentulous; another 25 million have lost half of their teeth. If dentures do not fit well or have not had proper repairs, chewing becomes difficult or impossible. Chewing (or mastication) is an essential first step of the digestive process. Problems with this first step can lead to a diet that leaves out harder to chew foods. This in turn can lead to undernutrition or obesity or various illnesses caused by dietary insufficiencies. The solution seems deceptively simple: sound preventive care, or at least properly fitted dentures. Unfortunately, many elderly persons are on fixed incomes that do not allow for the expense of dental care.

Lack of Mobility. Lack of mobility can contribute to an inadequate diet. The elderly adult who cannot drive or walk to a market comfortably or who cannot carry parcels home has to practice defensive shopping. Purchases must be economical and long-lasting. Often this means that the elderly person cannot buy fresh meat and produce. Instead, purchases may emphasize pastries or canned goods of lesser nutritional value. There are several ways that community services can help. Meals on Wheels programs ensure delivery of one hot meal daily to the elderly person who is unable to cook or who cannot get out to shop. Group shopping trips (often organized by voluntary agencies) provide transportation, companionship, and access to supermarkets in which the quality of goods may be better and prices lower than those in the elderly person's neighborhood.

The federal government has funded a nutrition program for the elderly under Title VII of the Older Americans Act. Although administered by different agencies in different states (department of health and public welfare), basically all agencies provide a quality diet prepared and distributed to the elderly at low or no cost in a community facility.

☐ ECONOMIC COMPONENT

The 1980 census report demonstrated that 15 per cent of persons 65 or over live below the poverty level (Statistical Abstract, 1985). (The average poverty threshold for a family of four was $7412 in 1979 [1980 census]). This means that of the 26 million elderly, 3.9 million live below the poverty level. The Ten State Nutritional Survey (conducted by the Centers for Disease Control, 1968 to 1970) demonstrated that as income decreases, the incidence of malnutrition increases. As inflation nudges prices upward, the elderly citizen on a fixed income has severely limited purchasing power. Ironically, the very foods that contain the most important nutrients—protein and calcium—are the most expensive. The survey clearly showed that malnutrition in persons over age 65 is caused by poor food choices and lack of money. Social Security is the only source of income for many elderly people. Although the benefits are increased from time to time, these increases do not necessarily keep pace with inflation.

Of the 3.9 million persons who are elderly and living below the poverty level, most did not become poor until they became old. Americans are retiring earlier and living longer on a minimal income. Ensuring an adequate diet is a challenge for society.

☐ PSYCHOLOGIC COMPONENT

Mrs. Taylor, 70, lives alone. She is in fairly good health. Her late husband's pension plan, supplemented by Social Security benefits, provides her with an adequate standard of living. For breakfast Mrs. Taylor has toast and coffee; lunch is usually soup or a sandwich. At supper time she may open a can of spaghetti or ravioli. Occasionally she varies this with scrambled eggs. When she forgets to eat lunch or supper, which happens now and then, she nibbles on pastries, cookies, or occasionally a candy bar.

Mrs. Taylor can comfortably afford a more varied, nutritionally sound menu. Why does she not include meat, fresh fruits, vegetables, and dairy products in her diet?

> When my two children were small, I used to love to cook. In fact, the first thing I did after they were off to school and my husband left for work was to make a special dessert for supper. When the boys grew up and married, I missed them with a real ache. But I still had my husband to fuss over. Now that he's gone, it just doesn't seem worth the trouble to cook for one person.

The loss of role in the family is a determining factor in undernutrition of the elderly. When Mrs. Taylor was no longer needed as mother and wife, she lost part of her identity.

Henry and Ada Marks were childless. When Mrs. Marks died last year, her husband was lost. He barely knew how to use a can opener because his wife had always taken such good care of him. Mr. Marks is a vigorous 69 but he exists on anything that "comes out of a can or box and doesn't need fussing." He's close to a fast food outlet and he patronizes it as a matter of convenience a few times a week. How much longer will this man be vigorous on such a limited diet? Lack of knowledge about how to shop and prepare food is a big stumbling block to many elderly, particularly if there is no motivation for learning.

Margaret and Alice Miller are retired school teachers in their late 70's. Margaret has edematous legs secondary to congestive heart failure. She is a semi invalid confined to the house. Alice tries to take care of the marketing chores, a difficult task, as she is obese and arthritic. She moves slowly and painfully down the five blocks to the supermarket. Once there, she selects ground meat, day-old pastries, and some canned goods. On the return trip, she stops at a liquor store. Alice is alcoholic, and three or four days a week she is in a stupor. Alcoholism, which can be a consequence of poor mental health, insecurity, or despair, is a common contributor to malnourishment in the elderly.

Emotionally caused malnutrition is not limited to a certain social class or income bracket. It can be difficult to motivate some persons to eat properly. Many elderly need to be convinced that money spent for food is money well spent. Others need reinforcement of a sense of self worth.

Eating has social connotations. We join friends for coffee, celebrate with a dinner. Most of us do not like to eat alone because we have always associated some social or family activity with food. This underscores the key role that sharing meals and companionship can play in maintaining satisfactory nutrition levels.

According to N.J. Grills,

> Most general complaints, i.e., fatigue, apathy, anorexia, nervousness, headache, irritability, dyspepsia, and depression, may be a sign of psychogenic originating disease. If nutritionally related, this can be simply and inexpensively relieved by improving the quality and quantity of nutrients. Sometimes symptoms disappear after the elderly are treated with multivitamins for several months. (Grills, 1977)

This statement certainly makes a strong case for developing cooking and marketing skills. Preparing balanced meals can be within the reach of most elderly who have the physical ability to get around and the knowledge about nutrition and budget-wise food preparation.

☐ *Energy Needs*

As discussed earlier, most researchers agree that nutrition has a role in the aging process: there is little agreement on what exactly that role is, however. Currently, there are no U.S. government recommendations for optimal nutrient intake by aged adults. The Recommended Dietary Allowances (RDA's) have been taken from the nutrient needs of younger (and healthier) adults. Therefore, they are not precise geriatric nutrition guides. There has been an attempt, however, to divide the elderly population into two groups in order to judge energy (caloric) needs: 51 to 75 years and over 75 years. Health professionals must remember that nutritional needs are based not only on physiologic changes associated with aging but also on a broad array of social and psychologic factors.

There is a decline in energy requirements for older adults. Two factors are involved in this decline: first, there is a natural decline in metabolism of 10 to 15 per cent after the age of 50. Second, most elderly persons decrease their level of physical activity. Reduced energy requirements means that calorie intake must decrease. When caloric intake is decreased, it is particularly important to verify that essential nutrients are not omitted from the diet. Specifically, there should be a reduction in fats and sweets eaten and an increase in nutrient-rich foods, e.g., whole grain breads and cereals, fruits and vegetables, and sources of protein.

☐ COMMON NUTRIENTS AND HOW THEY ACT

Protein	Builds, preserves, and restores body tissue.
Carbohydrates	Supply energy and fuel for the body.
Fat	Supplies twice as much energy and fuel as carbohydrates; also has twice as many calories. Essential fatty acids are necessary for certain body functions.
Minerals	Have essential building and regulating functions. Are found in all body tissues and fluids. Essential for bones, teeth, and red blood cell formation.

Vitamins   Act as body regulators, enabling carbohydrates, proteins, and fats to be metabolized by the body. Act as catalysts.

Protein. The precise protein requirements of the elderly have not been established, but 12 per cent of the total food intake is approximate. Older adults may need an increase in protein because they have more incidences of illness and multiple chronic diseases; and illness produces stress, which causes losses of protein. The caregiver monitoring the nutritional status of an elderly client should be aware that too much protein is hazardous. There can be urinary losses of calcium accompanied by a negative calcium balance following the ingestion of excessive amounts of protein. The nursing implication is that the protein needs of a healthy aged individual can vary dramatically from the needs of a sick older person. This fact reinforces the need for cooperation among disciplines in taking care of the elderly person.

Carbohydrates. Elderly individuals should plan on consuming almost 60 per cent of their total calories in carbohydrates. Appropriate foods include whole grain or enriched breads and cereals, rice, potatoes, beets, peas, lentils, corn, and beans. Canned and frozen fruits usually have added sugar and should be used sparingly. The syrup can be poured off canned fruit to reduce sugar content.

Fats. No more than 25 to 30 per cent of the total caloric intake in the form of fats is recommended. Many Americans consume up to 50 per cent of their daily calories in the form of fats. A high fat intake can cause indigestion and malabsorption because of a decline in the efficiency of the gastrointestinal tract and because of reduced pancreatic and liver function in old age.

Minerals

Calcium. An insufficient calcium intake over the years contributes to osteoporosis. An increase in calcium-rich foods retards bone loss. Between 800 and 1000 mg. of calcium daily has been the recommended amount for normal bone density. Some experts are now recommending that that amount be increased to 1000 to 1200 mg. daily for women. (An 8-ounce glass of nonfat milk contains 302 mg. of calcium and 90 calories; a 1-ounce slice of cheddar cheese contains 204 mg. of calcium and 115 calories.) Calcium supplements are also available; calcium supplements can be constipating, however. Elderly persons often have bowel problems due to a slowing down of peristalsis. Foods high in fiber or bran should be added to the diet.

Iron. Iron deficiency anemia is common among low income elderly persons, who have particular problems with adequate nourishment. Elderly women of all economic levels are not getting enough iron in their diets. The Recommended Dietary Allowance for elderly men and women is 10 mg. daily.

Iron-rich foods are meat, whole grain and fortified cereals, dried beans and peas, and eggs. (One large egg contains 1 mg. iron; 3 ounces of lean roast beef contains 3.2 mg. of iron.)

☐ Factors Influencing Geriatric Nutrition

1. Slowed metabolic processes due to decline in functioning cells.
2. Malabsorption; digestive disturbances may be secondary to chronic disease and may be due to reduced secretory ability of digestive glands and or a decrease in the production of hydrochloric acid.
3. Altered taste as the number of taste buds declines; upper denture covers much of the palate, which may also reduce taste perceptions. Careful oral hygiene can improve this situation.
4. Chronic disease, such as diabetes, atherosclerosis, or periodontal disease, because of the need to alter the diet.
5. Physical disability, such as impaired vision or arthritis. Physical handicaps may make food preparation difficult.
6. Dental problems. Fifty per cent of those over 65 have lost all of their teeth; others have poorly fitting dentures. Dental problems impair ability to chew.
7. Psychologic
   a. Organic, as in cerebral arteriosclerosis, Alzheimer's disease, multi-infarct disease. (Inappropriate choice of foods may result from psychologic problems.)
   b. Functional, as in anxiety and depression, which lead to less physical activity and anorexia, reduced intake. There may be incidences of overeating of comfort foods that are high in calories and low in nutrients.
8. Social isolation
   a. Decline of the extended family
   b. Death of spouse, friends
   c. Inadequate transportation (limits shopping trips)
9. Economics. Income decreases and medical expenses increase.
10. Drug and food interactions. Laxatives reduce nutrient absorption; some medicines alter taste perceptions and appetite.

☐ Suggestions for Improving Geriatric Nutrition

Ideally, improved nutritional practices beginning in childhood would ensure that elders are nutritionally sound. The next best thing, however, would be to improve the dietary status of the older adult. The following are ways of doing this:

Nutritional Education. Poorly educated elders are usually poorly nourished. Caregivers should evaluate vision and hearing before teaching about improved food selection and preparation. Motivation and disabilities caused by chronic illness also need to be assessed and included in the teaching plan. The habits of a lifetime do not change easily; therefore, when specific changes need to be made in an elderly person's diet due to a medical problem, it is important to adapt the person's eating habits rather than to introduce totally new ones.

Feeding Programs. The 1973 Older Americans Act, through the National Nutritional Program for the Elderly, authorizes a fund for group feeding programs at designated sites (e.g., schools, churches, senior centers) at low cost to the elderly and for "Meals on Wheels," home-delivered meals to homebound elderly persons.

Food Stamps. Persons on limited income may buy food stamps, which have a purchasing power greater than the amount that is paid for them. Elderly persons may fear negative social implications and thus not apply for food stamps. Others simply do not know how to go about applying for aid or do not know that they are eligible.

Homemaker/Home Health Aides. These persons are trained by community agencies or proprietary agencies to assist and maintain an older adult's independent way of life. In regard to nutrition, aides may help with menu planning, support food preparation, budgeting, and shopping, depending on the needs of the elderly person.

□ *Nutritional Management of the Acutely Ill Older Adult*

The elderly person who is acutely ill has a double problem: a decreased appetite and an increased requirement for nutrients. Malnutrition is a serious problem in the ill elderly, overlooked by many health care professionals, even in some of our best and most modern hospitals.

Hospital admission gives many people a false sense of security. "I'm in good hands," thinks the patient, settling back in bed. "He's getting the best of care," says the family with a collective sigh of relief. The unhappy truth is that malnutrition often exists through ignorance or through poor patterns of care.

Agnes Newell, 69, is a patient on an orthopedic unit. She is recovering from a fractured hip. A victim of organic brain syndrome, she was admitted from the nursing home where she had lived for 3 years. At mealtimes, a dietary aide serves her a tray and 45 minutes later two nursing assistants roll a cart down the corridor and, pressured for time, collect all the trays. No one is sure how much Mrs. Newell eats, or if she eats anything, and she is too confused to tell them.

Richard Marlow, 75, is in the hospital hoping to learn the cause of his abdominal pain. Yesterday he fasted for an upper GI series. The schedule was delayed, and by the time he got back to his room, lunch was over. Today he's having an IVP at noon. He'll miss breakfast and lunch, again.

The list of practices that interfere with or prevent optimal nutritional health for hospital patients are many: failure to observe and record food intake, failure to provide food after meals are missed because of diagnostic tests, absence of recorded height and weight. These practices are dangerous and objectionable. A well adult who consumes between 2000 and 3000 calories daily may need twice that amount when subjected to the stress of surgery and fever. Mrs. Newell is confused and she has had surgery on her fractured hip. While she cannot feed herself, it is a nursing responsibility to monitor her meals. Hunger will make her uncomfortable and frustrated. But more important, inadequate food intake will also slow down her convalescence and ultimate healing.

Mr. Marlow's problem is different from Mrs. Newell's, but it is no less serious. He has never paid much attention to his diet and his normal eating habits are irregular at home. In theory, hospitalization should guarantee him nutritionally balanced meals, but so far it has not worked out that way. He has only "picked at" food that has been served, and he has missed several meals because of his test schedule. Now he may need surgery. The caloric cost of that stress plus the nutritional demand in the subsequent cell and tissue repair will put enormous demands on his metabolism that may or may not be met. The way food substances are broken down and the way new cells are developed can be affected by these combined stress situations. His levels of hemoglobin and plasma protein will drop, as will his red blood count, if he is not consuming a well-balanced diet. He will be likely to have muscle weakness, pulmonary problems and cardiovascular insufficiency. In extreme cases, survival depends on the balance between the impact of stress and the mobilization of the body's protective mechanisms, namely, cell metabolism and function. Problems can be prevented when there is protein synthesis sufficient to enable the body to bear the stresses of illness and surgery.

In 1980, 38 per cent of inpatient days (in hospitals) were used by persons aged 65 or older. These persons had a higher average admission rate (400 per 1000 admissions) than did younger adults (136 per 1000). Moreover, of the persons aged 65 or older who were admitted, 25 per cent were readmitted at least once during the same year (Evashwick, 1982). If past trends continue, the growth of the aging population between 1980 and 1989 will result in a 12 per cent increase in the number of inpatient days, with the elderly accounting for 60 per cent of that increase (Evashwick, 1982).

The significance of the malnourished hospitalized patient has been referred to in recent nursing journals (AORN Journal, 1984; Aust Nurses J,

1983). In an editorial in the March, 1985, American Journal of Nursing entitled "Food for Thought," it was reported that 25 to 50 per cent of those hospitalized for 2 weeks or more had been found to be malnourished and in need of intensive nutritional support.

Some of the consequences of nutritional deficits in the older adult include impaired cardiovascular function, impaired liver function, decreased digestive and absorptive capacities, and depressed cellular immunity, leading to slow healing, infection, decubitus ulcers, and bowel fistulas. Nutritional assessment and prompt intervention can help to reverse such life-threatening changes. In addition to medical and nursing histories, a comprehensive nutritional evaluation is needed. This will include a diet and weight history, physical examination, and biochemical and immunologic testing as necessary.

□ NUTRITIONAL REQUIREMENTS OF THE ILL ELDERLY

Factors that affect basic nutritional requirements are stress, hypermetabolism, and malnutrition. Generally, for weight maintenance, 33 calories per kilogram of ideal body weight are required and for weight gain, 44 calories per kilogram of body weight are required. In times of stress, this figure may double. Protein needs increase also. For example, if the average daily protein intake is 1 gram/kilogram of ideal body weight, under moderate stress the need increases to 2 grams/kilogram of ideal body weight. Under severe stress, such as surgery or illness, 4 grams/kilogram of ideal body weight may be needed.

It is important to establish a baseline intake and then determine what nutritional support is needed. Many factors can contribute to a patient's hospital-induced malnutrition: the illness itself, fasting for diagnostic tests, and therapies that interrupt mealtimes. The older clients who are most at risk are those undergoing chemotherapy, radiation therapy, hemodialysis, or surgery. Medically prescribed restrictive diets such as low sodium, diabetic, and low cholesterol diets may depress a patient or limit food choices to such an extent that he or she eats inadequately.

Medications can adversely affect appetite and the absorption of nutrients. Some examples of such medications are sedatives, anti-inflammatory drugs, hypotensive drugs, and antibiotics.

□ HOW TO ENCOURAGE ADEQUATE ORAL INTAKE

1. Try to make the eating environment pleasant, e.g., comfortable temperature in the room, absence of odors, unpleasant sights covered or screened.
2. See that the patient is comfortable: pain free, any incisional site dry and clean, sheets clean and wrinkle free.
3. Encourage good oral care and adequate water intake.
4. Avoid clinical procedures close to mealtimes.

5. Position the patient so that he or she can see and smell foods.
6. Encourage families to bring favorite foods (as medically allowed) and to assist with eating or feeding if necessary.
7. Assess the patient's reaction to pureed foods and recommend to the dietician or physician that they be limited. Purees are often overused. There is no tempting aroma; taste is bland; the patient may feel that eating them is an infantilizing experience and reject them. Soft diets are often just as suitable and are much more palatable.
8. Therapeutic multivitamins and minerals may be ordered if food intake is inadequate. In addition, if protein and caloric intake is inadequate, oral supplements may be given in 250 ml. amounts three or four times a day. When food supplements are prescribed, let patients "test taste" and select their preferred supplements. If patients participate in choosing, compliance is more likely.

Malnutrition in the hospitalized elderly can be dealt with successfully only if health care professionals know how to find its causes. They must accurately assess the present condition of the patient before they can determine why he or she is poorly nourished. Then they must calculate the nutrients missing and supply the calories, protein, vitamins, or electrolytes, as needed.

The root causes of malnutrition are complex. Sometimes dentures are not

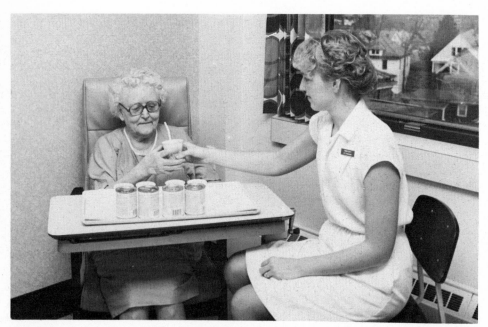

Figure 8–1 ☐ The elderly person who needs food supplements should have a chance to sample various flavors and choose favored ones. (From Poleman and Capra, p. 216.)

fitted properly. Sometimes the patient has difficulty swallowing or digesting food. In hospital situations, the nurse can help correct these problems. Estimating and providing nutrients requires the joint effort of physician, nurse, dietician, and patient.

□ THE NURSE'S ROLE

Why is the nurse the likely person to become involved with the nutritional state of the patient? Initially, the physician prescribes for the dietary needs. The dietician plans meals to fill the needs and explains the diet to the patient. The physician is concerned with the plan of treatment and the patient's physical recovery, response to medications, and diagnostic tests. The dietician may be responsible for from 75 to 100 patients. Neither professional may observe the patient's eating habits as closely as does the nurse. The nurse is in the best position to note the patient's height and weight, intake and output, and eating habits and to observe that the patient is eating the diet prescribed. Equally important, the nurse can let the patient know that substitutions are available for food that he or she does not, or cannot, eat. The nurse is the valuable reinforcer of the plan for nutritional therapy.

□ *Labeling*

The food industry and the Food and Drug Administration (FDA) developed nutrition labeling in order to provide the general public with nutrition information. Elders, like any other consumer group, should read labels.

In the United States, Recommended Dietary Allowances (RDA's) were formed by the FDA for use in nutrition labeling. RDA's replace the minimum daily requirements (MDR's), and they are set at a value high enough to meet the needs of most healthy adults in the United States. Generally speaking, RDA's apply to most older adults.

Reading nutrition labels permits the consumer to
1. select foods that are major sources for important nutrients
2. evaluate the nutrient composition of a variety of foods
3. select foods that offer the best nutritional value for the price
4. select foods that have the best nutrient to calorie ratio (elders require fewer calories, not fewer nutrients)
5. calculate the nutritional adequacy of daily food intake
6. make appropriate adjustments if the diet is nutritionally inadequate
7. choose foods for therapeutic restrictions, i.e., low sodium diets and diabetic diets

Elders who practice reading labels will become thrifty and discriminating shoppers, improving their health and their budgets.

The following information appears in a standard design and in the same order on all labels:
1. nutrition information for single servings
2. the size of a single serving
3. protein, carbohydrate, and fat in grams
4. protein as to percentage of the United States RDA
5. seven vitamins and minerals and their percentage of the United States RDA
6. OPTIONAL: 12 other vitamins and minerals
7. OPTIONAL: the percentage of calories from fat and amounts of fatty acids, cholesterol, and sodium

As many elderly are often not in good health and may not have access to a wide variety of food sources, the RDA may not be the appropriate guideline of dietary adequacy. RDA's were developed as general guidelines and not as precise nutritional benchmarks.

☐ General Facts Relating to Geriatric Nutrition

- It is a common, widely held myth that in order to be properly nourished, additional vitamins are necessary. The truth is that a diet that does not include the basic four food groups and is supplemented with vitamin concentrates may be lacking in protein, minerals, and other nutrients. Vitamin concentrates do not take the place of food. If a vitamin deficiency exists, however, supplements should be prescribed by a physician in order to be sure that the needed vitamin is ingested in the correct amount.
- Caloric needs of the older adult decline because of a lower metabolic rate and a decrease in physical activity. This fact is of special interest to women who can use very little more than the basic four food groups if nutritional requirements are to be met without weight gain. A woman 65 or older needs 300 to 400 fewer calories a day than does a younger woman at the same level of activity.
- Older adults may prefer four to six small meals daily rather than three large meals.
- Dentures can cause problems with eating habits. Dentures may have to be rinsed during a meal, meat may have to be cut into very small pieces, and the denture wearer may have to return to the dentist to have dentures refitted.
- Adding bulk and more liquid to the diet can help older adults avoid constipation, a common geriatric problem. Two tablespoons of bran may be added to the morning cereal. Raw vegetables, rich in fiber, can be put into a blender. Although this does not look appetizing, it does add flavor and variety to the diet. The addition of cellulose (fiber) to the diet can eliminate the need for laxatives and stool softeners.

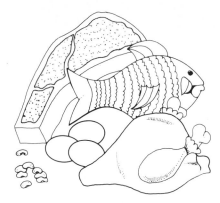

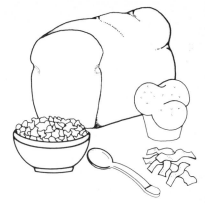

THE PROTEIN GROUP (Meat, Poultry, Fish, Beans)
<u>2 servings daily</u>
One-half servings is
  1 to 1½ ounces lean, boneless, cooked
    meat, poultry, or fish
  1 egg
  ½ to ¾ cup cooked dry beans, peas,
    lentils, or soybeans
  2 tablespoons peanut butter
  ¼ to ½ cup nuts or sesame or sunflower
    seeds

THE BREAD AND CEREAL GROUP
<u>4 servings daily</u>
1 serving is
  1 slice bread
  ½ to ¾ cup cooked cereal or pasta
  1 ounce ready-to-eat cereal

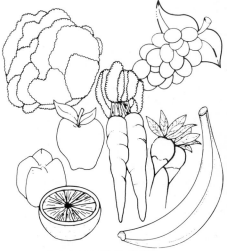

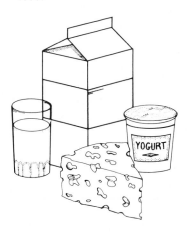

THE MILK-CHEESE GROUP
<u>2 to 4 servings daily</u>
One serving is
  1 cup milk or yogurt
  1⅓ ounces Cheddar or Swiss cheese
  2 ounces processed cheese food
  1½ cups ice cream or ice milk
  2 cups cottage cheese

THE VEGETABLE AND FRUIT GROUP
<u>4 servings daily</u>
1 serving is
  ½ cup cooked vegetable
  a small salad
  a medium-sized potato
  an orange
  ½ cantaloupe
  ½ grapefruit
  (have citrus fruits, melon, berries,
  or tomatoes daily and a dark green or dark
  yellow vegetable frequently)

Figure 8–2 □ *A,* Milk/cheese group; *B,* protein group (meat, poultry, fish, and beans); *C,* bread/cereal group; *D,* fruit/vegetable group. (See instructions for each group.)

• Protein requirements do not decrease with age. The RDA remains at .8 gram per kilogram of body weight. The RDA for minerals is the same for older adults as for young adults with one exception: premenopausal women need 18 mg. of iron; postmenopausal women need only 10 mg.

Physical changes related to malnutrition in the elderly are often attributed to "old age" and thus viewed as normal. The obese older adult may be just as malnourished and apt to be lacking essential protein intake and other nutrients as the thin elder. An admission note reading "WDWNF," well-developed, well-nourished female, is not helpful. It states nothing useful. A common nutritional myth is that elderly people need fewer nutrients than do younger adults. The older adult may believe that his or her intake is adequate, even when serious deficiencies actually exist. Remember that although the elderly person may need fewer *calories*, her or his need for protein, vitamins, minerals, and most other nutrients remains the same.

☐ Solving Nutritional Problems

Problem. Inadequate Protein Intake.

Solution. Although most elderly adults recognize that a hot meal consisting of meat and vegetables is desirable and is a good way of getting protein, not all are aware that there are easy and inexpensive ways to increase the protein value of foods. Here are some ways that this can be done:

Protein Packed Milk. This is actually double-strength milk made by adding 1 cup of dried milk to 1 quart of liquid whole milk. (Ordinarily you would add dry milk to water.) One cup of this will provide twice as much protein as whole milk or skim milk.

Protein packed milk can be flavored by the addition of pureed fruits, fruit syrups, chocolate syrup, vanilla, and so on. It can also be used in cooking, e.g., in soups, cereals, puddings, creamed foods (tuna, chicken), meat loaf, mashed potatoes, and scrambled eggs.

High Protein Milk (½ cup equals 8 grams of protein). To 1 quart of whole or skim milk, add ½ cup of skim milk powder. Mix thoroughly and chill. To be used as double-strength milk or taken between meals. There are more calories if it is made with whole milk.

The American Dietetic Association recommends .8 gram of protein per kilogram of body weight. Multiply the number of pounds a person weighs by 2.2 to determine the corresponding weight in kilograms. (140 lbs. equals 308 kg.)

A woman over the age of 51 requires about 44 grams of protein per day. A man the same age requires about 48.

Note. If snacks are to be used in daily diets, make them high-protein quick snacks. Some examples would be yogurt, cheese, peanut butter, nuts, luncheon meats, precooked sausage, prepared sandwich fillings.

Sample Foods and Their Protein Content		Daily Meals
8 oz. milk (whole or skim)	8 grams	8 grams
1 oz. meat, fish, poultry		
1 egg		
2 tablespoons peanut butter	7 grams	28 grams (4 servings)
1 oz. cheese		
¼ cup cottage cheese		
1 serving starch (grains,		8 grams (4 servings)
cereals, bread)	2 grams	
½ cup vegetables	2 grams	4 grams (2 servings)
TOTAL PROTEIN INTAKE		48 grams

Problem. Obesity, Heart Disease.

Solution. Low fat, low sodium diets. In addition to reducing caloric intake, a person troubled with obesity will benefit from a low fat diet, i.e., a diet in which the main modification in the nutrient content is that the fat content is reduced. Dairy products are permitted but are limited to skim milk, buttermilk, yogurt, uncreamed cottage cheese, and a limited amount of butter or margarine.

Appropriate meats are chicken, turkey, and veal. Fish is permitted.

The low fat diet must be monitored in order to prevent a possible vitamin A deficiency.

A low sodium diet is prescribed in order to prevent edema, an accumulation of water, and sodium in the body tissues that results in a swollen appearance and occurs in cardiovascular disease. The diet is not 100 per cent free of sodium because traces of this element are found in water and most foods. However, by restricting salt, a tolerable sodium level is maintained. Sodium regulates water balance in the body.

A problem with this type of diet may be a lack of flavor. Herbs and mild spices may be used to enhance food tastes.

The following publications are available free from your local Heart Association chapter or from the National Heart Association office:

Save Food $$ and Help Your Heart, 50-032A
Eat Well but Wisely to Reduce Your Risk of Heart Attack, 51-005A
A Guide to Weight Reduction, 50-034A
In addition to these publications, free booklets of low-sodium recipes are put out by the Campbell Soup Company. Write to:
Low Sodium, GH Box 288 CC
Collingswood, New Jersey 08108

Reduction of caloric intake while maintaining adequate nutrients in the food can be accomplished in the following ways:

1. Develop a variety of foods from which to choose the recommended servings in the basic four food groups (two servings from the milk group, two servings from the meat group, four servings from the grain group, and four servings from the fruit and vegetable group).
2. Cut down on fat; trim excess from meats. Avoid any fried foods.
3. Substitute low fat or skim milk for homogenized milk. Buy low fat cheese.
4. Use fresh fruits for desserts or eat less than half the portion.
5. Omit creamed foods. Use scant servings of sauces and gravies.
6. Drink water between meals and just *before* meals.
7. Eliminate or sharply reduce alcoholic beverages.

Problem. Dental Deficiencies.

Solution. When chewing is a problem, whether because of poorly fitted dentures or lack of dentures, it may be necessary to use a soft diet. This type of diet includes finely diced meats or ground meats and pureed fruits or vegetables in addition to a vast number of soft foods—enough to provide a satisfactory variety and a well-balanced diet. In fact, the only restrictions are tough, fibrous meat, whole meat or poultry, whole frankfurters, shrimp, scallops, hard cheeses, hard fried eggs, course bread or rolls with seeds, raisins, nuts, and all the raw fruits or vegetables the person cannot chew.

Problem. Physical Handicaps.

Solution. Older adults with handicaps, whether living independently or not, can benefit from the following suggestions:

1. Plan the texture, consistency, and size of food pieces so that they are handled comfortably, using either fingers or self-feeding devices.
2. Use deep plates or food guards that fit 9- or 11-inch plates.
3. Grasp can be secure when using lightweight mugs or terrycloth covers.
4. Foam rubber curlers can slip over handles of utensils for improved grip.
5. Suction cups or dampened cloths can be used to help anchor bowls and plates.

In a hospital or nursing home, the following are measures that can aid in self feeding:

1. Is the patient wearing his or her eyeglasses? Are they clean?
2. Cut meat, open sealed containers as needed.
3. Be sure the patient is rested. Fatigue will interfere with eating.
4. Evaluate any swallowing problem.
5. Check dentures for fit.
6. Adapt utensil handles as needed (see 4 in the previous list).
7. Chopped or mashed foods are more palatable than puréed. Purées should be used sparingly. Even stroke patients with swallowing problems can usually tolerate thickened liquids rather than juices, broth, and so on.

Problem. Constipation.*

---

*Adapted from Ross Laboratories' Dietary Modifications, Ross Laboratories Division of Abbott Laboratories, Columbus, OH.

Solution. The following suggestions may be used as a guide in encouraging the patient to choose foods that will help correct or avoid constipation.

Foods that dieticians refer to as "high residue," "bulky," or "fibrous" are often helpful to the person troubled with constipation. They are not used completely by the body and so they provide bulk in the large intestine. This bulk encourages evacuation.

Although fruits and vegetables are often recommended for bulk, not all are useful. If the patient may have high-residue foods, he or she should be encouraged to select the following items from the menu or tray:

salads of *raw* fruits or vegetables

vegetables with long fibers (greens, kale, cabbage, celery)

whole fruits with skin rather than peeled fruits or juices

stewed prunes, apricots, or figs

dried fruits (apricots, figs, dates, prunes)

cereals and bread with part of the whole grain in them

Whole grain cereals and dark bread provide bulk since the grain covering is not digested by the body. The following foods and menus will help overcome constipation.

Suggested Foods	Sample Menu
Breakfast	
fruit	prunes
whole grain cereal	oatmeal
bacon or egg	2 strips bacon
whole grain bread	1 slice whole wheat bread
butter	1 pat butter
cream, milk	as needed for cereal
coffee or tea	beverage as desired
Lunch	
soup	vegetable soup
meat, fish, fowl	Swiss steak
potato	mashed potatoes
vegetable	beets
salad (fr. or veg.)	gelatin fruit salad
whole grain bread	1 slice whole wheat bread
butter	1 pat butter
dessert	baked apple with cream
milk, coffee, tea	beverage as desired
Dinner	
meat, fish, fowl, eggs	cold meat
potato, rice, macaroni	Spanish rice
vegetable	buttered carrots
salad	vegetable salad
whole grain bread	1 slice whole wheat bread
butter	1 pat butter
dessert	tapioca pudding
milk	1 glass milk
Snacks	
3 PM, fruit juice	
8 PM, fruit juice	

If necessary, more vegetables, fruits, and fruit juice may be added.

Problem. Anorexia.†

Solution. Various techniques to encourage oral intake:

1. Patients complaining that foods have lost their taste should be encouraged to experiment with a variety of flavors and *aromas*. Flavoring extracts and a variety of herbs enhance the flavor of foods. People can be taught that various food aromas help stimulate appetite and improve mental attitude.
2. Patients experiencing anorexia and early satiety should be advised to eat small, frequent meals.
3. Relatives should be cautioned against developing the "eat a little more" syndrome, and they should be encouraged to create a natural, pleasant atmosphere during meals.
4. Fruit juices or other high caloric beverages can be substituted for coffee, tea, or water.
5. Fresh fruits may make ice cream, milk shakes, puddings, custards, and commercial food supplements more appealing.
6. Between-meal supplements can be encouraged to add to daily protein and calorie intake.
7. Diet should be modified in texture and consistency (bland, soft) to accommodate individual needs.
8. Meticulous oral hygiene should be carried out. Scrupulously clean teeth and mouth enhance the taste of food.

Elderly people often have changes in their tastes, appetites, or food interests in general that can interfere with good nutrition. Here are some ways to stimulate food intake:

1. When preparing foods, vary colors, flavors, textures, temperatures, and shapes.
2. Select appropriate herbs with which to season foods.
3. Improve oral hygiene.
4. Eat regularly.
5. Experiment with new foods occasionally.
6. Do not mix foods haphazardly on the plate. Arrange food attractively.
7. Include hot and cold foods at the same meal.
8. Exercise.
9. Have occasional meals with friends.
10. Serve small portions.
11. Add a flower or colorful placemat to the tray or table.

Problem. Nutrition for the Elderly Diabetic.

Solution. As explained in Chapter 17, The Endocrine System, diabetes mellitus in the older adult is usually discovered as a result of an examination for some other problem. Glucose tolerance declines as aging progresses; therefore, a large number of elderly persons develop diabetes. Elderly women and

---

†Adapted from Ross Laboratories' Dietary Modifications, Ross Laboratories Division of Abbott Laboratories, Columbus, OH.

those elderly individuals who are overweight are more likely to develop diabetes.

The most important aspect of dietary treatment of maturity-onset diabetes is reduction of weight until ideal weight (or even weight slightly below the ideal) is achieved. Many endocrinologists agree that the ideal weight for a diabetic is 10 per cent less than the nondiabetic ideal weight. (Larger fat cells are more insulin-resistant than small fat cells so much higher levels of insulin are needed for glucose metabolism in an obese individual.)

The measured diet is felt to be the best choice of maturity-onset diabetics who are obese and thus require a fixed caloric intake. Total caloric needs are derived by multiplying body weight in kilograms by 25 calories. The carbohydrate allowance is usually between 45 and 55 per cent of total calories. In the past, carbohydrates were restricted. However, most endocrinologists support the idea that diabetics do best when consuming diets rather higher in carbohydrates and lower in fats. Protein intake should make up about 15 per cent of the calories, with fat at 30 to 35 per cent.

These nutrients are the foundation of the simple food exchange system that divides all foods into four basic exchanges: meat, bread and cereal, fruit and vegetables, and milk groups. For example, one small apple is one fruit exchange, one slice of bread is one bread exchange, and 1 ounce of meat is one meat exchange.

The diabetic's diet is controlled by having him or her eat the same number of calories and the same food exchanges each day. This does not mean that a patient must eat the same foods each day. Rather, it means that the patient cannot substitute a fruit exchange for a bread exchange.

It is important to design a diet, based on the physician's prescription, that meets the patient's needs, because it is not realistic to give the patient a diet that he or she will not follow.

Problem. Economic Restrictions.

Solution. Low-budget balanced diet. Plan meals using the basic four food groups. Some of the following ways to keep food costs down are simple and practical:

1. Buy foods according to their use. Buy small, less attractive fruits if planning to cut them up.
2. Use less tender cuts of meat whenever possible. Learn how to cook less tender pieces.
3. Buy large pieces of meat and plan meals around leftovers.
4. Buy "house brands" and generic brands instead of advertised brands whenever possible.
5. Buy foods in season.
6. Shop at large supermarkets instead of convenience stores.
7. Use a list when shopping.
8. Plan meals around "specials."
9. Avoid impulsive buying.
10. Never shop when you are hungry.

11. Use store coupons only if the product will actually be cheaper than house or generic brands. Look for double coupon days.
12. Find out if you are eligible for food stamps. If so, use them.

   Problem. Loneliness.

   Solution. Group dining. This is a way to ease the isolation of eating alone day after day. Most senior centers serve a daily hot meal for a nominal cost. The companionship is as important as the nutrients ingested. Perhaps occasional meals can be shared with a friend or neighbor. Churches, lodges, nondenominational clubs, and even some schools provide for group dining.

☐ *The Role of Dieticians*

Dieticians are professionals who assess nutritional status. They may consult with other disciplines in evaluating problems and implementing nutri-

---

Basic Rules for Diabetic Food Preparation

1. Understanding the food exchange lists is the key to cooking or selecting delicious foods for the diabetic diet.

2. Spend enough time planning meals. Read your local newspaper ads to keep up with foods in season and those featured at special prices. Plan your meals by the week and shop accordingly. Select your main dish from the meat list on your diet and then choose vegetables, salad, fruit, bread, or substitute to go with it.

3. You should not need to buy a great many special diet foods. You will find that you will be able to eat the same meats, vegetables, salads, and fruits as your family most of the time. The amount of fat added in preparation should always be considered in your diet. Your neighborhood grocer can supply you with food that is nutritionally adequate in every way. You do not need organically grown foods or other unusual items. If you are eating a variety of foods, you may not need added vitamin supplements. If you have a special need for them your doctor will prescribe or suggest them.

4. Provide yourself with good cooking utensils, measuring cup, spoons, and possibly scales. You deserve to pamper yourself a little by using a variety of spices and selected seasonings.

5. You may adapt recipes from standard cookbooks to your own eating pattern.

6. You do need to buy good meats, vegetables, and fruits. If you are using these foods in the proper amounts and eliminating those you should not use, you may be buying *less* food.

7. Don't tempt yourself by keeping many "forbidden" foods around the kitchen. The better job you do with the diabetic diet, the less they will interest you.

8. A good rule for all "cooks": Remember that an attractive and simple meal served in a happy and congenial family atmosphere is more important to everyone than the number of heavy, overly rich foods served at the table.

tional care plans. Often they educate patients and families in determining needs and suggesting appropriate dietary measures.

Nurses can work cooperatively with dieticians by noting certain factors that indicate potential nutritional problems, such as:

- lives alone
- recently widowed
- handicapped
- inadequate income
- substance abuse
- anorexia
- habitual use of prescription or OTC drugs
- post surgery
- weight loss of 10 per cent or more; weight more than 20 per cent above desirable weight
- nutrition-related illness (diabetes, hypertension, cancer)
- below normal hemoglobin (lower than 10 mg/100 ml for women, 12 mg/100 ml for men)

Professional intervention probably will not be necessary in each case. However, cooperation between the two disciplines, nursing and dietetics, can help establish baseline information on patients who are problem free and will recognize possible problems and allow for developing solutions.

Chapter 8 □ Review Questions

MULTIPLE CHOICE

1. Osteoporosis is a disturbance of
   A. bone formation and maintenance
   B. cardiovascular function
   C. thrombolytic enzymes
   D. vertebral bodies
2. When physical activity in the older adult decreases,
   A. there is an increase in energy requirements
   B. caloric intake should decrease
   C. disability increases
   D. energy requirements are unchanged
3. Excessive amounts of protein
   A. are excreted daily without ill effect
   B. are water soluble
   C. can contribute to negative calcium balance
   D. have a negligible effect on metabolism
4. Iron deficiency anemia is
   A. rare in the female population
   B. caused by pancreatic dysfunction
   C. often found among low-income elderly
   D. corrected with the addition of bran to the diet

5. A suggestion for improving geriatric nutrition for the frail elderly would be to
   A. puree most foods
   B. arrange for Meals on Wheels, a home-delivered meal program
   C. increase oral fluids
   D. weigh all foods before cooking them
6. Generally speaking, for weight gain, 44 calories per kilogram of body weight is required. In times of stress,
   A. this figure may decrease
   B. this figure may increase
   C. the requirement is unchanged
   D. the requirement is unchanged for females only
7. Hospital-induced malnutrition is
   A. confined to confused patients
   B. rare if patients have I.V. therapy
   C. caused by diagnostic tests
   D. a factor in slow convalescence and poor healing
8. A low sodium diet would be prescribed to
   A. prevent edema
   B. prevent osteoporosis
   C. enhance liver function
   D. avoid constipation
9. An example of a high-residue, fiber-rich food would be
   A. creamed soup
   B. eggs
   C. canned peaches
   D. raw vegetables
10. When planning a diabetic diet, it is important to
   A. be realistic and give the patient a diet he or she can follow
   B. plan to substitute fruit exchanges with bread exchanges
   C. limit caloric intake to 1200 calories
   D. recognize that regular cookbooks can no longer be used

MATCHING

_____ 1. laxatives   A. builds body tissues

_____ 2. milk   B. necessary for utilization of food

_____ 3. dry skin   C. provides empty calories

_____ 4. proteins   D. provides calcium

_____ 5. carbohydrate   E. reduce nutrient absorption

_____ 6. alcohol

_____ 7. osteoporosis

_____ 8. minerals

_____ 9. vitamins

_____ 10. whole grain cereals

F. vitamin A deficiency

G. provides iron

H. supplies energy, fuel for the body

I. calcium deficiency

J. essential for bones, teeth, red blood cell formation

K. protein deficiency

☐ REFERENCES

Blackburn, G., et al.: Nutritional and metabolic assessment of the hospitalized patient. J Parenter Nutr Ent Nutr, 1(1):11–22, 1977.

Evashwick, C.: Long term care: New role for hospitals. Hospitals, 56:51–53, 1982.

Grills, N.: Nutritional needs of elderly women. Clin Obstet Gynecol, 20(1):137–143, 1977.

Harrill, I.: Observations on food acceptance by elderly women. Gerontics, 16(4):394–399, 1976.

Klinger, J.: Mealtime Manual for the Aged and Handicapped. Institute of Rehabilitation Medicine, New York University Medical Center, Essendess Special Editions, New York, 1970.

Krause, M., and Mahan, L.: Food, Nutrition and Diet Therapy. Philadelphia, W.B. Saunders, 1984.

Lecos, C.: Diet and the elderly. FDA Consumer, 18:22–25, 1984.

Lewis, C.: Nutritional Considerations for the Elderly. Philadelphia, F.A. Davis, 1978.

Lichtenstein, V.: Care of the acutely ill older adult: Nutritional management. Geriatr Nurs, 6: 386–391, 1982.

Lipton, M.: Nutritional fads and the search for mental health. University of North Carolina, Bulletin 21, Autumn, 1985, pp. 4–10.

Mayer, J.: Human Nutrition. Springfield, IL, Charles C Thomas, 1979.

National Dairy Council: To Your Health in Your Second Fifty Years. Rosemont, IL, National Dairy Council, 1974.

Natow, A., and Heslin, J.: Geriatric Nutrition. Boston, CBI Publishing Company, 1980.

1980 Census of Population. U.S. Department of Commerce, Bureau of the Census, U.S. Government Printing Office, Washington, DC.

Organ, C., and Finn, M.: The importance of nutritional support for the elderly surgical patient. Geriatrics, 32(5):77–84, 1977.

Palmer, P.: Malnutrition: Reversing the trend in the surgical patient. AORN J, 40:347–352, 1984.

Poleman, C., and Capra, C.: Nutrition Essentials and Diet Therapy. Philadelphia, W.B. Saunders, 1984.

Schrier, R.: Clinical Internal Medicine in the Aged. Philadelphia, W.B. Saunders, 1982.

Short, E.: Peri-operative starvation: An often unrecognized condition. Aust Nurses J, 13:47–49, 1983.

Statistical Abstract of United States, 1985. 105th ed. U.S. Department of Commerce, Bureau of the Census, U.S. Government Printing Office, Washington, DC.

Ten State Nutritional Survey. Center for Disease Control, DHEW Pub. No. (HSM) 72-8130-34, Atlanta, GA.

Todd, B.: Can osteoporosis be treated? Geriatric Nurs, 6:359, 1985.

Yen, P.: Special help for eating problems. Geriatric Nurs, 4:257, 1983.

Yen, P.: Nurse Dietician Teamwork. Geriatric Nurs, 4:49, 1983.

Objectives

After completing this chapter, the student should be able to

- [ ] name and explain the five stages of dying
- [ ] describe the philosophy of the hospice movement
- [ ] describe four signs of impending death
- [ ] identify two ethical issues facing nurses in care of older adults
- [ ] explain the meaning of active and passive euthanasia
- [ ] define the term *living will*

Vocabulary

ethical
euthanasia
hospice
thanatology

CHAPTER 9

Death and Dying

Chapter Outline

About 25 years ago Dr. Elisabeth Kübler-Ross began research on the emotions and attitudes people experience when facing death. At first her research was hampered by doctors and nurses who refused to acknowledge that their hospitalized patients were dying or to discuss how the patients and they themselves as caregivers dealt with the facts of death. Through painstaking investigation and the publication of several books, Kübler-Ross focused attention on *thanatology* (the study of death) and improved understanding and communication among patients, families, and caregivers.

Kübler-Ross identified five stages that patients experience when they learn they are dying. The stages are identified as *denial, anger, bargaining, depression,* and *acceptance.* Not all professionals agree that there are five stages that progress in just this order, but it is agreed that Kübler-Ross brought a neglected and feared subject out of obscurity and did so with great compassion and skill.

Nursing has moved from a detached and aloof attitude that was once considered "professional" when caring for the terminally ill to an emphasis on meeting the total needs of the patient and significant others. Careful assessment of the attitudes, beliefs, and experiences of dying patients contributes to the development of therapeutic and individualized support.

□ Stages of Dying

Denial. When an individual learns that he or she is dying, a common initial reaction is to reject the possibility. "Doctors make mistakes" and "the lab reports may be wrong" are some comments that indicate denial. With denial, however, the patient is allowed time to slowly absorb and adjust to the news that he or she has a terminal condition.

The nurse should be sensitive to the need of the individual to discuss approaching death while at the same time denying that it is happening *to him* or *her.* Acceptance of the patient's reaction without judging its value and encouraging open and honest communication are the most important factors for the nurse to remember at this time.

Anger. After denial comes anger. Anger at the fact that it is happening *to him* or *her;* anger at the fact that life is not fair. This is an extremely challenging time for nurses and caregivers. The patient may show dissatisfaction with everything that is being done for him or her and may be impatient and angry with all those people who are trying to be comforting and supportive. Families experience guilt and embarrassment along with their grief. Nurses struggle with the feeling that the patient's anger is a personal affront to them.

To be able to remain supportive, the nurse needs to assess the situation in light of what the patient is experiencing. Accept the anger, thus giving the patient permission to express his or her feelings. Try to anticipate the patient's needs. Use interpersonal communication techniques that allow and encourage expression of feelings.

Bargaining. The patient bargains for more time. Bargaining often takes the form of the patient expressing a desire to see a child graduate, to live through one more wedding anniversary, or for one more Christmas with the family. Even patients who have had no religious inclination will promise God to be good or to do something in exchange for more time. What they promise is insignificant. These patients may try to involve their caregivers in these agreements.

The most important thing the nurse can do at this time is to encourage the patient to share his or her feelings and thoughts. The attitude of acceptance and understanding without value judgments lets the patient know he or she is a person worthy of respect, yet it does not raise false hopes.

Depression. As illness progresses and improvement ceases, the reality of death takes hold. The devastation at the loss of family, friends, and career may overwhelm the patient, and he or she may respond with silence or quiet weeping.

The nurse must be sensitive to the spiritual needs of the dying patient. Many hospitals have pastoral care available for patients and their families. The nurse can let the patient know that there is support available. The nurse should understand and can reflect to the patient that the depression is a period of growth during which there is preparation for the final stage, *acceptance*.

Acceptance. The patient finally accepts what he or she cannot change. This is not a happy stage, but the patient recognizes that his or her time is very close and consents to the fact. For some, there is relief.

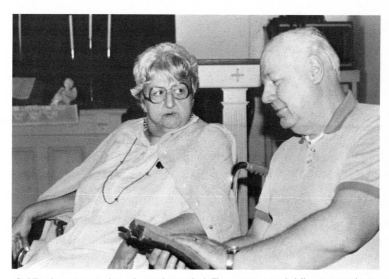

Spiritual care may be of great comfort. The nurse can let the person know that pastoral visits are available in the hospital or nursing home.

Unnecessary environmental stimulation can be reduced for the patient who wants calm and withdrawal. Touching, comfort measures, and, most of all, the presence of family or some caring person are the most important factors in this final stage.

Not all dying persons pass through all these stages. Some may go through only a few or may move back and forth through several stages at different times. The nurse's role is one of support and encouragement, being there whatever the needs of a patient at a particular time.

☐ Ethical Questions

Death is the ending of all vital functions. Caregivers, by virtue of their specialized training, are oriented toward the maintenance and restoration of health. The reality is, however, that the professional must deal with the entire process of death and dying. This total experience includes clients, family, and friends, all who are involved with the dying individual.

☐ THE CAREGIVER'S ATTITUDE

In earlier times, the two most important events in a person's life—birth and death—occurred at home. Advances in medicine gradually found death occurring in the sterile, frequently alien, environment of the hospital. The physical needs of the dying patient were met, but health professionals were unable or unwilling to meet emotional needs. Visitors, families and friends, were frequently treated as intruders. The professional had to deal with first, the patient who was not getting well, and thus was frustrating the professional's mission of healing, and second, the visitors who intruded into the professional's domain and perhaps at times even dared question his or her decisions.

The focus on cures and healing has made it extremely hard for caregivers to deal with what many regard as failure—the death of a patient. The whole issue of death forces one to acknowledge the fact of mortality and the negative emotions that accompany this situation. Nurses and colleagues can help each other by offering support when the need arises and by being aware of reactions that might interfere with a therapeutic nurse-client relationship.

☐ RESUSCITATION

Many physicians and nurses are reluctant to resuscitate patients who obviously will not benefit from, or who may not wish, cardiopulmonary resuscitation (CPR). Many physicians, threatened by legal consequences, are unwilling to write a do not resuscitate (DNR) order on a medical record. As a result, the unwritten slow code "order" has evolved. For example, the physician may request to be called if the patient has a cardiac arrest. An order like this can have the effect of a DNR order because of the delay in obtaining orders *after* the physician is notified. There is a twofold effect: (1) the resuscitation effort is delayed and (2) the patient's chances of survival are reduced. There is an important distinction. The nurse who follows a written DNR order is within the law. The "slow code" situation is illegal.

The consequences of choosing to follow a slow code "order" are very serious for the nurse. In choosing to follow a slow code order, the nurse will have to decide how much of an effort to exert in resuscitating the patient. This forces the nurse to make a *medical* decision. Such a decision may cause the nurse to face prosecution and even license revocation.

Carried further, if a patient dies because of the so-called slow code order and the nurse's efforts are judged to be inadequate, the nurse might be held on a more serious charge of manslaughter.

The risks are obvious and serious. Therefore, most hospitals' written policies state that the physician must designate any patient who is not to be resuscitated. This means that the order is written in the patient's medical record and that it is documented in the progress notes, which will indicate that the physician has discussed the decision with the patient or the family, or both.

When a DNR order does not exist, the nurse must initiate CPR and call a code on a patient who arrests, regardless of the patient's or the family's wishes.

The nurse must know what the hospital policy on resuscitation says, where it is kept, and who drafted and adopted it. If any part of the policy is unclear it should be rewritten so no one can misunderstand its intent (Merkel, 1985).

□ INFORMED CONSENT

Most health professionals would say that informed consent is good and necessary. Reasons range from self interest (i.e., protection from lawsuits) to a knowledge of ethical and legal principles involved.

A critical factor is how much information is enough. On the one hand, the health professional's first duty is to do no harm. On the other hand, if ensuring patients' rights and maintaining the adult patient's autonomy are significant, then there is the obligation to tell the patient what he or she wants to know.

A case is cited of a 90-year-old woman who was admitted to the hospital with the diagnosis of intestinal obstruction. She asked for and received an honest appraisal of the risks. After thinking it over she told her surgeon that considering her slim chance of surviving surgery, she had decided against it. The surgeon immediately ordered a psychiatric consultation. If she had agreed to surgery, the surgeon probably would not have requested a psychiatrist because he would have seen her decision as the "right" one.

It is a gamble when information is imparted to patients. It permits people to act autonomously and to make decisions that caregivers may find difficult to accept. For example, health professionals might believe that complex technology is the best treatment for a terminally ill patient, but the patient might not agree. The chance that patients will disagree with health professionals should not lead to the withholding of information from patients and their families. Informed consent may be hazardous, but this does not excuse health professionals from the obligation of providing adequate information in a manner understandable to the patient (Davis, 1985).

☐ EUTHANASIA

Originally, the word *euthanasia* was taken from the Greek vocabulary meaning good or happy death. It has come to signify mercy killing, death with dignity, peaceful death, or the deliberate easing of pain with sometimes irreversible fatal effects. Basically, euthanasia may be active or passive.

Active euthanasia indicates a positive act deliberately done to hasten death. Most of Western culture regards this as murder. Passive euthanasia, however, denotes the failure to take the type of action that would prolong life.

Euthanasia may be viewed from two legal premises: the right to privacy and the right to refuse treatment.

The actual definition of death has become a highly technologic issue. Caregivers must give thought to several factors: under what conditions or artificial supports should the patient have to live? What value or quality will the life extended have? Will the benefits of treatment and the costs to patient and family outweigh the alternatives? Exploration of these and similar questions will assist clients and support persons to cope with illness, disability, and dying.

☐ LIVING WILLS*

Within the last few years the possibility that some functions of life can be maintained by sophisticated life support systems has prompted many individuals to insist on their own right to control the nature of their deaths as much as possible.

Questions such as to how many times to resuscitate terminally ill aged patients and when to turn off life-sustaining respirators when comatose patients have no hope of regaining consciousness have prompted legislatures to act. Twenty-two state legislatures have responded to these types of ethical dilemmas by enacting living will legislation that offers guidelines and legal protection for health professionals when they participate in decisions about life and death.

---

*From The living will—where it stands. Geriatr Nurs, 6:18–20, 1985.

In some states, any adult can write his or her own living will directives, yet in other states, legislative language specifies strict guidelines for *all* adults. Such legislation may be called "living will," "natural death," or "right to die" legislation.

Nurses are cautioned to refer to their health-care employers, state nurses' associations, and state attorney generals' offices for further guidance and policy statements.

□ *Hospice*

In recent years, there has been a movement to offer the terminally ill an environment in which death can occur with dignity and peace.

The term "hospice" originally meant shelter, a house of rest for pilgrims and travelers. Today, hospice represents a *philosophy of care* that provides physical, emotional, and, sometimes, spiritual care to terminally ill persons and their families. With hospice support a dying person may be able to remain at home. Many hospice programs are sponsored by home health agencies, which use the same health professionals to provide home health care and hospice care.

The primary aims of hospice programs are to
- decrease the pain and discomfort of the patient
- accent making life full and meaningful
- offer support for patient, family, and friends

Hospice care today is given in a client's home, in a free standing structure, or in a special unit in a hospital. In whatever the surroundings, the basic philosophy is the same: to help the patient live as fully and as constructively as possible.

Hospice care is available 24 hours a day, 7 days a week. If hospice care is ordered by a physician and is provided by a certified home health agency, costs may be partially covered by Medicare or Medicaid.

It may be of interest to student nurses to know that one of the pioneers in the hospice movement was Rose Hawthorne Lathrop, the daughter of Nathaniel Hawthorne. More than 85 years ago, Rose Lathrop and a small band of cancer nurses (who later formed a religious congregation) opened their first hospice, a residence for the poor and incurably ill. There remain today the same two criteria for admission to any of the hospices these Dominican nuns maintain across the United States: the patient must be terminally ill and the patient must be unable to afford the medical care. On her visit to St. Rose's in Fall River, Massachusetts, Dr. Elisabeth Kübler-Ross described it as "a hospice for indigent, terminally ill patients, run by Dominican Sisters in the most loving, caring manner that I have ever witnessed in this country (Kübler-Ross, 1978)."

Another important name in the hospice movement is Dr. Cicely Saunders, who opened St. Christopher's Hospice in England in 1967 to provide compas-

---

My Living Will
To My Family, My Physician, My Lawyer
and All Others Whom It May Concern

Death is as much a reality as birth, growth, maturity and old age—it is the one certainty of life. If the time comes when I can no longer take part in decisions for my own future, let this statement stand as an expression of my wishes and directions, while I am still of sound mind.

If at such a time the situation should arise in which there is no reasonable expectation of my recovery from extreme physical or mental disability, I direct that I be allowed to die and not be kept alive by medications, artificial means or "heroic measures". I do, however, ask that medication be mercifully administered to me to alleviate suffering even though this may shorten my remaining life.

This statement is made after careful consideration and is in accordance with my strong convictions and beliefs. I want the wishes and directions here expressed carried out to the extent permitted by law. Insofar as they are not legally enforceable, I hope that those to whom this Will is addressed will regard themselves as morally bound by these provisions.

(Optional specific provisions to be made in this space — see other side)

DURABLE POWER OF ATTORNEY (optional)

I hereby designate _____ to serve as my attorney-in-fact for the purpose of making medical treatment decisions. This power of attorney shall remain effective in the event that I become incompetent or otherwise unable to make such decisions for myself.

Optional Notarization:

"Sworn and subscribed to

before me this _____ day .

of _____, 19_____."

_____
Notary Public
(seal)

Signed_____

Date _____

Witness _____

_____
Address

Witness _____

_____
Address

Copies of this request have been given to _____

_____   _____

(Optional)   My Living Will is registered with Concern for Dying (No. _____)

Distributed by Concern for Dying, 250 West 57th Street, New York, NY 10107 (212) 246-6962

A living will. (From Concern for Dying, New York, pp. 696–697.)

sionate physical care while meeting the psychologic and social needs of the terminally ill patient and his or her family.

Dying at Home. When illness has been confirmed and the diagnosis is such that recovery is unlikely, the family and the patient may decide in favor of home care instead of hospital care. Once this decision has been made, there are several steps the responsible family member has to make.

Will there be dressings, treatments, and so on, for the family to attend to? What will be the reaction of the patient? What type of instruction will the caregiver at home need in order to function? Will the caregiver be responsible for mouth care, bladder and bowel care, ostomy care? Visiting nurses and other professionals in the field of health care will be especially helpful. There are also organizations that can provide educational materials and low or no cost equipment to families (The American Cancer Society, the American Heart Association, and so on) who are caring at home for a terminally ill person.

Good communication between patient and family is essential. However, communication need not always be verbal. Touching, stroking, just being there is emotionally satisfying.

□ *Care at Death*

□ Signs of Approaching Death

There are certain indications that death is near. Reflexes are absent and the patient does not move. Respirations may become labored. Cheyne-Stokes respirations may occur, that is, the characteristic breathing of the dying, apnea lasting from 10 to 60 seconds followed by gradually increasing respirations. The skin will become mottled and this will be followed by faint cyanosis. The skin will feel cold and clammy. Pulse will accelerate and blood pressure will decrease.

It is important for the nurse to monitor vital signs and make general observations frequently. Skin care, oral hygiene care, hydration, nutrition, and general comfort care are important. It is also important to keep the room clean and odor free and to allow familiar items and objects near at hand as the patient wishes.

□ Signs of Death

Generally speaking, breathing ceases first and the heart stops beating shortly after. Death is said to occur when respirations and heartbeats have ceased for several minutes. The nurse should note the exact time the heart stops beating and that respirations cease. A physician should pronounce the patient dead, according to the laws of the particular state.

When death occurs at home, the most important thing is for the family to do what seems to be natural for them at this time: stay near the body, cover it, hold it. Some may prefer to leave the room until professionals come in to help. Whatever feels natural and comfortable for them at that time is correct.

Depending on the laws in the particular area, the home caregiver may have to notify a county coroner, sheriff, or physician to make an official pronouncement of death. As soon as the appropriate official visits the home to make the pronouncement, the body may be moved to a mortuary.

When death occurs in the hospital, aftercare is usually a nursing responsibility. The body is placed in supine position the head slightly elevated. The body should be positioned immediately after death before rigor mortis sets in. Since relatives may wish to view the body, it should appear clean and at peace. The room should be neat and all unnecessary equipment should be removed.

Hospital policy regarding dentures varies. Some institutions want dentures inserted; others recommend that dentures be sent along to the mortician. Rings should be taped in place and documentation to this effect is made on the chart.

Since muscles relax after death, the nurse will apply pads to the perineal area. Blood or drainage should be washed and fresh dressings applied.

☐ The Nurse

Nurses need to analyze their attitudes toward death. How do religious philosophy, culture, family concepts, and personal experience influence a nurse? How can a youth-oriented culture allow for a balanced perspective? The nurse's experience with death may be limited to formal readings in an educational setting. Death may provoke feelings of defeat and inadequacy. Colleagues should assist the nurse who is involved with the dying patient to explore troubling personal reactions. Professional resource persons are also valuable in providing emotional support to the nurse who is caring for the dying individual.

Chapter 9 ☐ Review Questions

Multiple Choice

1. A terminally ill patient receiving care through a hospice program will most likely
   A. be cared for in a hospital that specializes in oncology
   B. experience a remission of symptoms

    C. be cared for at home and allowed to spend his or her last days among relatives and friends

    D. receive care from nonprofessionals who are poorly trained to deal with the dying

2. A sign of approaching death is
    A. mottling of skin followed by cyanosis
    B. delerium accompanied by hallucinations
    C. extreme pain requiring large amounts of narcotics
    D. rapid respirations

3. A factor that might be used to describe living wills is that they
    A. are never contested
    B. are always legally binding in all states
    C. always prevent heroic measures from being taken with patients
    D. have enabled many individuals to control the nature of their death

4. Passive euthanasia
    A. indicates an act deliberately done
    B. denotes failure to take action that would prolong life
    C. always is followed by prosecution
    D. usually occurs in a hospital setting

5. Do not resuscitate (DNR) orders are
    A. illegal
    B. are freely written by physicians
    C. must be carefully documented in both the patient's medical record and the progress notes
    D. must be cosigned by two physicians

6. One reason health professionals say informed consent is needed is that
    A. it encourages a knowledge of ethical and legal principles involved
    B. it can guarantee that patients understand clearly their prognosis
    C. it prevents unsuccessful surgery
    D. it prevents lawsuits

7. Health professionals are reluctant to resuscitate patients
    A. unless all the proper equipment is at hand
    B. who are over 60 years of age
    C. who may not be mentally competent
    D. who may not benefit from it or may not even wish it

8. A nurse may be prosecuted if
    A. she makes a medical decision
    B. she administers CPR
    C. she does not meet the patient's emotional needs
    D. her license lapses

9. Kübler-Ross is a pioneer in the study of
    A. informed consent
    B. ethical decisions
    C. thanatology
    D. depression

10. When an individual learns he or she is dying a common initial reaction
    is
    A. depression
    B. denial
    C. acceptance
    D. bargaining

DISCUSSION QUESTIONS

1. Your neighbor has just learned that he has a terminal illness. He has asked
   you to help him avoid heroic measures that will prolong his life. How will
   you respond to him?
2. Mr. and Mrs. Williams are elderly friends of yours. Mrs. Williams has been
   treated for several months for a terminal disease and now she, her husband, and the physician have agreed that nothing more will be done. Mr.
   Williams insists on caring for his wife at home. What are some ways you
   can advise this couple? List agencies they may contact as resources, practical aspects of care that might be involved, and specific situations Mr. Williams should be prepared to meet.
3. What are the laws in your community regarding living wills?
4. You are visiting an elderly relative in a nursing home and she says to you,
   "What is the easiest way to commit suicide?" Bearing in mind that your
   relative is alert and aware in spite of her advanced years, what would you
   reply?

☐ REFERENCES

Benoliel, J.Q.: Nursing research on death, dying, and terminal illness: Development, present state,
    and prospects. Ann Rev Nurs Res, 1:101–130, 1983.
Brucker, E.: Expanded Medicare-Hospice coverage: A checklist for nurses. Home Health Nursing,
    2(3):47–48, 1984.
Byrne, C.M.: An assessment of the need for hospice services in a rural area. J Community Health
    Nurs, 1(1):59–64, 1984.
Castledine, G.: When life moves on . . . how to deal with death and dying. Nurs Mirror,
    158(17):22, 1984.
Corr, D.: The hospice movement. Nurs Mirror, 159(16):19–22, 1984.
Curtin, L.L.: Death quota and PRO's . . . hospital death rates. Nurs Management, 15(9):7–8, 1984.
Davis, A.J.: Informed consent: How much information is enough? Nurs Outlook, 33(1):40–42,
    1985.
Death Education: The media exchange: Annotated bibliography. Death Education, 7(4):401–404,
    1983.
DeKornfeld, T.J.: The terminally ill patient: Ethical and legal considerations. Curr Rev Respir
    Ther, 6(15):115–118, 1984.
Gillis, B.: Hospice: Life to its fullest. Am Health Care Assoc J, 10(1):14, 16–17, 1984.
Graham, H., et al.: Dying as a diagnosis: Difficulties of communication and management in el-
    derly patients. Lancet, 2(8351):670–672, 1983.
Haultain, J.: Hospice care in a general hospital. NZ Nurs J, 76(11):22–23, 1983.
Kliban, M.G., et al.: Bereavement counseling in groups . . . hospice care includes followup care
    for survivors. Caring, 3(9):12–18, 1984.

Kübler-Ross, E.: To Live Until We Say Good-Bye. Englewood Cliffs, NJ, Prentice-Hall, 1978, p. 141.

Merkel, M.E.: The slow code dilemma. Nurs Life, 5(2):23–25, 1985.

Mor, V., et al.: Burnout among hospice staff. Health Soc Work, 9(4):274–283, 1984.

Mullins, L.C., et al.: The effects of a short term death training program on nursing home nursing staff. Death Education, 7(4):353–368, 1983.

Novak, N.: "Natural Death Acts" let patients refuse treatments. Hospitals, 58(15):71–73, 1984.

Pizzi, M.: Hospice and the terminally ill geriatric patient. Am J Occup Ther, 38:252–257, 1984.

Ritchie, N.D.: Nurses and hospice administration. J Nurs Admin, 14:14, 1984.

Rodek, C.F., et al.: Hospice legislation: A new trail . . . Medicare reimbursement. Cancer Nurs, 7(5):385–390, 1984.

Sheehan, C.J., et al.: Analysis of the Medicare/Hospice program: Rural application. Home Health Nurs, 2(5):38–40, 1984.

Smith, H.L., et al.: New Management strategies help solve unique challenges of terminal care. Hosp Top, 62(4):18–21, 48, 1984.

Nursing Life: Special poll report on the right to die . . . a survey of 3504 nurses. Nurs Life, 4(3):47–53, 1984.

Thompson, L.M.: Cultural and institutional restrictions on dying styles in a technological society. Death Education, 8(4):223–229, 1984.

Utley, O.E., et al.: Coping with loss: A group experience with elderly survivors. J Gerontol Nurs, 10(8):8–9, 1984.

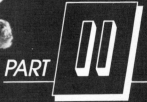

PART II

Geriatric
Nursing
Skills

Objectives

After completing this chapter, the student should be able to

- ☐ list the age-related changes in the integumentary system
- ☐ name some common skin problems found in elderly persons
- ☐ discuss the principles of proper skin hygiene
- ☐ identify factors that contribute to compromising skin integrity
- ☐ list therapies for decubitus ulcers
- ☐ evaluate effectiveness of nursing interventions for decubitus ulcers
- ☐ describe hair care for the bed-bound patient

Vocabulary

axilla
coccyx
decubitus ulcer
epidermis
Fowler's position
incontinence
keratosis
leukoplakia
perineal area
podiatrist
pruritus
sacrum
sebum
subcutaneous

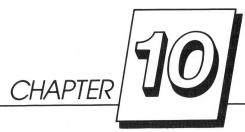

CHAPTER

The Integumentary System

Chapter Outline

☐ Anatomy Review

☐ STRUCTURES AND FUNCTIONS

Epidermis. The outermost layer provides a protective physical barrier. It is continually being shed and replaced.

Dermis. Beneath the epidermis, the dermis is a tough but elastic support structure that contains the blood vessels, nerves, and skin appendages.

Exocrine Glands. These glands discharge their secretion through ducts, e.g., sweat glands, which help regulate body temperature by excreting sweat onto the surface of the skin, from which the cooling process of evaporation takes place. Cf. endocrine glands, which are ductless, e.g., pituitary glands.

Sebaceous Glands. The sebaceous glands produce an oily substance termed *sebum* that may serve as a skin moisturizer.

Hair Follicle. Hair follicles are small sacs that contain the hair roots. Hair serves a protective function in most mammals but in humans is largely decorative.

Nails. Nails are made of keratin, a tough protein. They protect the ends of the fingers and toes.

Subcutaneous Fat. A layer of subcutaneous fat lies between the dermis and underlying muscles. The layer of fat helps insulate the body from cold, protects deep tissue from trauma, and serves as a reserve source of food.

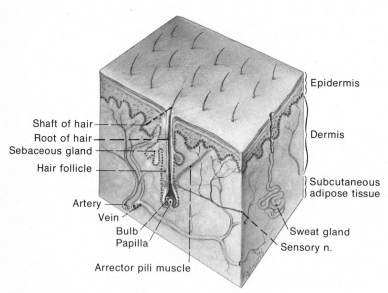

Figure 10–1 ☐ Three-dimensional view of the skin. (From Jacob, Francone, and Lossow, p. 77.)

□ Age-Related Changes

Wrinkles. Wrinkles are the characteristic sign of aging skin. They are caused by decreased subcutaneous fat and loss of collagen and elastic fibers.

Dry Skin. As skin ages, it looses moisture and softness and may feel leathery. The skin becomes dry as the production of sebum, nature's lubricant, by the sebaceous glands decreases.

Thinner, More Fragile Skin. As the skin becomes less elastic, it becomes more easily damaged. Damaged skin heals less quickly because blood supply to the skin is reduced and the replacement of cells in the epidermis is slowed down.

Pigmentation and Growths. In Caucasians, brown spots (sometimes called liver spots) appear. They do not indicate any disorder but are often upsetting to the person because of their appearance. Also, a reduction in the number and functioning of melanocytes (the structure that enables the skin to tan) means that the elderly person is more sensitive to sunlight.

Several types of benign growths typically appear on the skin after age 50. Skin tags (soft, pedunculated, flesh-colored growths) and seborrheic keratosis (darker, scaly growths) are very common and pose no medical problems. Less common, more serious lesions are described under Age-Related Disorders.

Brittle Nails. Fingernails become ridged and brittle. They should be kept short and smooth. The color may change, turning yellowish or grayish.

Hair. The hair of the elderly person is generally thin due to reduction of the activity of the hair follicles. Dryness may be a problem because of reduced sebum production. Loss of pigmentation of the hair shaft results in graying and white hair. Hair patterns vary in different racial groups; therefore, changes with aging also vary. Among Caucasians, older women often develop facial hair.

□ Age-Related Disorders

Itching. Itching (pruritus) that accompanies dryness is a common complaint of the elderly person. Pruritus can be a symptom of disease or drug reaction also. Therefore, complaints should be investigated. Humidification of the environment and additional moisturizing of the skin will help alleviate itching due to dry skin.

Premalignant and Malignant Lesions. Since premalignant and malignant lesions of the skin frequently develop as a result of years of exposure to the sun, changes in the skin should be noted by the nurse and referred to a physician. Among the disorders seen are *actinic keratosis* (scaly, rough growth, without clear margins; reddened or light brown), *squamous cell carcinoma* (a scaling plaque or nodule that sometimes bleeds or ulcerates; most commonly seen on areas exposed to the sun on fair-skinned people), and *basal cell carcinoma* (malignant growth that is the most common type of skin cancer; it has several different types of appearance; therefore, unusual growths on the skin should be referred to the physician).

Leukoplakia is a whitish gray plaque lesion that affects mucous membranes, particularly the lower lip, tongue, and hard palate. It is sometimes seen on the vulva and labia. This is a premalignant condition and needs treatment.

Most elderly are on several medications for a variety of problems; therefore, drug-induced skin reaction must first be ruled out. Many systemic disorders, e.g., cancer or diabetes, show symptoms on the skin. In addition, grief and depression often cause skin eruptions, and emotional reactions may delay the patient from seeking treatment.

Decubitus Ulcers. Decubitus ulcers frequently occur in the elderly person confined to bed or wheelchair. The thinner, more fragile skin of the elderly person is more susceptible to decubitus ulcers, but with good nursing care they can be prevented. This topic is covered in greater detail later in this chapter.

☐ *Nursing Interventions*

☐ THE BED BATH

In health care facilities, much "AM care" time is devoted to giving bed baths. Done correctly, they leave the patient comfortable, relaxed, and refreshed in body and spirit.

Bathtime is an excellent time to assess a patient. The nurse can observe the skin for color, texture, rashes, or scars. Equally important is that the bath giver has an opportunity to know the patient. Because the skin of the elderly person is dry, a full bath may not be given on a daily basis. Often, only a partial bath is given daily.

The cleansing bed bath, given by someone else, offers only passive exercise. So the sooner the patient is able to bathe himself or herself, the sooner he or she benefits from active exercise and a sense of independence.

Purposes

to bathe patients who cannot get out of bed
to identify skin abnormalities

Equipment

bath blanket	gown	deodorant
basin	wash cloth	lotion
bath towel	soap	powder
face towel		

Sequence

1. identify patient; introduce self; explain procedure
2. see that room temperature is comfortable; many elderly persons are especially susceptible to chilling. Be sure the room is warm enough for the patient, not just for the caregiver.
3. insure privacy with screens, curtains, or draping
4. check dressings (change as indicated)
5. replace top sheet and spread with the bath blanket
6. remove gown, eyeglasses, wristwatch, and so on
7. fill basin three-fourths full of 110°F water (use bath thermometer)
8. place patient in low Fowler's position, near to the side of the bed
9. lay small hand towel on top of bath blanket over chest
10. ask if soap is used on face; wet cloth, wring out
11. make a mitt out of cloth by clasping the corners between thumb and fingers

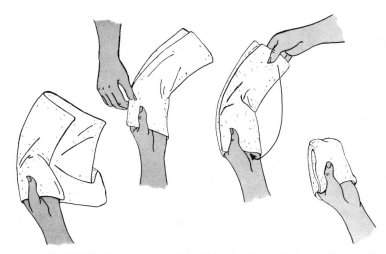

Figure 10–2 □ Making a washcloth mitt for bathing. This type of bath mitt covers the ends of the fingers and protects the patient from being jabbed with sharp fingernails. (From Leake, p. 40.)

12. wash and rinse face, neck, ears; blot dry
13. uncover *far* arm: wash and rinse, using long, smooth strokes; dry arm and axilla; apply deodorant
14. repeat with near arm
15. let patient place hands in basin if possible; wash, rinse, dry hands; clean nails
16. place bath towel over chest; fold bath blanket to waist; wash, rinse, and dry; observe for excoriations in skin folds under pendulous breasts of obese females; treat according to policy of the facility
17. wash *far* leg using long, smooth strokes; if possible, place basin on the bed, flex patient's knee, cup your hand to support heel and lower foot into basin; wash, rinse and dry; repeat for other leg; care for toenails according to institution's policy
18. change bath water
19. turn patient and wash and rinse back; back rub may be given at this time or after bath is completed

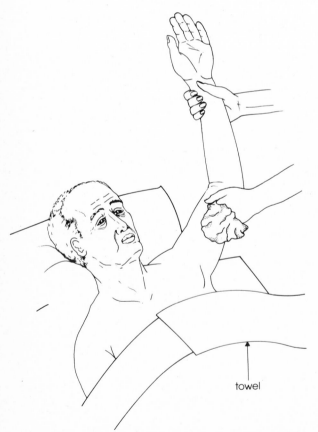

Figure 10–3 □ Wash the arms. (Modified from Rambo and Wood, p. 340.)

towel

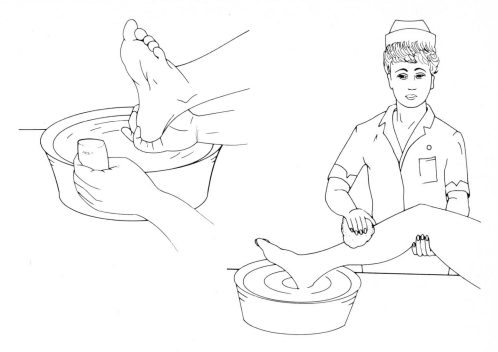

Figure 10–4 □ Wash the feet and legs. (Modified from Rambo and Wood, p. 340.)

20. place patient again in low Fowler's position; place equipment near patient; tell him or her to complete personal bath (genital area) if he or she is able, or complete bath for helpless patient

Notes. When giving perineal care to the incontinent, uncircumsized male patient, retract the foreskin (prepuce) while washing the penis in order to remove secretions that can cause odor and irritation. When genital hygiene is complete, draw foreskin back over the penis. Turn patient on his side, lift buttock, wash anal area, rinse and dry.

The female patient benefits from being placed on a bedpan and having a pitcher of warm water poured over the vulva. The labia must be separated carefully to give genital hygiene to the female patient.

Improper draping and screening of patients violates not only their dignity but also their rights.

□ THE TUB BATH

Immersing hands or feet in a basin of water adds considerably to the enjoyment of the bath. When a person is able to get into a tub of warm water and soak, the bath becomes a doubly pleasurable experience.

The nurse must take precautions against skids and falls (for the nurse as well as for the patient!). A nonskid tub mat is as important as a dry floor. The door is not locked even for the alert, reliable self-care person. Plan to check on the patient within 5 minutes. Point out the emergency call light to the patient.

Purpose

to bathe in a bathtub safely and effectively.

Equipment

bath blanket	soap	bath mat
two bath towels	tub mat (or towel)	chair
wash cloth		

Sequence

1. identify patient; introduce self; explain procedure
2. inspect tub to be sure it is clean; fill half full of 110°F water
3. have person test water before getting into tub
4. place mat or towel in tub
5. caution patient to use handrail; assist as needed
6. assist with bath or leave person alone as situation indicates
7. indicate call signal to patient; return in 5 minutes; wash back, observe skin for abnormalities
8. assist patient out of tub, dry and help dress as necessary
9. clean tub and leave it presentable for next patient

It may be necessary to use a mechanical lifting device for some patients. If using a Hoyer lift, for example, use the following precautions:

1. check the device to be sure it is working properly
2. explain the procedure to the patient
3. have enough assistance available for a difficult patient (i.e., one who is uncooperative, contracted, or extremely obese)

☐ THE BACK RUB

Giving a good back rub is as satisfying for the nurse as getting a good back rub is for the patient. The actual "laying on of hands" reinforces the nursing role of comforter. At the end of the back rub, the patient should feel comfortable, relaxed, and cared for.

If the patient can tolerate it, he or she should lie on his or her abdomen. Otherwise, the side-lying position is used. Beginning at the base of the spine, the nurse uses long, smooth strokes that travel up the back, part at the base of the neck, and then glide downward so the hands meet at the coccyx.

Purposes

to relieve tension.
to promote circulation of the skin and help prevent decubitus ulcers.

Equipment

towel   lotion   powder   gown

Sequence

1. identify patient; introduce self; explain procedure
2. screen patient
3. open back of gown
4. pour small amount of lotion into palm of hand to take chill off lotion; rub hands together
5. place hands together, palms down on coccyx
6. slide hands up backbone, exerting pressure
7. separate hands at neck; slide hands down back
8. inspect skin for reddened areas
9. massage coccyx area to stimulate circulation
10. continue back rub for from 3 to 5 minutes
11. blot dry with towel
12. powder sparingly, if desired; replace gown
13. reposition patient

☐ HINTS FOR HOME CARE

• Substances other than soap and water can be alternated with the tub or bed bath. Lotion, for example, or a no-rinse cleansing agent can be gently rubbed on the skin. This stimulates circulation and lubricates skin, thus preventing skin breakdown
• Use equipment available to make tub bathing easier and safer. Some examples are: tub rails, safety mats, adhesive strips for tub, bath bench, hydraulic lift
• A shower chair may be used in the shower. A hand-held shower attachment is another useful device.

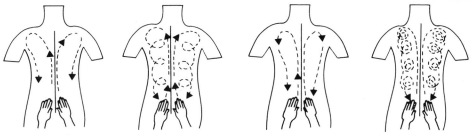

Figure 10–5 ☐ The back rub. Arrows indicate direction in which hands move. Circles indicate areas to massage. The sacral area requires extra massage.

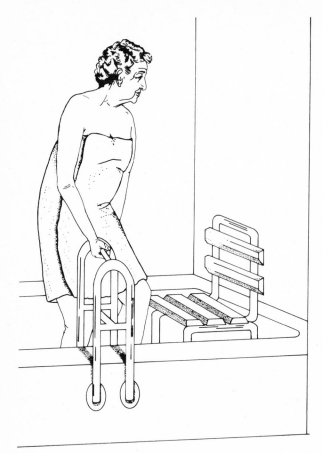

Figure 10–6 ☐ In the home, many safety devices can be installed to increase safety for the older adult. A shower seat and a tub rail can make it possible for the older adult with some impairment of mobility to bathe alone.

- If the patient uses a wheelchair, roll the wheelchair to the tub's edge, ease patient's legs over the side, *lock* wheels, and assist the patient into the tub (A straight-backed chair can be made mobile by attaching casters to the legs.)
- The bath, whether in the tub or in the bed, is a time to encourage range of motion exercise. These exercises can improve joint mobility in some and maintain mobility in patients with limited range of motion.

Note. Never leave a weak or confused patient alone in the bathtub. Always leave the bathroom door unlocked.

☐ THE SITZ BATH

There are special tubs designed so that patients sit in them and only the rectal, buttock, and perineal areas are bathed. There are also portable basins that may be used to administer sitz baths in the home and in the hospital.

A sitz bath is usually prescribed by a physician to relieve pain and encourage wound healing when someone has had rectal surgery. Occasionally, they are ordered to relieve urine retention. Warm water 110°F to 115°F produces maximum effects within 15 minutes.

Purposes

to relieve rectal or perineal pain and promote healing

Equipment

towel or air ring for tub	bath mat	chair
towel for drying patient	bath blanket	

Sequence

1. identify patient; introduce self; explain procedure
2. draw bath for patient; test temperature of water; place towel or air ring in tub
3. drape bath blanket around patient's shoulders
4. maintain proper body alignment while patient is sitting in tub
5. aftercare, dressing change as per physician's order
    A sitz tub is better than a regular bathtub because there is more concentration of heated water on the anal-pelvic region. The nurse should observe carefully for patient's weakness, color change, or dizziness while soak is being given.

□ PREVENTION AND CARE OF DECUBITUS ULCERS

The word *decubitus* refers to lying down and the word *ulcer* means that the integrity of the skin is compromised. A decubitus ulcer, or *pressure sore*, is the result of great pressure for a short period of time or continuous pressure for a long period of time.

What actually happens in either situation is that the pressure on the skin and underlying tissue causes cells to die because the circulation is blocked. Cellular necrosis (dead tissues) is, therefore, produced where there is lack of blood flow.

Healthy people do not get pressure sores because they move around all the time. They shift weight and change position whether sitting, standing, or lying down. Even when asleep, the healthy person changes position several times during the night.

Who, then, is likely to develop pressure sores? Generally speaking, the person who moves too little, or not at all, and is poorly nourished is susceptible to decubitus ulcers.

Decubitus ulcers are always unpleasant and often dangerous. They prolong illness, retard recovery, increase the cost of health care, and in some cases, can cause death.

The following patients are those who are at risk for decubitus ulcers:
- acutely ill with a rapidly deteriorating condition
- elderly and confined to bed
- thin, cachetic
- obese, and therefore placing more pressure on overburdened joints
- regularly sedated
- paralyzed
- malnourished
- incontinent
- have impaired circulation
- wear casts; are in traction
- have neurologically debilitating problems (Parkinson's disease, cerebrovascular accident [CVA], multiple sclerosis)

The previous list is a partial one. Any ill or disabled person who spends time in a bed or wheelchair can develop a decubitus ulcer.

Most pressure sores can be prevented, however. The nurse must first identify the patient who is at risk, examine the patient daily, and implement a preventive regimen.

Measures to Prevent Decubitus Ulcers

1. turn patient at least every 2 hours
2. maintain skin cleanliness; lubricate and massage bony prominences
3. use alternating pressure pad, egg crate mattress, sheepskin underpad

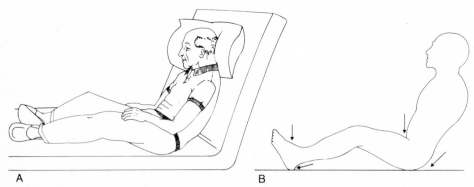

A   B

Figure 10–7 ☐ A, Poor position often assumed by a person in bed with back rest elevated. Note flexion of neck, curve of back, compression of chest, external rotation of hips, and foot- and wristdrop. Also observe the areas of the body bearing the patient's weight, thus being prone to development of pressure sores. B, The shearing force exerts a downward and forward pressure.

4. use bed cradle to keep linens off feet
5. use sheepskin heel and elbow protectors (must be removed every 8 hours to check skin integrity)
6. encourage fluids, therapeutically adequate diet (sufficient protein to repair and build tissues)
7. avoid "shearing" force of position in bed or chair (Fig. 10–7)
8. encourage movement, mobility where possible
9. "bridging" to reduce or eliminate pressure; trochanter rolls

Common Local Therapies

Numerous treatments are available for application to the site of a pressure sore. Some of the more common measures are

Karaya products	granulated sugar
Gelfoam	debriding agents
Mylanta	exposure to air, ultraviolet lights
beaten egg whites	tincture of benzoin

Covered foam rubber pillows and firm cushions are also successfully used to provide "bridging" of pressure-prone areas of the skin from contact with other surfaces. These devices can support the body in proper alignment and help to eliminate pressure from the entire area of the body.

Whatever method or device is used, it is essential that all shifts observe continuity of care and that all personnel document what is being done for the patient.

Hints for Home Care

The home caregiver should check bedsheets for crumbs and wrinkles, as these can irritate skin. Avoid harsh laundry detergents and be sure that all bed linens are thoroughly rinsed. An irritating residue can cause skin problems.

The following devices can be purchased at a surgical supply store:
1. sheepskin, Kodel, synthetic fur pads (use tape or velcro to fasten); cut to fit the area to be protected
2. heel and elbow protectors. *Be sure to remove these every 8 hours to check the skin*
3. specially designed mattresses

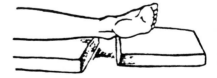

Figure 10–8 □ "Bridging" for the prevention or treatment of decubitus ulcers. (From Talbot, p. 13.)

4. a cut-out carton to place over knees and lift linens off patient
5. overhead trapeze to help the patient to position himself or herself

Summary: Decubitus Ulcers

Etiology	Immobility Debilitation Pressure over bony prominences Poor circulation
Symptoms	Redness of skin over pressure points Mottled skin Blistering, broken skin
Prevention	Frequent position change Cleanliness Massage Alternating pressure pads, sheepskin

The responsibility of the nurse in the initial assessment cannot be over-stated. When skin is examined, compromised areas measured, and the appropriate documentation done, then the common effort of all nurses in developing the care plan will produce the desired effect.

Assessment of decubitus ulcers must indicate stage and size. For example:

STAGE I	area is pink; skin is unbroken but blanches on touch; feels warm and dry
STAGE II	skin is cracked, blistered, broken; surrounding area is reddened
STAGE III	skin is broken with deep decubitus ulcer; tissue involvement; drainage is present
STAGE IV	skin is broken; deep decubitus ulcer involving tissue, bone, and muscle

Decubitus ulcers should be measured at the time of assessment and *three times a week* (e.g., Mon., Wed., Friday). Document stage and size in inches as to diameter and depth.

CARE OF THE HAIR

Encourage patients to comb their own hair. Many elderly in hospitals and nursing homes are able to do their own hair if positioned in front of a mirror and given their own combs and brushes. The benefits are many, including good range of motion exercise to arms, increased self esteem, and growth of independence. Appearance is an extremely important aspect of geriatric care.

Follow the next procedure for patients who are unable to care for their own hair.

Purposes

to keep hair and scalp clean and healthy
to improve the patient's appearance
to encourage a feeling of well being through grooming

Equipment

comb   towel
brush   hairpins or rubber bands (if patient is female)

Sequence

1. place towel over the patient's shoulders
2. brush or comb small sections of hair at a time, starting at the *ends* of the hair and working upwards
3. alcohol may be applied to snarls of oily hair; Vaseline may be used on the snarls of dry hair
4. observe the scalp for lesions and the hair for parasites (lice, nits)
5. long hair may be braided and secured with elastics

   Note. Hair is never cut by a nurse except in emergency situations.

□ SHAMPOO IN BED

Many hospitals and nursing homes have beauty salons on the premises. However, the majority do not. If the patient cannot shampoo his or her own hair, a caregiver must do this for the patient.

A bed shampoo may be a physician's or a nurse's order. Determine which at your own facility.

Although no-rinse shampoo products are available, the bed shampoo is very simple and effective when an unused bedpan is used. (Of course, that bedpan is reserved for giving shampoos only!) Place a bath towel under the patient's head and shoulders, pad the narrow end of the bedpan that the neck will rest on with another bath towel and use pitchers of water and shampoo as necessary. The hair will be clean, the patient refreshed, and the caregiver pleased at how easy and fast the whole procedure is.

An alternative to a bed shampoo might be to get the patient on a stretcher and into the utility room where a shampoo may be given over a sink or hopper. The ambulatory patient may comfortably be shampooed at the bathroom sink or, in some cases, if the sink is too high, over the toilet. The nurse should observe the patient carefully for signs of weakness. If this occurs, the shampoo is stopped and the patient is returned to bed.

☐ HAIR CARE FOR THE BLACK PATIENT

The liquid shampoo generally used on white patients may not be suitable for the naturally dry, coarse, very curly hair of the black patient. The nurse should determine whether there are any allergies to oil or alcohol. Then, with the patient's and physician's permission, a mixture of one part alcohol to four parts mineral oil can be massaged into the scalp and hair, and toweled off. A wide-toothed afro comb can then be used to arrange the hair suitably. Consult the patient or patient's family about preferred hair care products. Ingrown hair is a problem for blacks. Hair follicles in black persons are curved. When the hair grows out of a curved follicle, it can re-enter the skin and cause an inflammatory reaction. This in turn, predisposes the black patient to chronic folliculitis and possibly even keloid formation.

☐ CARE OF THE NAILS

Included in daily hygiene is care of the fingernails and toenails. Fingernails may be cleaned with an orangewood stick after the bath. Rough or jagged nails should be smoothed with an emery board.

The toenails of the elderly patient are more difficult to care for. They may be thickened and brittle and hard to cut. If, after giving the patient a thorough footsoak and using an emery board to smooth the toenails, the nurse finds that the elderly patient needs more attention than the nurse can give, a podiatrist should be sent for. Bandage scissors are unsuitable and toenail clippers are risky to use on an elderly patient, and the podiatrist has the special instruments and skill with which to solve the problem.

☐ THE FOOT SOAK

After the bed bath has been given, if the patient's condition permits him or her to be out of bed he or she should be allowed to sit in a chair and soak his or her feet. A towel or newspaper is spread on the floor under the basin of warm water. The patient can soak his or her feet while the nurse makes the bed. Then the feet are thoroughly dried, lotion is applied, and socks or slippers are put on. This makes up in a small way for not being able to take a shower or tub bath!

Diabetic Precautions. Poor circulation is a problem among diabetics and foot care is part of patient teaching if the nurse is caring for a diabetic patient. Meticulous skin care is mandatory and it should consist of washing, drying between each toe, and keeping the toenails trimmed straight across. Footwear must be scrupulously clean. Above all, the diabetic must avoid treating corns, calluses, and so on with any home remedies. The only one competent to care for these foot problems is a podiatrist.

All elderly persons, whether diabetic or not, should have their feet properly protected with the correct type of shoes when they are up and walking about.

Chapter 10 □ Review Questions

MULTIPLE CHOICE

1. The outer layer of the skin is called
   A. follicle
   B. tubule
   C. epidermis
   D. sebum
2. The bed bath is an excellent time to
   A. explain hospital policies
   B. assess skin abnormalities
   C. lower body temperature
   D. use cold water for rinsing
3. Improper draping and screening
   A. irritates physicians
   B. confuses patients
   C. violates patients' rights
   D. reduces effective evaluation of nurses
4. When administering a back rub, the nurse should
   A. verify the physician's order with the supervisor
   B. pour a small amount of lotion into her hands to take the chill off the lotion
   C. follow the back rub with plenty of powder
   D. put the patient in Sims' position

MATCHING

＿＿＿	1. sitz bath	A. can incorporate passive exercise
＿＿＿	2. decubitus ulcer	B. relieves pain after rectal surgery
＿＿＿	3. sheepskin pads	C. caused by sustained pressure on the skin and underlying tissue
＿＿＿	4. back rub	D. permit circulation of air to the skin
＿＿＿	5. bed bath	E. stimulates circulation and relieves tension

DISCUSSION QUESTIONS

1. In what ways might shampooing and grooming the hair of a black patient differ from caring for the hair of a white patient?
2. What are some common useful means of preventing decubitus ulcers?
3. How does the skin of an elderly person differ from that of a young adult?
4. What are the precautions the nurse can teach to a diabetic patient concerning foot care?
5. Describe some general factors about the skin of older people that must be taken into consideration when diagnosing and treating their skin problems.

□ REFERENCES

Boulton, S.W., et al.: Evaluating disposable briefs . . . treating incontinence. Am J Nurs, 84(11): 1413–1431, 1984.

Buchanan, G.: Light fantastic . . . psoralen plus ultra violet light. Nurs Mirror, 159(11):26–27, 30, 1984.

Byrne, N., et al.: Overcoming the red menace: preventing and treating decubitus ulcers. Nursing (Horsham), 14(4):55–57, 1984.

Care of the ingrowing toe nail: guidelines in technique. Hosp Med, 20(8):134–135, 1984.

Cowie, V.: Incontinentia pigmenti: Jervell and Lange Nielsen syndrome. Nurs Mirror, 158(5): inside back cover, 1984.

David, J.: Tissue breakdown . . . a pressure sore survey. Nurs Mirror, 158(1):i–ii (Clinical Forum), 1984.

Doty, C.: Pressure sores . . . the role of nutrition. Commun Outlook, Feb., 1984, p. 70.

Dotz, W., et al.: Dry skin: aids that preserve hydration and mitigate its loss. Consultant, 24(8): 46–48, 53, 56–57, 1984.

Dotz, W., et al.: Skin and cancer: signs that indicate internal malignancies. Consultant, 24(10):268–275, 279, 1984.

Fraser, M.C., et al.: Skin cancer's early warning system . . . dysplastic nevus syndrome (DNS). Am J Nurs, 84(10):1232–1236, 1984.

Getting the Wrinkles Out of Aging. Your Life Health, 97(4):19, 1982.

Kuhn, J.K., et al.: A multidisciplinary team approach to decubitus ulcer care. Nurs Homes, 33(1):29–33, 1984.

McClemont, E.J.M.: No pressure—no sore. Nursing (Oxford), 2(21):1–3, (Pressure Sores Suppl), 1984.

Milliard, L.G.: Dermatology in pigmented skin. Nursing (Oxford), 2(16):274–278, 1983.

Shannon, M.L.: Five famous fallacies about pressure sores. Nursing (Horsham), 14(10):34, 1984.

Slahetka, F.: Dakin's solution for deep ulcers. Geriatr Nurs, 5(3):168–169, 1984.

Smith, I.: Pressure sores: heel aids. Nurs Times, 80(36):35–39, 1984.

Staging care for pressure sores. Am J Nurs, 84(8):999–1003, 1984.

Tooman, T., et al.: Decubitus ulcer warfare: product vs process. Geriatr Nurs, 5(3):166–167, 1984.

Whitney, J.D., et al.: Do mattresses make a difference? . . . prevention of pressure sores. J Gerontol Nurs, 10(9):20–21, 24–25, 1984.

Wright, E.T.: Skin deep. Your Life Health, 98(11):8–9, 1983.

Objectives

After completing this chapter, the student should be able to

☐ describe the anatomy and physiology of the lungs and related respiratory organs
☐ identify common respiratory problems and describe appropriate interventions
☐ assess and document a client's ability to do breathing exercises
☐ identify relevant principles in the planning and implementation of nursing interventions to minimize a client's anxiety, collect sputum specimens, ensure adequate oxygen intake, and maintain patency of a patient's airway

Vocabulary

alveolus
aspirate
COPD
cyanosis
dyspnea
emphysema
expectorant
flowmeter
hypoxemia
kyphosis
mucous
mucus
nebulizer
uvula

The Respiratory System

Chapter Outline

☐ Anatomy Review

Breathing is essential to life. It is so important that we call it vital. That is why timing respirations (counting the rate at which a person is breathing) is called taking a vital sign.

☐ FUNCTIONS

The word "respiration" means an exchange of gases between an organism and the environment in which it lives. The respiratory system involves internal and external respiration.

External Respiration. Oxygen is delivered to the cells of the body by way of the bloodstream. Carbon dioxide, a waste product, is carried away by the same means. The actual process works this way: a person inhales; air enters alveoli, which are air sacs in the lungs; oxygen from that air passes through membranes that line the sacs and joins the red blood cells. The bloodstream carries oxygen along to the heart, which then distributes it to the rest of the body by means of its ceaseless pumping action. At the same time, carbon dioxide leaves the blood and gets collected briefly in the alveolar sacs until the person exhales.

Internal Respiration. This type of respiration takes place in the *cells*. Through a series of complex changes, the food we ingest is oxidized (burned). Oxygen is used to free the energy from our food. Some of this energy is used to stabilize body temperature and some of it is used directly by muscle cells.

☐ STRUCTURES

Lungs. Lungs are paired, triangular organs located in the thoracic cavity. The tip of the triangle is called the apex. The bottom is called the base. The lungs rest on the diaphragm, the muscle that serves as a partition between the thoracic cavity and the abdominal cavity. The right lung has three lobes (sections) and the left has two.

Lungs are spongy and are enclosed in a membrane called pleura. This membrane is double because it not only covers the lungs but also lines the thoracic cavity. It secretes a fluid that prevents friction between the two layers.

Alveolus. An alveolus is an air sac enclosed in a membrane richly supplied with capillaries.

Bronchiole. A stemlike entrance to the alveolus. It branches to form larger bronchi.

Bronchus. A large tubular structure; extends to bronchioles.

Trachea. The trachea channels air to the thorax. It is framed with cartilage rings.

Diaphragm. This is the floor of thoracic cavity. It curves upward. It contracts with each inspiration.

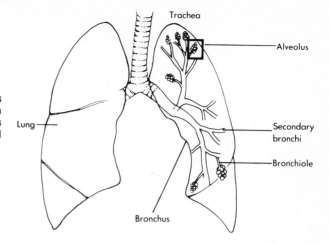

Figure 11–1 ☐ Major structures of the lungs. The small air sac in which exchange of gases takes place is the *alveolus*. (Modified from Dugas, p. 373.)

Intercostals. The external muscles between ribs. They raise the ribs and enlarge the thorax upon inspiration.

Ribs. The 12 pairs of ribs form a bony cage that protects lungs and heart.

This system is best visualized as a series of tunnels. We inhale air through the nose, which is lined with a warm, moist, mucous membrane that warms and moistens the air we breathe in.

The air continues down the pharynx, past the larynx (voicebox), and into the trachea. The trachea is the trunk of the bronchial tree. The trachea then branches out to a right and left bronchus. "Twigs" of these bronchi are *bronchioles*, minute tunnels in a system of tunnels that end in microscopic air sacs called *alveoli*. Alveoli are surrounded by a rich network of capillaries. A comparison might be a blossom (the alveoli) on a stem (the bronchiole). It is in the alveoli that the exchange of gases takes place. The air we breathe in has a higher concentration of oxygen than does the blood in the capillaries surrounding the alveoli. Therefore, the oxygen passes from the alveoli to the capillaries. The reverse is true of carbon dioxide. As blood circulates, carbon dioxide leaves the cells and enters the bloodstream. The carbon dioxide in the capillaries in the lungs passes into the alveoli to be exhaled.

☐ *Age-Related Changes*

The aging process brings about changes in the skeletal and muscular systems that can adversely affect the respiratory system. These include the following:
1. The rib cage becomes rigid as the costal cartilages calcify.
2. Osteoporosis and kyphosis (humpback) cause a stooped posture that decreases the ability of the chest to expand with each inspiration.

3. The abdominal muscles usually become weaker and lack tone, and then the diaphragm, an important organ of respiration, is affected.
4. The lungs lose some of their elasticity. Bronchioles and alveoli enlarge and decrease in number; their walls become thin and less elastic.
5. Arteriosclerosis prevents the forceful circulation of the blood; thus it is harder to circulate blood through the lungs.

All of these changes contribute to poor exchange of oxygen and carbon dioxide in the lungs and make respiratory diseases more serious in the elderly adult. Despite this, however, older people are usually able to breathe quite normally.

Chronic obstructive pulmonary disease (COPD) occurs more frequently in the older age group. Emphysema and chronic bronchitis are examples of COPD.

☐ Age-Related Disorders

☐ LUNG CANCER

There is an increased incidence in lung cancer among elderly persons because of the longer exposure to the carcinogen. (Lung cancer in general is increasing.) Some facts about lung cancer are as follows:
1. Eighty per cent of the cases seen are caused by smoking and are, therefore, largely preventable.
2. Chronic exposure to pollutants, e.g., asbestos, coal gas, and radioactive dusts, is also responsible for this lung disease.
3. Dyspnea, coughing, chest pain, wheezing, and fatigue (symptoms often overlooked because smokers are so used to them) should be investigated.
4. Many older women are at risk for developing lung cancer. In many areas of the country, lung cancer has surpassed breast cancer in incidence in women. The cause is directly attributed to the increased numbers of women smoking.

Diagnosis of lung cancer is confirmed by X-ray examination, sputum cytology, bronchoscopy, biopsy, and lung scans. Prophylactic radiation therapy to areas where obstruction might occur and to relieve pain is the usual form of treatment.

☐ EMPHYSEMA

In this condition, the alveoli are overdistended and filled with air. This distends the lungs and the heart must work increasingly harder to push blood through the lungs.

Causes. smoking; exposure to pollutants in air; chronic asthma.

Symptoms. expectoration of thick sputum, especially in the morning; shortness of breath; wheezing; coughing; large "barrel" chest.

Treatment. bronchodilators to relieve bronchospasm; postural drainage; antibiotics to combat infection; use of nebulizers to help liquefy secretions; breathing exercise; intermittent positive pressure breathing therapy.

The patient who has emphysema needs tremendous emotional support. The disease is progressive and exhausting. The patient leans forward in a chair with his or her shoulders hunched, neck muscles contracted, and lips pursed as he or she tries to conserve the strength and effort that make breathing, which is normally an involuntary function, very difficult. Eating is exhausting and he or she has little appetite. Weight loss is inevitable. The person soon becomes an invalid and death usually occurs as a result of secondary infection or enlargement of the right ventricle of the heart. The heart fails because the lungs cease to function. Right-sided heart failure due to diseases of the lung is called *cor pulmonale.*

☐ CHRONIC BRONCHITIS

This condition frequently progresses to emphysema or bronchiectasis.

Causes. irritants (including cigarettes); infections; hereditary factors.

Symptoms. coughing and expectoration of profuse, thick mucous secretions, especially early in the morning; dyspnea upon exertion; cyanotic lips; abdominal breathing.

Treatment. bronchodilators; postural drainage; chest physiotherapy (percussion, vibration); increased fluid intake; prevention of infection.

☐ *Nursing Interventions*

☐ POSTURAL DRAINAGE

Postural drainage is achieved by positioning a patient so that secretions can drain from the respiratory tract. The head and chest should be lower than the hips. This way the force of gravity helps drain secretions from the smaller bronchi into the trachea, where they are removed either by coughing or by suctioning. Once positioned, the patient remains in the position for 5 or more minutes. The patient should be carefully watched during postural drainage for fatigue, dyspnea, or cyanosis.

Chest physiotherapy consists of percussion and vibration. Percussion is done by hitting the thorax with cupped hands over the affected area. Hands *never slap* the chest wall. Vibration is done by applying firm pressure with the fingers and then moving them as in a tremor to help free mucus. It is difficult to do correctly and requires practice and supervision.

Aftercare includes collection of a specimen if ordered and proper disposal of the sputum, tissues, paper bag, and so on, as well as thorough oral hygiene for the patient. Documentation should include color, amount, and consistency of sputum and tolerance of the procedure.

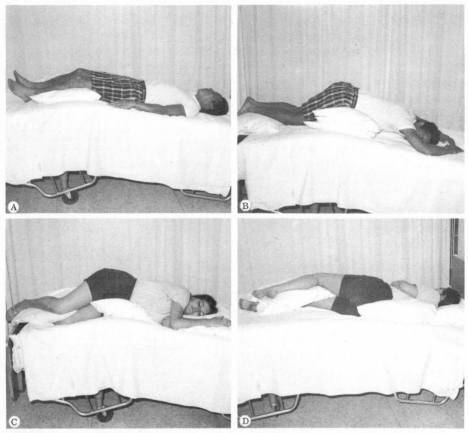

Figure 11–2 ☐ Postural drainage positions. The older adult who is weak or ill needs close supervision. Stop the procedure or change the patient's position if he or she becomes tired, cyanotic, or dyspneic. (From Kottke, Stillwell, and Lehmann, pp. 780–781.)

☐ BREATHING EXERCISES

Breathing, the act of inhaling and exhaling, and coughing, the clearing of the air passages, are two acts we generally take for granted. However, physical changes in the aged may make either or both actions difficult and ineffective. If an elderly person has COPD, breathing exercises will be prescribed. The problem is that these patients tend to breathe rapidly and shallowly from the upper chest. They need to be taught how to breathe so as to empty the lungs, place less strain on the abdominal muscles, and promote relaxation. A good time to do this is right after the patient has engaged in postural drainage. For example,

1. place the patient in a sitting position with his or her trunk slightly forward, feet on the floor, and knees and hips flexed to take strain off abdominal muscles

2. tell patient to breathe in slowly and deeply through the nose
3. tell the patient to cough while breathing out and to exert pressure with his or her hands on the abdomen with each cough

Another simple exercise for any elderly person to improve breathing efficiency is the following:

1. breathe through the nose in any position of comfort (sitting, standing, lying down)
2. breathe slowly and deeply to allow complete filling and emptying of the lungs
3. concentrate on having a rhythm, a pattern of breathing

Poor abdominal muscle tone can affect the efficiency of the diaphragm, an important accessory organ of respiration. An exercise that strengthens the diaphragm follows:

1. the patient is seated in a chair, feet on the floor
2. the patient's right hand is placed on the stomach, the left hand on the chest
3. while inhaling slowly through nose, the patient distends his or her abdomen as much as possible
4. the patient then exhales through pursed lips, with both hands pressing in and up on the abdomen while trying to keep abdomen contracted
5. repeat as often as ordered if tolerated comfortably

It is worth emphasizing that effective coughing clears air passages of secretions. Since many elderly people have arteriosclerosis and decreased cardiac reserve, these conditions, plus increased rigidity of the rib cage, can make most coughing ineffectual. The patient simply becomes exhausted and the cough is not beneficial. This is why simple instructions and an actual lesson in coughing are so important. The patient must make a conscious effort to activate this "cleansing" mechanism of the body.

□ INHALATIONS

The discomfort of chronic cough can often be eased by the use of steam inhalations. Electrically operated steam vaporizers are used in many health care facilities and in many homes as well. Sometimes the physician will order a drug to be added to the vaporizer. Careful reading of instructions is important, as there are many different models of inhalators on the market.

Purposes

to relieve cough and bronchial spasms
to loosen secretions
to soothe irritated and inflamed mucous membranes of the respiratory tract

Equipment

electric steam vaporizer
medication as ordered

Sequence

1. identify patient; explain procedure
2. add medication (as ordered) to medicine cup of machine
3. fill water container according to manufacturer's instructions
4. keep windows and doors closed during treatment
5. time treatment; observe and record effect on patient
6. empty and clean equipment after it has cooled
7. be sure patient is dry, warm, and out of drafts
8. give oral care as necessary

Notes. Electric vaporizers are a potential source of danger because they get very hot. The patient as well as health care personnel should be alerted to this possibility. The usual precautions in using such appliances prevail, e.g., checking for frayed cords, defective wiring, broken plugs, and so on.

Elderly patients should be encouraged to dispose of sputum and used tissues in suitable containers. Carelessness in this respect is usually due to weakness, poor eyesight, or fatigue. When offering oral care after these inhalations, the nurse should also give the patient an opportunity to wash his or her hands.

Cool mist vaporizers are often used for inhalations. Remember that both steam and cool mist cause condensation in rooms; bed clothes and floor coverings will become damp. The pans of water in humidifiers and vaporizers should be changed daily to prevent the growth of bacteria and the formation of mildew.

When humidity therapy is being used, whether steam inhalations or cool mist, the equipment should be explained to the patient and he or she should be encouraged to breathe in the water vapor deeply. This is also an appropriate time to remind the patient to expectorate mucus and to provide him or her with a container for the sputum.

☐ COLLECTION OF SPUTUM SPECIMENS

A sputum specimen may be ordered in almost any disease in which coughing is a symptom. Examples include tuberculosis, lung cancer, pneumonia, lung abscess, bronchiectasis, asthma, and chronic bronchitis. The patient needs to be informed of the difference between sputum and saliva. Sputum comes from the bronchi or lungs—it is not secreted in the mouth as is saliva, although it may be mixed with saliva. Although a sputum specimen may be collected any time, the best times are early in the morning just after the patient has awakened and after postural drainage.

Sputum specimens are ordered for diagnostic purposes. The sputum is collected in sterile sputum cups or sterile plastic sputum traps that attach to the breathing apparatus used by respiratory therapists.

Equipment

sputum container   emesis basin   tissues

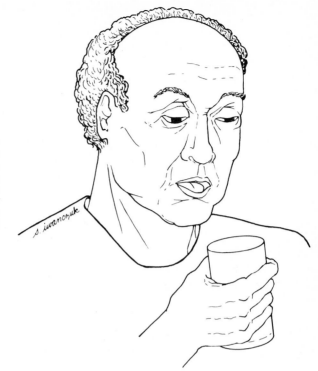

Figure 11–3 □ Obtaining a sputum specimen. Sputum is the mucus coughed up from the lungs, not the saliva in the mouth. Early morning may be the best time to obtain a specimen, as the person clears his or her lungs of material collected during the night.

Sequence

1. identify patient; explain procedure, screen unit
2. be sure mouth is free of food particles
3. have patient take several deep breaths, then cough deeply and expectorate into container
4. label container; check to see that there is no sputum on the outside; cover container
5. nurse and patient both wash hands
6. dispose of tissues properly
7. give oral care as required

Notes. It is important that the specimen be delivered to the laboratory as soon as possible. It is also helpful for the nurse to describe the specimen as to color, amount, consistency, and odor. The amount may be scant, moderate, or large; the color may be clear, yellow, rusty, greenish, blood-tinged; the consistency may be thick or thin; and the odor may be foul or odorless.

□ OXYGEN THERAPY

Oxygen is used to treat the effects of *hypoxemia* (insufficient oxygenation of the blood). Administration of oxygen does not cure the underlying disease.

It does, however, alleviate the harmful and often lethal effects of hypoxemia, decrease symptoms, and increase the patient's sense of well being.

Oxygen may be used in acute and chronic conditions.

Acute   airway obstruction, pulmonary edema, acute respiratory failure, shock

Chronic   chronic respiratory insufficiency, cardiac disorders, metabolic disorders, chronic obstructive lung disease

Oxygen therapy is ordered by the physician and is administered by nurses, just like other medications.

Some of the symptoms of hypoxemia are restlessness, anxiety, and dyspnea. The skin has a blue cast (cyanosis) and the patient usually feels weak. Since breathing difficulties are so extremely frightening, these patients need as much emotional support as physical care.

Most hospitals and nursing homes have wall outlets near the patients' beds that are connected with a central oxygen supply. An individual flowmeter on the wall controls the rate at which oxygen flows to the patient. The rate is prescribed by the physician, depending on the patient's condition. Others provide oxygen in cylinders or tanks.

Oxygen—colorless, odorless, and tasteless—is something we cannot live without. Yet we have to be careful when living with it. Because it supports combustion, most agencies have specific rules about oxygen that have to be observed in order to avoid fires. For example, a "No Smoking" sign must be prominently displayed in a patient's room and on the door. If two people share a room and only one is receiving oxygen therapy, *no one* may smoke in that room. This is true even if the oxygen is used only as needed. There are

---

Principles of Oxygen Needs

1. Oxygen is essential to life.
2. Survival without oxygen is possible for only a few minutes.
3. Insufficient supply impairs functioning of all body systems.
4. Irreversible brain damage usually results from periods of prolonged oxygen deprivation.
5. Cerebral cortex cells begin to die when deprived of oxygen.
6. The body's ability to meet its oxygen needs depends on the proper action of cardiovascular and respiratory systems.
7. A *patent* (open) airway is necessary to normal respiratory functioning.
8. Dyspnea causes anxiety.
9. Coughing, sneezing, and swallowing are means by which the body tries to expel foreign bodies from the respiratory tract.

many such rules and the nurse should check the policy of the agency to be sure that all necessary precautions are taken.

Oxygen is drying to the mucous membranes, and therefore it is passed through sterile distilled water before it is administered. Breathing masks, cannulae, and plastic tubing are used for one patient only and are frequently changed because of the possibility of infection.

There are several ways of administering oxygen: nasal cannula, nasal catheter, face mask, and the patient in a "tent" are the most common.

Mechanical ventilation is not discussed in this text. Refer to a medical-surgical nursing text for this information.

When oxygen therapy is ordered, the nurse's functions are to administer the oxygen as ordered, to provide proper care for the patient receiving oxygen, to provide reassurance, and to use adequate safety precautions.

Nasal Cannula

A nasal cannula is a plastic tube with two prongs that fit into the patient's nostrils. It is secured around the patient's head with an adjustable elastic. This is a simple and comfortable way to administer oxygen.
1. turn on oxygen at ordered rate
2. place prongs in nostrils
3. adjust elastic, being sure it is not too tight or causing pressure on an ear
4. clean at least once per shift
5. clean nostrils as needed
6. oral care when necessary

Nasal Catheter

A catheter is used for continuous oxygen administration. It is more efficient than a cannula but not quite as comfortable. A lubricant is used on the catheter and it is passed through the nostril until it can be seen just below the uvula.
1. check that oxygen is on at rate ordered
2. remove catheter and replace it during each nursing shift, alternating nostrils if possible
3. cleanse nostril as needed with applicator moistened with water; oral care when necessary
4. observe for kinking of tubing

Face Mask

Lightweight plastic masks that cover the patient's nose and mouth are used extensively. The mask provides oxygen concentration of about 50 per cent. Also available are rebreathing masks that provide an oxygen concentration of as much as 95 per cent.

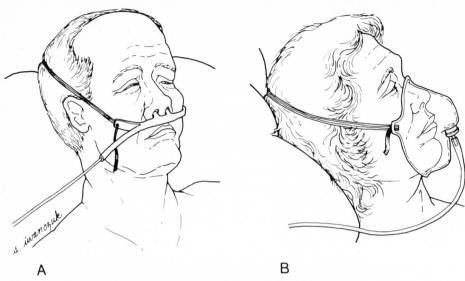

A   B

Figure 11–4 ☐ A, Nasal cannula for oxygen delivery. B, Plastic face mask.

A face mask is useful for administering high concentrations of oxygen. Use the following procedures:
1. check to see that flowmeter is set at ordered number of liters per minute
2. fit mask to patient comfortably
3. help patient relax and breathe normally
4. clean mask on each shift
5. wash patient's face; give oral care as necessary

Tent

Tents are seldom used but they are efficient when a high concentration of oxygen is needed. The biggest drawback to a tent is that it isolates the patient. It is frightening to patients and to families. The advantage of the tent is that it allows for free movement of the patient without altering the concentration of oxygen he or she receives, and tents are generally used if a high concentration is going to be used for an extended period of time.

Review of General Clinical Measures

1. Position patient correctly in order to maintain patent airway.
2. Encourage productive coughing.
3. Suction if necessary.
4. Give oral and nose care every 4 hours or more often if necessary.

5. Change patient's position periodically.
6. Give skin care.
7. Inspect equipment and obtain needed maintenance as needed. Follow safety rules.
8. Give appropriate emotional support to patient and provide patient teaching where indicated.
9. Teach patient self-care measures, as appropriate.

Safety Factors During Oxygen Administration

1. Proper grounding of all electrical equipment.
2. Strict enforcement of no smoking rules.
3. Inspection and replacement of any electrical wiring beginning to fray. Prohibition of extension cords in patient's rooms.
4. Prohibit use of electric razors.
5. Avoid use of any oils (e.g., hair dressings) or flammable solutions (e.g., alcohol) in patient's environment. Use water-based products only, e.g., K-Y jelly, if a lubricant is needed.
6. Prevent static electricity (e.g., wool blankets).

□ INTERMITTENT POSITIVE PRESSURE BREATHING

Intermittent positive pressure breathing (IPPB) is a method for forcing air and medication into the respiratory tract. It is commonly administered by a respiratory therapist for patients who need aerosol therapy or patients who need help in expectorating their secretions. Many people with COPD have trouble raising mucus from the respiratory tract and they benefit by the use of the antibiotics, expectorants, or bronchodilators used with IPPB. Respiratory therapy may combine IPPB with postural drainage, percussion, and vibration in order to relieve the breathing difficulties of these patients.

□ ORAL SUCTIONING

Suctioning, the aspiration of secretions, is done to remove secretions from the nose, mouth, or tracheobronchial tree. It is also done to stimulate productive coughing.

Whenever a nurse is assigned a patient who may need suctioning, the first thing to do is to check the equipment. Is there a suction kit? Does the pressure gauge work? (Do you know how to turn it on?) A patient who needs suctioning usually needs it right away and the nurse must be prepared.

Equipment

suction tip, cup, glove (sterile kit)   sterile distilled water

Sequence

1. identify patient; introduce self; explain procedure
2. screen patient
3. place patient in high Fowler's position unless contraindicated
4. turn on pressure gauge after checking to see that there is enough distilled water in vacuum bottle under gauge
5. pour sterile water into cup from sterile kit
6. glove hand that will be touching suction tip
7. attach tubing to suction tip
8. using suction, dip tip in water to lubricate it and to see if it works (to create suction, cover opening of aspirating catheter with finger)
9. with suction *off*, gently slide aspirating catheter along side of tongue and down pharynx
10. with suction *on*, rotate catheter; suction only as long as is necessary to remove secretions
11. remove catheter while continuing suction intermittently
12. clear catheter with sterile water and repeat
13. suction as few times as possible, just enough to maintain airway

Notes. Suctioning is irritating to pharyngeal mucosa. It stimulates secretions. It should be used sparingly. Oral care should be administered after suctioning is done.

There are several different kinds of oral suctioning apparatus. Although it is a clean technique, many hospitals and nursing homes use a sterile kit and discard it after each episode of suctioning. The principles do not change, but the nurse should use the method approved where employed.

☐ TRACHEOSTOMY SUCTIONING

A tracheostomy is an incision into the trachea by a surgeon in order to create an airway. It is done to remove an obstruction caused by a foreign body, malignancy, trauma, or respiratory disease such as croup. A tracheostomy can be permanent or temporary. The patient who has one is very apprehensive and needs a great deal of reassurance and emotional support.

A tracheostomy set has three parts: the outer cannula, the inner cannula, and the obturator.

The obturator is a guide that is placed in the outer cannula and smoothly facilitates the introduction of the outer cannula into the incision. When the surgeon is satisfied that the outer cannula is in place, the obturator is replaced by the *inner* cannula. Tracheostomy twill tape is threaded through the two slots in the outer cannula and secured around the patient's neck. During routine, periodic tracheostomy suctioning, the inner cannula remains in place. The technique used is described in the section on oral suctioning. When the inner cannula is to be cleaned (according to physician's order and when necessary), then the equipment and sequence are as follows:

Equipment

sterile suction kit
tracheostomy gauze
tracheostomy twill tape
suture set
two sterile basins

hydrogen peroxide
sterile water
special tracheostomy brush
sterile gloves
sterile applicators

Sequence

1. identify patient; introduce self; explain procedure; screen patient
2. unlock and remove soiled inner cannula; place in basin of hydrogen peroxide
3. remove soiled dressing as necessary and clean the area
4. put on sterile gloves; clean incision with sterile applicators and sterile water
5. use suture scissors to prepare trach gauze; place gauze at wound site
6. scrub inner cannula with trach brush; rinse with sterile water in separate basin
7. pass trach gauze through inner cannula with Kelly forceps from suture set to dry inner cannula
8. before the inner cannula is replaced, the patient should be aspirated
9. replace and lock inner cannula
10. replace twill tapes as necessary; clean around outer cannula
11. chart time of procedure, nature of secretions, patient's tolerance of procedure

In Addition ...

keep spare tracheostomy set at bedside for emergency
keep signal cord, writing materials at bedside
use heated mist or heated aerosol for patient
make sure patient is adequately hydrated
use only lint-free gauze for tracheostomy cleaning
chart respirations

Notes. Although the mouth is not sterile, the suctioning procedure is being done under surgical aseptic technique more and more frequently. The trachea is mainly free of bacteria and is *always* suctioned under the precaution of sterile technique. Another significant difference is the fact that the suction catheter is introduced only the distance of the *tracheostomy* tube, unless specifically ordered otherwise. A maximum of 15 seconds of suctioning is a good rule for both oral and tracheostomy suctioning.

Chapter 11 ☐ Review Questions

MULTIPLE CHOICE

1. The structure of the lung in which oxygen and carbon dioxide are exchanged is the
   A. trachea
   B. bronchiole
   C. alveolus
   D. pleura
2. The partition between the thoracic cavity and the abdominal cavity is
   A. the pleura
   B. the brochioles
   C. the costal cartilages
   D. the diaphragm
3. The intercostals
   A. decrease the size of the thorax upon inspiration
   B. increase the size of the thorax upon inspiration
   C. do not affect the size of the thorax
   D. are tubular structures leading to the bronchioles
4. Emphysema is characterized by
   A. tumor growth
   B. pus in the pleural cavity
   C. overdistended alveolar sacs
   D. weight gain
5. The purpose of postural drainage is
   A. to increase blood flow to the brain
   B. to increase relaxation
   C. to clear secretions from the lungs
   D. to improve the elderly person's posture
6. The major cause of emphysema is
   A. infection
   B. smoking
   C. poor nutrition
   D. the natural aging process
7. Which of the following is *not* a symptom of hypoxemia?
   A. anxiety
   B. cyanosis
   C. leg cramps
   D. dyspnea

DISCUSSION QUESTIONS

1. Describe four ways of administering oxygen.
2. What does IPPB mean?

3. What is the first thing the nurse should do if assigned to a patient needing suctioning?
4. What are two disadvantages to suctioning?
5. What type of technique is used when suctioning?
6. List safety rules for the use of oxygen therapy.
7. Name five principles of oxygen needs.

□ REFERENCES

Acee, S.: Helping patients breath more easily . . . non-invasive nursing measures. Geriatr Nurs, 5(6):230–233, 1984.

Alexander, M.R., et al.: Therapy of chronic obstructive lung airways disease. Drug Intell Clin Pharm, 18(4):279–291, 1984.

Avoiding threats to your breathing . . . you have chronic obstructive pulmonary disease. Patient Care, 18(1):186–187, 1984.

Braun, S.R., et al.: Predictive clinical value of nutritional assessment factors in COPD. Chest, 85(3):353–357, 1984.

Brodoff, A.S.: Helping the COPD patient help himself. Patient Care, 18(11):177–180, 183–184, 1984.

Cockram, P.: Anesthesia and the aged. AANA J, 52(2):156–163, 1984.

Coping with COPD. Patient Care, 18(11):185, 1984.

D'Agostine, J.S.: Teaching tips for living with COPD at home. Nursing (Horsham), 14(2):57, 1984.

Demarest, C.B.: COPD: when bronchodilators aren't enough. Patient Care, 18(20):85–89, 91, 94, 1984.

Exercise, diet, and COPD. Patient Care, 18(20):123, 125, 129, 1984.

Higgins, M.: Epidemiology of COPD: state of the art. Chest (Suppl.), 85(6):3S–8S, 1984.

Learning the basics about COPD . . . patient education aid. Patient care, 18(9):159–160, 1984.

Light, K.E.: Review of the aged respiratory system. Phys Occup Ther Geriatr, 3(1):5–15, 1983.

Moscher, L.D.: Helpful exercises for your COPD patient. RN, 47(6):33–35, 1984.

Phillipson, E.A., et al.: Breathing during sleep in chronic obstructive pulmonary disease: state of the art. Chest (Suppl.), 85(6):24S–29S, 1984.

Reid, W.D., et al.: Ventilatory muscle strength and endurance training in elderly patients and patients with chronic air flow limitation: a pilot study. Physiother Can, 36(6):305–311, 1984.

Rogers, R.M., et al.: Nutrition and COPD: state-of-the-art mini review. Chest (Suppl.), 85(6): 63S–66S, 1984.

Sexton, D.L.: The supporting cast: wives of COPD patients. J Gerontol Nurs, 10(2):82–85, 1984.

Stockdale-Woolley, R.: The effects of education on self care agency . . . individuals with COPD who attended group education classes. Public Health Nurs, 1(2):97–106, 1984.

Stoll, B.: The aging lung. MSRT J, 18(1):25–27, 1984.

Swisher, C.M.: When older patients don't learn. Respir Ther, 14(1):73–76, 78–79, 1984.

Zack, M.B., et al.: Ventilatory and non-ventilatory muscle exercise in COPD rehabilitation. Respir Ther, 14(5):41–42, 44–45, 1984.

Objectives

After completing this chapter, the student should be able to

- [ ] describe the anatomy and physiology of the digestive system
- [ ] name the age-related changes in the digestive system
- [ ] describe age-related disorders of the digestive system
- [ ] explain the difference between gavage feedings and hyperalimentation
- [ ] give examples of bowel problems of elders and list appropriate solutions
- [ ] identify bowel disorders that benefit from a bowel retraining program
- [ ] list key factors in a bowel retraining program
- [ ] explain the principles of colostomy irrigation

Vocabulary

atrophy
chyme
edentulous
hypertonic
impaction
ingestion
metastasis
mucosa
peristalsis
proctoscopy
residue
rugae
sordes
stoma

CHAPTER *12*

The Digestive System

Chapter Outline

☐ *Anatomy Review*

The gastrointestinal tract is a continuous tube of mucosa about 4.5 meters (15 feet) in length from mouth to anus. It has four functions: ingestion, digestion, absorption, and elimination. There are mechanical and chemical components to these functions. The gastrointestinal tract is composed of the mouth, pharynx, esophagus, stomach, and small and large intestines.

During the process of digestion, food and fluids taken into the body are mixed and processed, nutrients are selected and absorbed for utilization of body tissues, and the waste products of digestion are excreted.

Mouth. The mouth contains teeth, tongue, and salivary glands. Teeth grind food; the tongue helps to move the food about during chewing and swallowing. Saliva is secreted by parotid, submaxillary, and sublingual glands. This valuable body fluid contains mucus to offer lubrication for swallowing and the starch-splitting enzyme, ptyalin, to initiate digestion of starches and other carbohydrates in the food.

Pharynx. The muscular tissue of the pharynx contracts to direct food and fluid into the esophagus, closing off the openings to the larynx and nasal passages.

Esophagus. The esophagus is a section of the digestive tube that connects the pharynx with the stomach. It has rhythmic movements called peristaltic waves that help propel food down into the stomach.

Stomach. The stomach is a readily expandable sac lined with rugae. Its function is to continue digestion of food, change the consistency of the food bolus into chyme, and store chyme for gradual release into the small intestine. Enzymes in the gastric juice cause chemical changes to take place.

The distal opening of the stomach (pyloric sphincter) controls the passage of chyme into the small intestine.

Small Intestine. The small intestine connects the stomach with the large intestine. Here digestive secretions act upon starches, sugars, proteins, and fats.

Large Intestine. The cecum, colon, and rectum compose the large intestine. Chyme becomes feces, semisolid or solid consistency, and feces pass into the rectum, eventually to be eliminated from the body through the anus. The two major functions of the large intestine are absorption and conservation of water and elimination of digestive wastes.

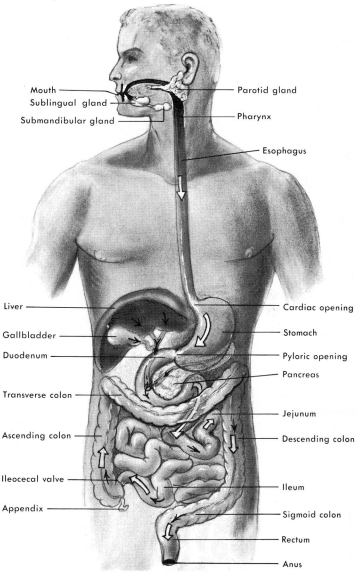

Figure 12–1 ☐ The digestive system. (From Dienhart, p. 184.)

☐ *Age-Related Changes*

Loss of Teeth. By the age of 65, two-thirds of all people in the United States have lost most of their teeth or are edentulous (without teeth). Changes in the gums and underlying bone do occur with age; and because of its prevalence, loss of teeth is listed here as an age-related change. However, it is important to note that *loss of teeth is not inevitable and with proper oral hygiene and regular dental attention, it could be prevented.*

Why don't people take care of their teeth? Some people accept the loss of teeth as a natural occurrence. Dental care is expensive and many elderly living on fixed income cannot afford to, or are reluctant to, spend money for something they consider nonessential. However, the loss of teeth or dentures that do not fit properly make chewing difficult and contribute to poor nutrition.

Hypochlorhydria. As we age, the activity of the digestive glands in the gastric mucosa decreases. The important substance that decreases at this time is hydrochloric acid, a secretion that prepares protein for absorption, retards the growth of bacteria, and encourages other digestive enzymes to function. Hypochlorhydria, the name given to this lessened secretion, encourages bacterial growth in the stomach and upper intestine. This may result in the increase of flatus (gas) or diarrhea.

Atrophy of the Stomach. The aging stomach actually shrinks a bit in size and that is why small amounts of food seem to "fill up" an elderly person. Frequent small feedings may be the best way of seeing that such a patient gets all the nutrients he or she needs.

Slower Peristalsis. Think of some elderly patients you have heard complain of "gas." You already know that a decrease in hydrochloric acid secretion may be at fault. But the blame must be shared by another digestive change we will all experience if we live long enough—the slowing down of peristalsis. Therefore, it is very important to ward off that threat to good bowel hygiene by reminding the elderly patient of the importance of adequate fluid and fiber intake and reasonable exercise.

Decline in Number of Taste Buds. As we age, the tiny groups of cells that respond to the food they come in contact with on the tongue diminish in number. Things truly "don't taste like they used to." The decline in the number of taste buds can contribute to a decrease in appetite.

Decrease in Saliva Production. Decrease in saliva production contributes to dry mouth and tongue and possibly to decreased sensations of taste (Steffl, 1984).

☐ *Age-Related Disorders*

Oral Lesions. These go undetected because people do not see a dentist at regular intervals. Common among these are irritations from broken or jagged teeth and poorly fitted dentures. In the person who smokes a pipe, a sore on the lip can be produced by the steady contact of the warm pipe stem on the lip. These sores frequently become malignant.

Leukoplakia. This condition of the oral cavity is common to the elderly. It appears as elevated white patches on the oral mucosa and is considered a precancerous lesion.

Diverticulosis and Diverticulitis. It is estimated that between 20 and 25 per cent of the population over the age of 40 has diverticulosis, a condition marked by the outpouching of the wall of the intestines. Tiny areas of weakness develop in the intestinal wall and these areas protrude by the hundreds. If any bowel content becomes trapped in these pockets, infection and inflammation result. Then the condition is called *diverticulitis*. Diverticulosis may be present without symptoms, and in fact it was once considered harmless. However, the possibility for obstruction is always there, and diverticulitis is painful and potentially serious.

Diverticulosis is treated by some physicians with a high residue, low roughage diet. Vegetables and fruits that can cause gas are omitted, as are nuts and bran. Patients may be on antispasmodics and other medications to reduce the growth of bacteria in the bowel. The overall plan is to produce a fecal mass that is soft and will not irritate the inflamed part of the bowel. The newer thinking is to place the patient on a low residue diet, monitor progress, and then advance the patient to a regular diet as tolerated.

Diverticulitis requires a bland, low residue diet. If there is pain, bed rest will be ordered along with antispasmodics, tranquilizers, and stool softeners. The patient will be closely observed for exacerbation of symptoms (abdominal distention or pain, fever, and nausea), as perforation of the bowel is always a possibility with diverticulitis.

Hemorrhoids. Dilated blood vessels in the anus, called hemorrhoids, may be internal or external. Nearly everyone experiences them at one time or another. Constipation can make them very uncomfortable, but relief may be obtained by using stool softeners, witch hazel compresses, and sitz baths.

Cancer of the Colon and Rectum. Colon cancer is a common type of cancer among the elderly population. Unfortunately, malignancies of the large bowel often go undiagnosed. *Change in bowel habits, cramps, and abdominal distention all too often are accepted as the consequences of old age.* Even bleeding, a startling signal to most people, is shrugged off as being caused by "piles," the lay term for hemorrhoids. The longer these symptoms are treated by home remedies, the less the chance that medical diagnosis and treatment, when they are finally given, will lead to recovery. The American Cancer Society recommends an annual rectal examination for those over age 40. Preferred by many physicians because of its simplicity is the hematest for occult blood, where a small particle of stool is placed on a disposable slide, a drop of reagent is added, and the specimen is read as being positive or negative according to a color chart.

More than 70 per cent of patients with cancer of the colon and rectum can be cured if it is diagnosed before metastasis occurs. But these people must be seen by a physician for a diagnosis to be made.

Cancer of the Esophagus. Older adults are more commonly afflicted with this cancer. The incidence is higher in males, blacks, and alcoholics. Some contributing factors are poor oral hygiene, chronic irritation from alcohol, and tobacco. Early symptoms are dysphagia, thirst, and hiccups. Gradually, anemia due to chronic bleeding ensues.

Hiatus Hernia. Elderly females are more frequently liable to develop hiatus hernia than are elderly males. In all probability, more than half of older adults have the disorder, which is characterized by dysphagia, heartburn, regurgitation, and vomiting. Symptoms are more severe when the patient is lying down. There may be pain and bleeding. Weight reduction, if the client is obese, bland foods, and several small meals usually bring about improvement. Elevating the head of the bed is also helpful.

Constipation. Constipation is one of the oldest and most common medical problems and humans have constantly sought means of correcting it. Legend suggests that the enema, for example, was in use long before recorded time by the ancient Chinese, Babylonians, and Egyptians. Many of the drugs and formulas used by ancient civilizations for laxatives are not very different from those we use today.

In simple terms, constipation means infrequent or difficult evacuation of feces. Remember, however, that "infrequent" is relative to the individual patient. Although a daily bowel movement is normal for most people, two or three times a week or even weekly may be normal for others.

It is possible for some persons who have a regular daily movement to rarely or never have a complete evacuation. Therefore, the frequency of bowel action alone is not an adequate criterion of constipation.

Constipation exists when
1. The period between bowel actions is too long—when the interval between movements is greater than that which is normal for that individual.
2. The fecal volume is too small—when any significant amount of feces re-

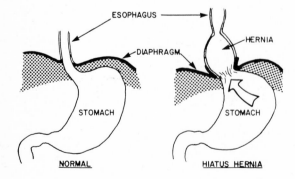

Figure 12-2 □ Hiatus hernia. The mechanism of a diaphragmatic hernia is shown. With age, the diaphragmatic muscle weakens and results in imperfect closure of the hiatus around the esophagus. Reflux of the stomach contents into the esophagus may occur, resulting in heartburn, regurgitation of acid fluid, a feeling of fullness, and shortness of breath. (From Howard and Herbold, p. 351.)

mains in the rectum after defecation, even though bowel action may be frequent.
3. The fecal consistency is too hard—so hard that the patient experiences difficulty and pain in passing the feces.

□ *Nursing Interventions*

□ ORAL CARE

Keeping the teeth and mouth clean slows the growth of disease-producing microorganisms, stimulates a flagging appetite, and refreshes the patient. Besides such a common oral problems as infection and decay, the nurse may also observe bleeding, sordes, and irritation due to improperly fitted dentures or jagged teeth. These observations should be recorded and reported so the proper action may be taken.

Most of us take brushing our teeth for granted. But for a patient confined to the hospital, particularly a geriatric patient, this activity of daily living requires modification.

Purposes

to keep the teeth and mouth clean
to stimulate appetite
to refresh the patient

Equipment

face towel	paper cups	water
toothbrush	mouthwash	emesis basin
dentifrice		

Sequence

1. identify patient; introduce self; explain procedure; screen patient
2. raise bed to comfortable position
3. place towel over top bedding
4. wet toothbrush; apply dentifrice
5. assist patient as needed, brushing upper teeth in a downward motion and lower teeth in an upward motion
6. use dental floss if available
7. have patient rinse with water, then with mouthwash (use emesis basin for this)
8. dry mouth and chin with towel; replace equipment after cleaning

If the patient is very weak or is unconscious, special oral care is needed. The equipment may be modified to include a padded tongue blade and a lemon/glycerin swab or toothette if a brush bruises the gums. (Caution: observe patient closely to see that the toothette is not bitten off!)

The sequence is the same as in steps 1 through 4. Of course, the patient cannot rinse his or her mouth, so several moistened swabs or a few padded tongue blades may have to be used to thoroughly clean and rinse the mouth. After the mouth and chin are dried, lubricant is applied.

Special mouth care should be administered several times a day to prevent sordes, the accumulation of brown crusts on the lips and teeth.

☐ DENTURE CARE

Dentures should be brushed the same as teeth—after early AM care, after each meal, and before bedtime. Since many people are self-conscious about dentures, privacy is important. If the patient is giving himself or herself oral care, simply draw the curtain and see that the necessary equipment is at hand.

Equipment

denture brush

commercial denture cleanser
   (regular dentifrice may be substituted)

emesis basin

small towel

paper cups

water

mouthwash

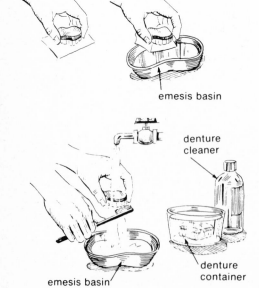

emesis basin

denture cleaner

emesis basin

denture container

Figure 12–3 ☐ Care of dentures. One may need to remove dentures and clean them for a person unable to do so. (From Rambo and Wood, p. 333.)

Sequence

1. identify patient; introduce self; explain procedure; screen patient
2. place patient in comfortable position; cover top bedding with towel
3. to remove dentures for helpless patient,
   hold upper denture between thumb and forefinger
   loosen denture gently to release suction and take out of mouth
   place in denture cup or emesis basin
   repeat for lower denture
4. carry dentures to sink and brush either over a basin of water or over a towel (a safety precaution in case nurse drops dentures)
5. use denture brush designed for small crevices
6. apply denture adhesive if needed
7. return dentures to patient either by way of denture cup or by handling with a paper towel
8. dry dentures are always moistened with cold water before placing them in a patient's mouth

Notes. Dentures are easily lost. Many times they have been placed in a pillow case or drawer or on a tray. Many nursing homes have instituted the practice of engraving names on dental plates to help identify them correctly. Dentures should always be placed in labeled denture cups when they are not being worn.

Some other aids to oral care are baking soda (bicarbonate) as a substitute dentifrice and sodium perborate or glyoxide for rinsing the mouth in severe cases of oral irritation.

□ ASSISTING WITH EATING

Independence in feeding oneself should be encouraged as much as possible. However, even people who can feed themselves may need some assistance if they are confined to bed. For example, before a tray is served, does a dressing need to be changed? Should oral care be given? Are the patient's hands washed? Is the patient in a position for a comfortable pleasant meal? Preparing a patient for mealtime includes mental as well as physical preparation. An uncluttered, tension-free environment is necessary because food is an important part of the overall care plan.

If the patient is to be fed, first check to see if he or she may receive a tray. Then verify that the diet to be served is the correct diet. Place the tray on an overbed table and raise the head of the bed as necessary. Protect the top bedding with a towel and place a napkin under the patient's chin. Prepare the foods by pouring hot liquids, buttering bread, and cutting meat. Permit the patient to hold the bread or to feed himself or herself if possible. Offer fluids and foods in a slow, relaxed manner. Conversation should be quiet and uncontroversial.

Blind patients who can feed themselves should have their trays explained to them, using the hands of a clock as fixation points. For example, "Your juice is at 12 o'clock, tea at 12:15," and so on. Encourage the patient's enjoyment of the meal by commenting that "the roll looks crispy" or "the soup seems tasty." If there are nuts in the cupcake, it's a good idea to say so. People like to know what they are eating.

Often, very old, regressed patients refuse to either suck from a straw or accept food from a spoon. Some agencies use a feeding syringe, a 20 ml. syringe with a 2-inch segment of rubber tubing on the end. This may be extremely hazardous and should only be used when other measures have proved unsuccessful and then with great caution.

□ GASTRIC GAVAGE

Gastric gavage, or *tube feeding,* is done through a tube that is inserted either through the nose or mouth into the stomach or directly (by way of a tube) into the stomach.

Gavage feedings become necessary when patients have serious problems that prevent them from eating normally. Some of these problems are stroke, coma, severe depression, and head and neck surgery. All these present obstacles to oral intake.

There are several categories of prepackaged diets: milk based, blended whole meals, elemental predigested diets, high nitrogen elemental diets, and semisynthetic diets are some examples of commercially prepared formulas. Some hospitals prepare their own. Many factors affect the desirability of one formula over the other; cost, shelf-life, total nutrient content, nutritional precautions, and nutrition omissions all must be evaluated by the physician before making a selection.

Commercial products save time in preparation, are purer, and are of known composition. The drawback is that they do not always meet the patient's needs. More physicians today are consulting with the registered dietician to ensure that all requirements are met. This is another example of interdisciplinary cooperation among health professionals.

The commonly used nasogastric tubes are the Salem sump and the Levin tube. These tubes are plastic and are inserted via the nose or mouth into the stomach. A gastrostomy feeding tube is a large Foley (No. 20 or 22 Fr.) or a Malecot catheter inserted directly into the stomach and secured by sutures.

Purpose

to provide nourishment when ordinary means of feeding are impossible

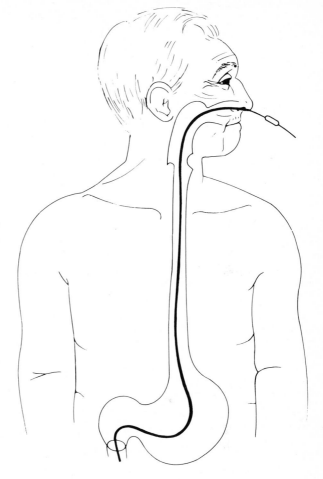

Figure 12–4 □ Positioning of the gastric tube used for gastric gavage.

Equipment

Asepto syringe or 50-ml syringe
towel

napkin
glass of warmed water (105° F)
prescribed feeding, warmed to 105°F

Sequence

1. identify patient; introduce self; explain procedure; screen patient
2. place patient in Fowler's position if he or she can tolerate this
3. protect gown and bedclothes with towel
4. remove clamp from nasogastric tube and with syringe aspirate a few ml. of gastric contents to ensure correct location of tube

5. using Asepto syringe or 50 ml. syringe allow 30-ml. water at room temperature to flow into tube *via gravity*
6. follow this with prescribed feeding, slowly; avoid introduction of air by keeping syringe full at all times and controlling feeding by raising and lowering syringe (about 30 ml. per minute is comfortable for the patient)
7. follow tube feeding with 30 ml. of water at room temperature in order to clear tubing.

If the patient has continuous gavage, the glass or plastic container is hung to the side of the patient at a level just above him or her. The nurse adjusts the rate of flow of the feeding as ordered. Frequent observation is essential in case the patient experiences any untoward results from the feeding.

Note. Many patients who have nasogastric tubes in place will try intentionally or otherwise to pull the tube out. Even when restrained, confused patients learn to cough the tube out of place. Nurses must be especially careful to observe these patients, check for tube placement, and carry out measures to prevent aspiration.

Tube Feeding Self-administered. Many patients learn to do their own tube feedings. It is important that the nurse assess the situation; even though the patient may be very old, there are many situations that allow for minimal assistance and modification of the procedure with patient compliance and success.

Patient control, independence, and dignity are some of the benefits beyond measure.

☐ TOTAL PARENTERAL NUTRITION (HYPERALIMENTATION)

Illness, trauma and surgery can seriously deplete the body of nutrients. When greater than normal amounts of nutrients are essential and oral intake is not possible, intravenous administration of hypertonic nutrient solutions (TPN—total parenteral nutrition) is used.

The solution is administered slowly through a central venous catheter directly into the superior vena cava. Infection is a great risk and sterile aseptic technique of the entire system is required. The presence or absence of sugar in the urine is usually tested regularly to determine if the infusion is running too rapidly for the body to metabolize glucose.

☐ *Prevention and Treatment of Constipation*

☐ COMMON CAUSES

Before undertaking a program for bowel retraining, the nurse should review the common causes of constipation, which are faulty personal habits, emotional factors, local and systemic diseases, muscular factors, inactivity, and diet.

Faulty Personal Habits. If the patient consistently refuses to heed the natural urge to defecate, awareness of rectal fullness becomes dulled and ultimately all natural periodic urge disappears more or less completely. This neglect may be the result of carelessness, demands of occupation, stress and rush of modern living, travel that requires abrupt adjustments to changes in time and food, and neurotic habit of delay (sometimes due to faulty childhood training). Laxative dependence and the chronic use of harsh laxatives also contribute to the problem. After the bowel has been emptied by a purgative, it generally takes 2 days for fecal material to accumulate in sufficient quantity to stimulate the desire for bowel action. If the purgative is repeated in the interim, and especially if the cycle is constantly repeated, this may lead to complete loss of natural, normal bowel habits.

Emotional Factors. Hypertonic colon, a condition that produces spastic constipation, is frequently associated with emotional disturbances, especially anxiety and tension. In some people the condition is so severe that the whole colon remains in a constant state of spasm. Occasionally, this is caused by inflammatory disease.

Neurotic persons, or those obsessed with "regularity," may upset evacuation by unnecessarily taking laxatives, cathartics, or enemas. This can lead to "the laxative habit."

Local and Systemic Disease. Painful lesions such as hemorrhoids, anal fissures, anorectal lesions, and local organic lesions either within or outside the colon or rectum can make defecation painful and this contributes to constipation.

Acute illness such as cancer of the large bowel, chronic dehydration, narcotic addiction, and lead poisoning may cause constipation.

Mechanical obstructions such as tumors often cause constipation. Certain drugs, e.g., narcotic analgesics, tranquilizers, and bismuth compounds, also cause constipation.

Muscular Factors. Weak or displaced abdominal wall muscles may lessen the ability to increase the pressure in the abdomen sufficiently to force out the feces. Defecation becomes more difficult.

The geriatric nurse often sees *atonic colon*—the condition of thin, weak colonic musculature and ineffective peristaltic contractions. It's quite common in the elderly and in those with chronic debilitating diseases.

The patient with chronic pulmonary emphysema cannot hold his or her breath long enough to cause the abdominal compression necessary for defecation.

Inactivity. Inactivity and lack of exercise also contribute to constipation. The older adult who is unable or unwilling to participate in some activity that requires vigorous movement, or even just regular walking, is going to experience defecation problems. Patients confined to bed for prolonged periods of time are inactive. Forced immobilization leads to muscle weakness and sluggish bowels, making complete evacuation difficult.

Diet. Food intake lacking in bulk or fluids can cause constipation. When food bulk is too small to cause normal distention, peristaltic movements become sluggish. Inadequate fluids cause the food residue to become hard and this is more difficult to move along the alimentary canal.

Persons on rigid reducing diets often suffer from constipation because there is a lack of bulk.

A patient who is to have nothing by mouth (NPO) as, for example, after surgery, usually will not have regular bowel movements until normal function of body organs occurs.

Some people (especially infants) become constipated from milk, since the large amount of casein in cow's milk tends to produce hard, firm stools. Milk products, e.g., cheeses, ice cream, and so on, can also be constipating in certain individuals.

☐ THE USE OF LAXATIVES

When food and good hygiene are not enough to establish and maintain good bowel habits, the physician may order thorough bowel cleansing, i.e., laxatives, cathartics, and enemas. These bowel evacuants work in different ways and have advantages and disadvantages. Enemas are discussed on page 212.

All laxatives and laxative suppositories should be used with caution. Read the package insert. These products are unpredictable, especially for older adults, and may cause incontinence.

Bulk Laxatives. The bulk laxatives may be divided into two groups: the saline laxatives and the hydrophilic colloids. All the bulk laxatives increase the bulk of the stool by increasing the water content. They reach this goal by different means, however.

The *saline laxatives* form a concentrated saline solution of high osmotic pressure in the intestine and actually draw fluid from the intestinal wall by osmosis. Examples include:

magnesium hydroxide (milk of magnesia)	magnesium oxide
magnesium sulfate (Epsom salt)	sodium sulfate
magnesium citrate	sodium phosphate
magnesium carbonate	

Saline laxatives may be violent in action; watery stools, colicky pain, and dehydration often follow their use.

The *hydrophilic colloids* simply absorb water from the intestinal contents. Generally, they are able to absorb amounts of liquid up to about ten times their own weight. They are more gentle in action but are seldom effective in relieving acute, severe constipation. Examples include agar, psyllium, manna, bran, and methylcellulose.

These laxatives require that the patient drink sufficient water to ensure effectiveness of the product.

Detergent Stool Softeners. Detergent stool softeners are essentially wetting agents. They promote both the retention of water and the emulsification of fats and are quite effective in ensuring a soft stool. Although they provide a soft stool, it is often necessary to take them for 2 or 3 days before having a satisfactory bowel movement. Some examples are dioctyl, sodium succinate, and propylene oxide.

Emollient Laxatives. These laxatives are simple lubricants—mineral oil and some vegetable oils. They have a mild effect; that is, they do not produce cramping. They are extremely useful in keeping the stool soft when straining could be hazardous, e.g. in aneurysm, in cerebral hemorrhage, and after rectal surgery.

A problem with the emollients is that there is sometimes embarrassing leakage through the anal sphincter. Also, habitual use of mineral oil may interfere with the absorption of the fat-soluble vitamins A, D, and K.

Contact Laxative. Bisacodyl (Dulcolax) is known as a contact laxative because of its particular mode of action. It takes effect when it comes in contact with the colonic mucosa, where it stimulates nerve endings in the intestinal wall. The nerve impulses produced reflexly stimulate peristaltic movement in the colon. This peristalsis propels the mass of wastes through the large intestine to the colon and rectum, where it brings about a natural urge to defecate.

As with any laxative, there may be some abdominal cramping.

Laxative and Evacuant Suppositories. Like the oral tablets, Dulcolax suppositories act when they come in contact with the colonic mucosa of the intestinal wall and produce evacuation in the same way. They are faster acting than the tablets, however, usually producing an effect within 15 minutes to 1 hour. Many nursing homes and hospitals use these suppositories before or in place of using enemas.

Glycerin irritates the rectum mechanically. The bowel attempts to eliminate the irritation by diluting it with a secretion of fluid. The fluid acts as a lubricant and liquefacient and a fecal discharge follows. Glycerin suppositories used occasionally are not harmful but if they are depended on habitually, they may injure the mucuous membrane.

Carbon dioxide suppositories release the gas in the lower part of the colon to create pressure and stimulate the peristaltic and defecation reflexes.

□ BOWEL RETRAINING

Bowel retraining is needed in many cases of chronic constipation.

Beginning the Program

1. obtain physician's order
2. gain patient's cooperation and understanding; explain program and encourage full participation
3. obtain a history of the patient's food habits, fluid intake, and use of laxatives (if any)
4. examine the rectum to check for impaction; remove according to institution's policy
5. evaluate associated factors, e.g., decubitus ulcers, dementia, motivation, acceptance
6. start the training with a clean bowel

Guidelines

1. establish a regular evacuation time (daily or on alternate days)
2. provide for maximum mobility of the patient; encourage exercise within limits permitted by the physician and tolerated by the patient
3. maintain complete records; record all results observed on each shift for each patient in the program
4. see that the patient takes adequate fluids
5. provide necessary physical facilities (privacy, commodes, toilet extenders, footstools, or anything else to make the patient comfortable)
6. persevere—anticipate lapses during the first 10 days
7. review the progress of the program with the physician, the staff, and the patient

Daily Procedure

1. the diet should be prescribed by the physician and should be well-balanced, with no food between meals; all meals should be served at a regular time each day
2. fluid intake per day should be 2500 to 3000 ml; prune juice, 2 to 4 ounces, is started on the first day without a stool or if the stool is exceptionally firm; output should be fairly comparable to intake
3. use of bowel evacuant;
   a) daily (after breakfast), depending on the pattern of the individual patient; insert Dulcolax suppository as high as finger will reach into the rectum past the internal sphincter. Be sure it is in contact with mucosal lining of bowel
   b) timing: note how much time elapses until the patient has a desire to evacuate; it will vary with each patient—usually from 15 minutes to an hour; *keep records*

   c) place patient on commode or assist him or her to bathroom; with non-ambulatory patient, use bedpan or diaper if necessary

   d) the presence of liquid stool or "oozing" is often a sign of impaction; check the patient digitally and follow the facility's procedures

   e) if liquid stools continue and no impaction is found, give 4 ounces tap water enema for 3 or 4 days until normal stools are obtained; report progress to physician

Termination of Program

1. continue daily training procedures for 14 to 21 days
2. gradually discontinue Dulcolax tablets or suppositories; goal of program is regular bowel habits for the patient without laxative support

No bowel training program would be complete without reinforcing the importance of nutrition. Dietary intake will affect all bowel functioning. A diet that contains adequate fluids and fiber will promote normal bowel functioning in most persons. Whole grain cereals, raw fruits, and vegetables are essential in order to provide sufficient bulk to stimulate peristaltic action of the intestines. The adult whose diet consists of highly refined foods usually has fewer bowel movements and the feces will be firmer and darker than one whose fiber consumption is appropriate. One to two tablespoons of bran should be added to breakfast cereal in order to supply needed bulk.

The water content of the body requires continual replenishment. Inadequate fluid intake will cause urine to become more concentrated and feces to become drier and harder than usual.

Bowel Functioning Principles

1. Elimination of waste products of digestion is the function of the bowels.
2. Efficient body functioning depends on normal bowel elimination.
3. Bowel malfunction can disturb fluid and electrolyte balance.
4. Bowel obstruction is serious.
5. Defecation urge results from stimulation of the rectal reflexes by distention of the lower colon and rectum.
6. Patterns of bowel elimination depend on dietary intake and activity.
7. Normal bowel elimination patterns vary in individuals from one bowel movement every 2 to 3 days to three bowel movements every day.
8. Bowel functioning is affected by stress and anxiety.
9. The attention of the elderly is frequently focused on their bowels, sometimes to the point of anxiety. Patience and understanding are needed. With a view toward avoiding dependency on enemas and laxatives, the nurse might create learning opportunities for patients by observing their eating habits and then by discussing the relationship of nutrition, adequate fluids, and reasonable exercise to healthful elimination patterns.

Fecal Incontinence

Despite the fact that fecal incontinence is not a true form of constipation, it should be mentioned here in relation to bowel retraining. In patients with spinal cord injury or CVA, bowel retraining is an important consideration in rehabilitation.

Where bowel retraining is impossible, regulation of bowel habit is usually possible. Many hospitals and nursing homes have found that their patients are helped by the administration of a suppository to bring about a daily bowel evacuation. In this way the patient does not have frequent, uncontrolled bowel movements during the day.

When the bisacodyl suppository is given after breakfast, it usually produces a response in 15 minutes to 1 hour. Bowel management can be completed in the morning.

□ ENEMAS

An enema is the introduction of fluid into the rectum. There are several reasons physicians order enemas: to relieve constipation, to cleanse the rectum and colon prior to examination, or to relieve fecal impaction.

Enemas stimulate peristalsis by irritation. Lubricating enemas help to make evacuation easier.

Cleansing enemas are given to remove feces from the colon. Soapsuds enemas usually contain 1000 ml. of soap solution; saline enemas contain 1000 ml. of normal saline, and tap water enemas contain about the same amount of common tap water. The volume of fluid distends the rectum and lower colon, which, in turn, stimulates the evacuation reflex.

There are commercial enemas that are commonly used in homes and health agencies. These disposable enemas contain a hypertonic solution, usually of sodium phosphate and biphosphate compounds. Their action is mainly irritating. The distention produced also helps to stimulate peristalsis.

Oil enemas may be given when the patient has a painful anal problem such as hemorrhoids or a rectal fissure or a painful lineal ulcer at the margin of the anus. Oil enemas are also used to lubricate dry, hardened fecal masses. Various oils such as olive or mineral oil may be used. The amount used is small (100 to 200 ml.), and the patient is encouraged to retain the enema for 30 to 60 minutes. A cleansing enema may be ordered to follow an oil retention enema.

Even though enemas have been popular for centuries, their use should not be taken lightly. It is a serious procedure. If the enema is too hot, the intestinal wall can be injured. Too much salt may cause inflammation of the colon, and even a soapsuds enema may cause some inflammation. *Laxatives and enemas should never be given when there is nausea, vomiting, or abdominal pain.*

Basically, there are two categories of enemas: retention and nonretention. The common retention enema is the oil retention enema. The nonretention enemas are the cleansing enemas, i.e., the tap water enema, the soapsuds enema, and the commercially prepared hypertonic solution in a plastic disposable squeeze bottle.

Oil Retention Enema

Purposes
to lubricate the rectum and lower bowel
to aid in the removal of feces

Equipment

lubricant	bath blanket
disposable protective pad	toilet tissue
bedpan	

Sequence
1. identify patient; introduce self; explain procedure; screen patient
2. fanfold top bedding to foot of bed, cover patient with bath blanket
3. place blanket in left lateral position, knees flexed
4. tuck protective pad under hips
5. lubricate enema tip, insert into anus about 4 inches
6. instill oil slowly, encouraging patient to mouth breathe and ask him to retain the oil for at least 30 minutes; apply pressure over anus for a minute or two after withdrawing enema tip; replace bed covers
7. record type of enema, amount of solution, and patient's reaction

The oil retention enema is usually ordered if a patient is severely constipated, has painful hemorrhoids, or has had a fecal impaction removed. In all cases, the nurse should be as gentle as possible in carrying out the procedure. Frequently the oil enema is followed, after a given period of time, by a cleansing enema. This is also ordered by the physician. The nurse then assists the patient to the bathroom if permitted, or positions him or her on a bedpan with the curtains drawn and with toilet tissue and a call light at hand. Aftercare is administered as necessary.

When bowel evacuation occurs, the nurse charts the time of the procedure and the amount and type of enema solution. Results of enemas should be documented: amount, color, consistency, and patient's reaction.

There are some adjustments that may have to be made in giving an enema to elderly people. For example, the preferred left-side lying position may be uncomfortable for someone with arthritis, contractures, and so on. The patient may have to be placed on his or her back and supported with pillows. If the patient is incontinent, gloves must be worn and the enema must be administered on the bedpan. Even if the patient is confined to bed, better results are achieved if an effort is made to get him or her up on a commode.

Cleansing Enema (Nonretention Enema)

A cleansing enema is given to rid the colon and lower bowel of feces. A physician's order is necessary for the tap water, soapsuds, or commercially packaged hypertonic solution. (This last increases the amount of fluid in the colon as it draws fluid from the body, which in turn stimulates peristalsis.)

It is unfortunate that most procedures are done at the convenience of the staff, not the patient. However, an enema should never be administered too close to mealtimes, visiting hours, or bedtime.

Purposes

to empty the rectum of feces

to relieve distention

Equipment

either tap water or soapsuds, according to physician's order, 105 to 110°F, plastic enema bag (or irrigating can with tubing and clamp)

lubricant

bed pan, toilet tissue

bath blanket

disposable protective pad

Sequence

1. identify patient; introduce self; explain procedure; screen patient
2. fanfold top bedding to foot of bed; cover patient with bath blanket
3. place patient in left lateral position, knees flexed
4. tuck protective pad under hips
5. lubricate enema tip, insert into anus about 4 inches
6. slowly introduce solution into rectum with the enema bag at a height of about 18 inches above the anus
7. instruct patient to take deep breaths during procedure and reassure him or her that if cramping is a problem you will stop the procedure until cramping subsides
8. when most of solution has been given, clamp off tubing and withdraw it
9. position patient on bedpan, leave toilet tissue and call light within reach, or
10. assist patient to bathroom and instruct him or her not to flush the toilet until contents have been observed
11. aftercare of patient as needed; use of room deodorizer as needed
12. record time of procedure; amount and type of solution used; reaction of patient; amount, color, and consistency of results of enema

Beginning students often ask, "Can I perforate the rectal mucosa by giving an enema from too high a level or by giving it too fast?" The answer is a qualified no. To be sure, the rectal mucosa of an elderly patient is probably thinner than that of a younger adult, but perforation will not take place unless there is a stricture or other type of anomaly in the rectum. Perforation might also take place if a hard or sharp instrument was carelessly used but not from the

Figure 12–5 ☐ Placement of a rectal suppository. The suppository must be inserted so that it rests against the inner surface of the rectum, rather than in the fecal mass. (From Rambo and Wood, p. 534.)

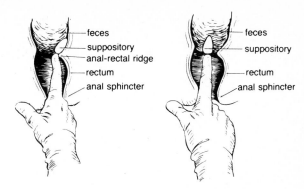

feces
suppository
anal-rectal ridge
rectum
anal sphincter

feces
suppository
rectum
anal sphincter

Correct placement.   Incorrect placement.

flow of water alone. However, if an enema is given too fast or too high, the patient will complain of abdominal cramping and most likely will not be able to hold the enema.

Never give an enema to a geriatric patient while the patient is sitting on a commode. The proper way is to have the patient lying on the left side (Fig. 12–5) and to have the bed thoroughly padded. The nurse should wear a disposable glove in the hand administering the enema as many elderly clients are unable to retain the fluid being administered for more than a few minutes.

☐ RECTAL SUPPOSITORIES

A suppository is a small cone-shaped semisolid containing a medication in a base (glycerin or cocoa butter) that melts at body temperature. Because suppositories melt so easily, they are usually kept in the refrigerator.

Rectal suppositories may be ordered to relieve pain, soothe the rectum or cause a bowel evacuation. The rectal suppositories that cause a bowel evacuation release a gas as they melt. This in turn stimulates peristalsis and eventually causes a bowel movement. Suppositories are alternatives to enemas.

Purposes

to cause a bowel evacuation
to relieve abdominal distention due to flatus and constipation

Equipment

disposable protective pad   suppository
finger cot or disposable rubber glove   lubricant

Sequence

1. identify patient; introduce self; explain procedure; screen patient
2. place patient in left lateral position, knees flexed
3. expose patient just enough to tuck protective pad under hips and visualize anus
4. put on finger cot or glove; lubricate suppository and index finger
5. insert suppository gently until pressure of the inner anal sphincter is felt upon the index finger; if fecal mass is felt, manually remove the fecal mass (inpaction) first before inserting suppository
6. apply external pressure over anus after suppository is inserted until the patient's urge to expel the suppository has passed
7. record time of procedure and results obtained

☐ *Colostomy Irrigation*

A colostomy irrigation may be compared to an enema. The difference is that the solution is introduced through an artificial anus called a stoma that has been created on the abdominal wall. Colostomy surgery is done to relieve obstructions or to rest the bowel, and the stoma may be temporary or permanent. Of course, the initial psychologic trauma is just as bad in either case when the patient actually sees the feces leaving his or her body by way of an abdominal stoma. A temporary colostomy may be "double barreled," that is, with two stomas. One of them is called the *distal* opening and the other the *proximal* opening. The physician indicates which stoma is to be irrigated. The stoma that is not irrigated drains some mucus.

Irrigations usually begin about the fourth or fifth day postoperatively. Although successful irrigations depend on several things, regularity and diet should be emphasized. Irrigations are best done after a meal because eating stimulates peristalsis and bowel evacuation. Diet will affect the functioning of a colostomy and the patient will simply note the foods that cause discomfort.

Postoperative colostomy dressings will have to be changed frequently. The attitude and attention of the nurse can affect the motivation of the patient,

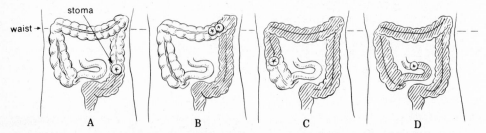

Figure 12–6 ☐ Stoma sites: *A,* descending colon; *B,* transverse colon; *C,* ascending colon, *D,* ileostomy stoma. (From Rambo and Wood, p. 536.)

as the odor and the distress of wet dressings and full colostomy bags are disheartening.

Purpose

to irrigate the bowels of a patient who has a colostomy

Equipment

commercial colostomy irrigation set
   or disposable enema bag
colostomy irrigating pouch
temporary colostomy bag
disposable protective pads
lubricant
finger cot
bath blanket

solution as ordered
dressings as needed
bedpan
tincture of benzoin spray
   (or other skin preparation)
paper bag for discards
two emesis basins

Chapter 12 □ Review Questions

MULTIPLE CHOICE

1. The wavelike movements that occur in the esophagus and small and large intestines are called
   A. rugae
   B. ptyalin
   C. flatus
   D. peristalsis
2. An obvious sign of aging is
   A. wrinkling of skin
   B. arteriosclerosis
   C. stomach atrophy
   D. achlorhydria
3. A useful step toward decreasing dependence on laxatives is
   A. increased fiber in diet
   B. decreased exercise
   C. increased bedrest
   D. periodic enemas
4. A patient who might have a swallowing problem would be
   A. a patient on bedrest
   B. a patient in traction
   C. a stroke victim
   D. a colostomy patient

MATCHING

_____ 1. rugae   A. bland, low residue diet

_____ 2. diverticulosis   B. aspiration risk

_____ 3. tumor   C. furrows in the stomach

_____ 4. tap water enema   D. without teeth

_____ 5. edentulous   E. can be caused by stress

_____ 6. bowel malfunction   F. test urine for glucose

_____ 7. constipation   G. outpouchings of intestinal wall

_____ 8. tube feeding   H. mechanical obstruction

_____ 9. TPN   I. chronic dehydration

_____ 10. diverticulitis   J. remove feces from colon

DISCUSSION QUESTIONS

1. Mr. B., 82, is a patient in a nursing home. He is confined to bed or wheel-chair and needs assistance with all activities of daily living. As the nurse prepares to bathe Mr. B., she notices fecal oozing. What is the probable cause of the oozing? What steps should the nurse take?
2. Linda M. is a student nurse participating in clinical experiences at a nursing home. Linda notices that many of the residents focus much attention on bowel problems. What are some reasons for this behavior of elderly persons?
3. As the nurse in charge of a unit of chronically ill older adults, you have decided to implement a bowel retraining program with selected patients. What are four key factors in bowel retraining?

☐ REFERENCES

Bender, M., et al.: Total parenteral nutrition: nursing implications ... home study program. AORN J, 40(3):354–359, 362–365, 1984.
Bourke, R.: Thriving with a stoma. Nurs Mirror, 159(9):v–vi (Clinics Forum), 1984.
Couchman, M.: A softer option ... more comfortable microenemas. Nurs Mirror, 159(7):39, 1984.
Evans, G.: The digestive system. Nurs Mirror, 158(15):23–25, 1984.
Hendrickson, D. R.: The complementary roles of the gastrointestinal assistant and the enterostomal therapist. S GA J, 5(2):12–14, 1982.
Mager-O'Connor, E.: How to identify and remove fecal impactions. Geriatr Nurs, 5(3):158–161, 1984.

Pringle, W.: Colostomy irrigation. Nurs Mirror, 159(8):29–31, 1984.

Quick guide to digestive disorders. Nursing (Horsham) (Can Ed), 14(8):15, 1984.

Steffl, B.: Handbook of Gerontological Nursing. New York, Van Nostrand Reinhold, 1984, p. 52.

Stoia, R.: Stress, food and the digestive system. Your Life Health, 98(8):10–11, 1983.

Sweet, K.: Hiatal hernia: what to guard against most in post-op patients. Nursing, 13(12):38–45, 1983.

Toga, C.J.: Gerodontics. J Hosp Dent Pract, 14(1):24–26, 1980.

White, L.: The elderly patient in the gastroenterology lab. SGA J, 5(1):52–53, 1982.

Objectives

After completing this chapter, the student should be able to

- [ ] describe the anatomy and physiology of the musculoskeletal system
- [ ] name three age-related changes of the musculoskeletal system
- [ ] name five age-related disorders of the musculoskeletal system
- [ ] describe mechanical aids to ambulation and their use
- [ ] describe range of motion exercises
- [ ] explain indications for restraints and related safety measures

Vocabulary

abduction
adduction
alignment
arthroplasty
articulate
atrophy
circumduction
contracture
degenerative
extension
facies
flexion
gait
lactic acid
osteoporosis
plantar
pronation
prosthesis
rotation
supination

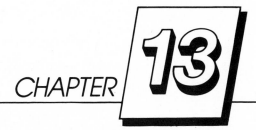

CHAPTER **13**

The Musculoskeletal System

Chapter Outline

□ Anatomy Review

Muscles. Muscles are generally classified as voluntary and involuntary. Voluntary muscles are also referred to as *skeletal muscles,* since they are attached to bones. They pull on the bones and make the body move. These muscles are constructed of striated muscle fibers.

Involuntary muscles (smooth or visceral muscles) make up the walls of the intestines, blood vessels, and abdominal organs. They are built of small, spindle-shaped muscle fibers and are not striated. The heart is made up of cardiac muscle, which is a type of involuntary muscle.

As skeletal muscles are used, *lactic acid,* a waste product, accumulates. This causes fatigue. Muscles that continually move the body and keep it in position become tired. Visceral muscles, however, work more slowly and steadily and are not affected by fatigue. This is the major difference between voluntary and involuntary muscles.

Bones. Two thirds of the material that makes up the bones consist of minerals, mainly calcium and phosphorus. The remaining third is fibrous protein. Bones are spongy on the inside and extremely hard (compact) on the outside. They provide the supporting structure for muscles, tendons, and ligaments.

Almost every bone in the body articulates with another bone; that is, each bone functions with another bone to produce movements. These articulations are called *joints.*

Cartilage. The articulations at the ends of the bones are covered with smooth cartilage, which provides flexibility. Cartilage is also found in the rib cage, where flexibility is very important to breathing.

Joints. Some joints, such as those in the skull, do not move, but most joints are freely movable. Movable joints are contained in a joint capsule made up of fibrous connective tissue that is lined with a slippery synovial membrane. This membrane secretes synovial fluid, which prevents friction during movement. The capsule covers the ends of the two articulating bones like a sheath.

Joints have two functions: to hold bones together and to provide for a range of movement between these bones. As we age, however, several problems may develop that bring discomfort and impaired function to our joints. Among them are the adhesions that form between the cartilage and overgrowth of bone at the joint edges.

□ Age-Related Changes

Joint Degeneration. More than 90 per cent of adults over the age of 65 have some degree of degenerative joint disease (arthrosis) as a result of the continuous wear and tear on the joints over the years. Usually, but not always,

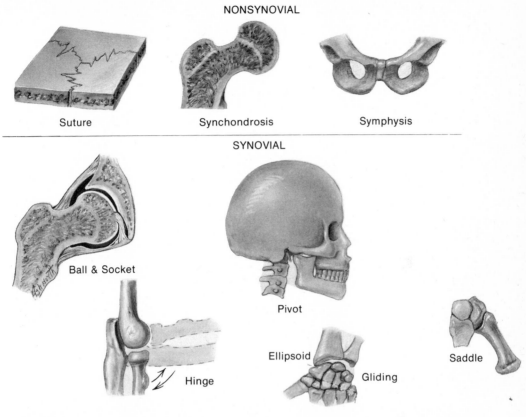

Figure 13–1 ☐ Movable joints are termed *synovial* joints. The surfaces that articulate are covered with *articular cartilage* and lubricated by *synovial fluid*. As a person ages, the cartilage undergoes wear and tear. It becomes softer and in some people actually disintegrates. Bony growths may form in its place, making movement of the joint more difficult and painful. (From Jacob, Francone, and Lossow, p. 150.)

joints become painful or stiff, or both. Cartilage thins, bones overgrow, spurs form, and the ultimate result can be limitation or even loss of function.

Degenerative joint disease primarily affects the weight-bearing joints. It is easy to see how the burden of obesity aggravates the problem. The more pressure on the joint, the more painful it feels. The obvious solution is weight reduction, but it is not a simple thing to reduce the overweight elderly, especially those who are fairly inactive. Weight reduction requires careful medical supervision and a high degree of motivation on the part of the obese person.

Degenerative joint disease is treated with analgesics, physiotherapy, anti-inflammatory agents, and heat. The positioning of the body is important and a bed board and firm mattress are advised. Canes, cervical collars, and foot supports are often used. In cases of disabling pain and severely impaired function, the physician may suggest surgery. Reconstructive joint surgery and prostheses have helped many people to increase their mobility and obtain relief from pain.

Osteoporosis. *Osteoporosis* is a disorder of bone mass related to calcium and estrogen deficiency. Millions of women are affected. There is a strong relationship between osteoporosis and hip fracture. In one study of hip fracture in women over 65, 34 per cent died within 6 months of sustaining a fracture because of the complications associated with treatment. The survivors were unable to take care of themselves and needed nursing care. The costs to the individual and to society are enormous. Hip fractures in this country cost several billion dollars a year.

Postmenopausal osteoporosis is preventable. The progression of the disorder can be halted by the administration of oral estrogens in low doses, oral calcium carbonate, and exercise (where practical). Some literature refers to the risk of endometrial cancer. Each patient must be investigated and individual protocols designed. The feeling among physicians and other health professionals is that prophylaxis is the solution to this major public health problem.

Osteoporosis is the result of demineralization of the bone. The chemical composition of the bone (calcium, phosphorus, and so on) does not change, but the amount of bone tissue diminishes, so that the bones become less dense and more porous. This weakens them and they fracture easily. Osteoporosis is present in 80 per cent of white women over the age of 65. The principal fracture is vertebral compression, a condition that exists in about 25 per cent of women over 65. Other sites for fracture in women with osteoporosis are head of the radius (Colles' fracture) and ribs. The most serious complication is fracture of the hip.

Much of the distressing back pain endured by elderly persons is caused by compression fractures of the lower thoracic and lumbar vertebrae. These fractures can occur as a result of sneezing or a coughing spell. In fact, back pain may be the reason a person visits a doctor and it may be then that the person first learns that she has osteoporosis. Also associated with osteoporosis are postural changes such as kyphosis and a gradual loss of height. Most elderly people are 2 to 3 inches shorter after the age of 75 than they were as younger adults.

Muscle Atrophy. The loss of muscle mass in the elderly is the cause of diminished strength. There is actually a gradual decrease in the number of muscle fibers. Most elderly people have enough strength to do what they want to do within reason. Since the loss of muscle mass happens quite gradually over a long period of time, they make adaptations to compensate for it.

☐ Age-Related Disorders

Contractures. Because contractures develop quickly in the inactive older person, physical exercise is encouraged. Active exercise is best, of course, but

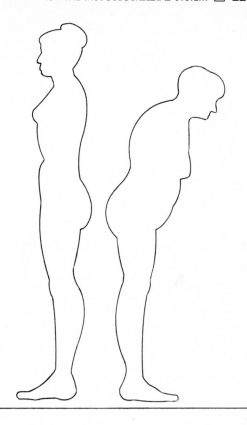

Figure 13–2 ☐ Osteoporosis contributes to the loss of height and stooped posture character-istic of many older women. Typi-cally, older adults are two to three inches shorter than they were in young adulthood.

if this is not possible, passive range of motion exercises should be given.* If the person is ambulatory, his or her shoes should be well-fitted, as they are important to help provide a firm base of support and to help the patient keep a good sense of balance, especially on uneven surfaces.

Accidents. Many deaths over the age of 65 are the result of accidents, most frequently a fall. Any or all of the following elements for an accident may be present in an elderly person: diminished muscle strength, loss of hear-

---

*Range of motion is discussed in detail at the end of this chapter.

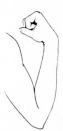

Figure 13–3 ☐ Contracture of the hand, wrist, and elbow. The joints are rigid and can be moved only slightly. (From Rambo and Wood, p. 237.)

ing, poor eyesight, awkward gait, difficulty in maintaining balance, and a slow reaction when changing the position of the body. If the elderly adult does not understand the obvious hazards of the bathroom (hard, slippery surfaces, poorly labeled medications), the bedroom (scatter rugs, light cords), and the stairs, then someone responsible must assess the danger potential and eliminate it.

Hip Fractures. Elderly persons, particularly women, are prone to accidents that result in fractures of the hip. Curiously, the precipitating cause, usually a fall, is often insignificant and makes one wonder which came first, the fall or the fracture. The end of the femur that engages with the acetabulum in the innominate bone for the "hip joint" is the site of intracapsular or extracapsular fractures.

Hip fractures in the elderly patient are usually complicated by a complexity of medical disorders common among the aged: diabetes, hypertension, peripheral vascular disorders, and neurologic disorders, to name a few.

The prognosis for those with hip fractures is much better today than it was 30 years ago. In fact, it was once regarded as a death sentence because of the long period of immobility it required. The aged patient who, with weakened physical defenses, was confined to bed often developed a hypostatic pneumonia and died. Hypostatic pneumonia is still a very real threat, but with frequent turning, deep breathing exercises, range of motion exercises, and early ambulation, the risk is decidedly less. In addition, better infection control, improved nutrition, and physical therapy allow for a much more favorable outlook.

The treatment of a patient with a hip fracture usually begins with traction

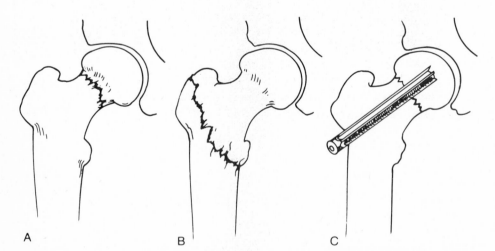

A   B   C

Figure 13–4 ☐ A and B, Typical sites of fractures of the proximal end of the femur. C, Internal fixation; a metal pin is inserted into the bone. This procedure generally allows a person to be mobile soon after surgery.

in order to prevent contractures, to relieve muscle spasm, and to prevent movement of bone fragments. A bed board is also used. The patient probably will be in a bed with a frame to which a trapeze has been attached to enable him or her to lift and move if possible. When surgery is indicated, internal fixation, using the insertion of pins or nails, fixation of screw plates and implantation of a prosthesis to replace the head and neck of the femur are usually the choices. Internal fixation often makes early mobilization possible soon after surgery. This is very important for older adults who are susceptible to the complications of immobility.

Leg Cramps. A common complaint of the elderly is that of severe leg cramps, usually in the calf, that most often occur at night. They may be caused by poor circulation or by fatigue, or by standing for long periods. They may also be caused by the excessive use of diuretics, a frequent medication of the aged patient. The condition should be investigated medically.

Rheumatoid Arthritis. The cause of rheumatoid arthritis, a chronic, systemic disease of the connective tissue, is unknown. Two or three times as many women are affected as are men. The disease often begins in young or middle adulthood, although acute initial attacks in the elderly do occur.

The symptoms are pain, heat, and swelling in the joints and stiffness of joints in the morning. Stiffness usually lasts 1 to 2 hours after the person arises. The patient usually suffers muscle spasms, contractures, and enlarged joints of the wrists, hands, and feet. The joints' cartilage and ligaments are gradually destroyed.

The disease is treated systemically with corticosteroids, anti-inflammatory agents, and analgesics. Local treatment consists of moist heat and massage. Good nutrition and a program of adequate rest and exercise are important. Mechanical aids can help the person overcome the disability. Some examples of aids include canes, walkers, chair leg extenders, and specially designed kitchen utensils.

Certain surgical procedures, too, are designed to relieve the severe disabling pain. Total joint replacement may offer relief in selected cases.

Both the patient and the patient's family need continuing emotional support, as the disease is progressive, although there are exacerbations and remissions.

☐ *Nursing Interventions*

☐ PATIENTS IN TRACTION

Traction means drawing or pulling. Traction is frequently used to pull the ends of broken bones, especially arm or leg bones, into proper alignment. In this way, the extremity may be immobilized and the bones kept in position for healing. Traction is also used in treating fractured vertebrae and for patients with muscle spasms.

Two kinds of traction are skin traction and skeletal traction. With skin traction, the force pulls on an extremity—a leg, for example—that has been prepared with adhesive or moleskin strips attached to a block positioned so there is no pressure on the side of the foot. The extremity is then wrapped in Ace or tensor bandages, whichever the physician orders. A rope is tied to the block, guided over a pulley, and fastened to a weight. With skeletal traction, the force is applied directly to a bone by means of pins or wires passed through the bone or by tongs (Crutchfield tongs are one type) anchored in the bone.

General Care of a Patient in Traction

1. ensure that the ropes are on the pulleys and are not frayed
2. ensure that the weights swing free of the bed and are not removed without a doctor's order
3. steady the weights when moving the bed
4. when a pillow is used to support the leg, check to see that there is no pressure on the heel or the back of the knee
5. inspect skin over all pressure points regularly
6. if skeletal traction is used, check for signs of infection around pin or wire site; cover sharp ends of pins with cork (guards) and be sure bed linen does not snag on pins or wires; change dressings when necessary and use recommended skin care preparations
7. encourage patient to use trapeze to lift himself or herself when using the bedpan or just to change position, if only for a few seconds—even a few seconds off the pressure areas permit circulation to the skin
8. encourage patient to actively exercise all joints and muscles not affected by traction; include coughing and deep breathing
9. when making the occupied bed of a patient in traction, change the linen from top to bottom instead of from side to side

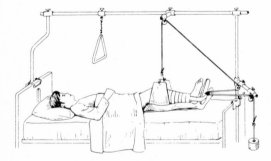

Figure 13–5 □ Russell's traction is an example of traction used for patients with a femoral fracture. Older patients, however, often cannot tolerate immobilization, and traction may be used for only a short period before surgery. (From Rambo and Wood, p. 359.)

10. provide for comfort by use of toe socks if a foot is exposed and inspect the bed covers to see that they do not interfere with traction
11. use foot support to prevent foot drop
12. check color and temperature of both feet every 4 hours

Note. Avoid pressure at danger points and prevent rubbing of skin by edges of elastic wrapping bandages. Rubbing can cause erosion sores. Danger points are

any bony prominence—elbow, wrist, ankle, back of heel, spine, shoulder blades, iliac crest, sacral areas
behind the knee where the peroneal nerve passes over the neck of the fibula
the elbow, where the ulnar nerve passes over the inner side

Another application of traction is called "balanced suspension." This is suspending an extremity or other part of the body so it "floats" independently of the other parts of the body.

There are numerous types of traction, and the preceding information is meant to acquaint the nurse with general information about traction. Each application of traction is done according to a specific physician's order. Although two patients may have exactly the same fracture in exactly the same extremity, the chances are that their specific orders will be different. One doctor may allow the patient to be transported to X-ray out of traction and another will insist that traction is to be maintained at all times. Orders will have to be verified.

□ PATIENTS WITH TOTAL HIP AND KNEE REPLACEMENT

Total hip replacement is a surgical procedure used in treating several conditions, including severe arthritis of the hip. It has provided dramatic relief from pain, correction of deformity, and increased mobility in selected cases.

The metal and plastic prosthesis is kept in place with screws or an intermedullary stem or with an acrylic cement.

The operation carries considerable risk. The patients are usually elderly, quite a lot of blood is lost during surgery, and postoperatively there is the possibility of dislocation of the prosthesis, thromboembolic sepsis, and infection. However, with careful nursing and medical management, the overall picture is optimistic, and the procedure is being done with increasing frequency.

Total knee replacement is a surgical procedure that may give the patient with degenerative knee disease or rheumatoid knees marked relief from pain and improved knee motion.

The prosthesis is made of metal and plastic and is anchored in place with a plastic cement. Patients begin weight-bearing with a walker, then crutches, and gradually progress to a cane. In time, if it is comfortable, they may walk unaided.

☐ CAST CARE

The reasons casts are used are
1. to immobilize, support, and protect a part during healing processes
2. to prevent deformities
3. to correct deformities

Casts are usually made of plaster of Paris, although there are some newer materials (fiberglass, for one) that are lightweight and will not deteriorate when wet.

A cast that has just been applied should be exposed to the air so it dries, a process that takes about 48 hours. A dry plaster of Paris cast is hard, white, and shiny.

Nursing care of the patient who has had a cast applied includes reassuring the patient that the heat felt when the cast is newly applied is normal and that this heat occurs only while the cast is drying. This uncomfortable feeling is short-lived.

CSM (circulation, sensation, and mobility) checks are made regularly. Listen to the patient's complaints and document and report them! Pain, swelling, tingling, numbness, inability to move fingers or toes, and bluish fingernails or toenails must be reported immediately because these observations may indicate pressure on a nerve, constriction of blood vessels, or swelling of the part enclosed in the cast, which may lead to paralysis or tissue necrosis.

Sometimes casts have to be split (bivalved) if circulation is constricted. A physician determines what action to take based on the information elicited from the patient and the nurse.

Continuous emotional support is imperative. The elderly person already has diminished muscular strength and casts are heavy. Pain may also be present. Add to this the anticipation of a long period of rehabilitation or physiotherapy, and it is no wonder that patients in casts become depressed.

The foregoing instructions apply to the care of all patients in casts. The nurse will need to check physicians' orders as they apply to individual patients.

☐ POSITIONING

A patient in bed may lie in three basic positions: on the back (dorsal), on the side (lateral), or on the abdomen (prone). Patients are sometimes put in variations of these three basic positions for various treatments and examinations. The nurse is responsible for knowing how to correctly position and drape the patient for examination and treatment.

Purposes

to prepare the patient for examination or treatment without unnecessary exposure
to provide comfort

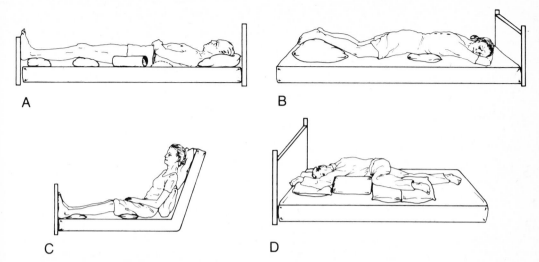

Figure 13–6 □ Positioning. *A,* Supine position with padding for support and to prevent pressure on bony prominences. *B,* Prone position. *C,* Fowler's position. *D,* Sims' position.

Types of Positions

1. *Horizontal Recumbent Position (Supine).* Used for comfort and examination. Patient lies flat on back with legs together and extended (sometimes slightly flexed to relax abdominal muscles); pillow under head; arms at side of body.
2. *Dorsal Recumbent Position.* Used for vaginal and rectal examinations and treatments. Patient lies flat on back with knees flexed, draped with a sheet or bath blanket that is drawn back for the examination.
3. *Lithotomy Position.* Used for vaginal and rectal examinations. Same as dorsal recumbent except that the legs are elevated and the feet may be placed in stirrups.
4. *Prone Position.* Used for examination of back, spinal surgery, and treatment of sacral decubitus ulcers. Patient lies on abdomen, head to the side, arms flexed beside head.
5. *Fowler's Position.* Used for comfort or when supine position is contraindicated. Head of the bed is elevated to a 45-degree angle. Variations: high Fowler's, low Fowler's.
6. *Sims' Position.* Used for rectal examination, enemas, inserting suppositories, taking rectal temperatures. Patient lies on left side with pillow under head, right knee flexed against the abdomen, left knee slightly flexed, left arm behind body, right arm beside head.
7. *Knee Chest Position (Genupectoral).* Used for rectal examination, vaginal exam, surgical procedures, and postpartum exercises. Patient on knees, chest on bed, arms in position of comfort, hips should be directly above knees, face to side.

8. *Trendelenburg Position.* Sometimes ordered for shock. Patient supine; head of bed is lower than foot so that the body is on an inclined plane slanting downward.

The position and arrangement of the parts of the body is called posture. Patients restricted to bed rest often have poor posture because they bend their backs while lying on the sides and flex their knees and hips. They may assume this position because they are cold or in pain. Good body alignment is a must for someone confined to bed for any length of time.

A firm supporting mattress is the first requirement for achieving good body alignment. A frequent complication of bed rest is foot drop. If the foot is resting unsupported, the muscles in the anterior leg stretch and the tendon of the calf muscles shortens. Foot drop can be prevented by using a padded footboard against which the patient can place his or her feet. A bed cradle, a frame designed to keep linens off the patient's feet, may also be used. When prolonged immobility keeps patients off their feet, many health professionals use street or tennis shoes on their patients in order to maintain the normal physiologic position.

Since many elderly have poor circulation to their extremities, their feet are often cold. Covering the feet with socks or booties is a welcome comfort measure.

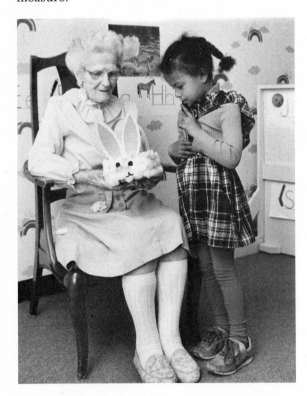

Figure 13–7 □ The older adult frequently has poor circulation in the extremities and appreciates warm socks to keep her or his feet and legs comfortable. (Courtesy of Ring Nursing Homes.)

Other means of providing support for the immobile patient include sandbags, trochanter rolls (rolled up bath blankets placed along the hip), and hand rolls. Hand rolls should have a firm center to avoid flexion contractures. When using the side lying position, a pillow or rolled bath blanket should be placed between the knees and one leg should be flexed.

Positioning the Bed Patient

Purposes
to make the patient comfortable while in bed
to prevent external rotation of hips
to prevent foot drop

Positioning Patient on Back
1. feet against footboard, under bed cradle, or supported by braced sandbags
2. bath blanket under hips, rolled at each hip to prevent external rotation
3. pillow under head; head of bed in Fowler's or low Fowler's
4. hand rolls if necessary

Positioning Patient on Side
1. pillow under head; head of bed in low Fowler's
2. pillow at back
3. top leg flexed, supported by pillow or folded bath blanket
4. arms in position of comfort
5. hand rolls if necessary

Positioning Patient Prone
1. rolled bath blanket under ankles
2. head on small pillow, to one side
3. shoulder rolls or small pillow under abdomen if advisable
4. hand rolls

☐ RESTRAINTS

Restraints are used for the protection of the patient and the safety of others. They are always ordered by the physician (except in cases of emergency) and should be used only as a last resort after all other attempts at calming or orienting the patient have failed. Note that *any limitation of movement is a restraint;* for example, a locked door, a patient secured in a geri-chair, or holding a patient with your hands. There are chemical as well as physical restraints. *Never use restraints as a threat or punishment.*

Since restraining a patient may be directly related to charges of false imprisonment, the nurse must be aware of the gravity of the action and the importance of keeping the clinical record.

Charting must include
1. the reason the patient was restrained
2. a description of the restraint used

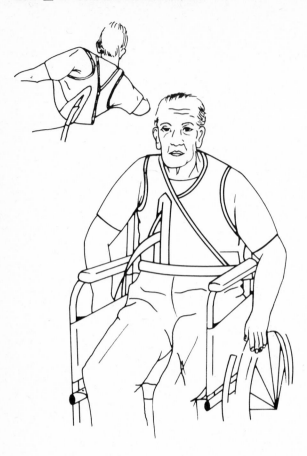

Figure 13–8 □ Older adults who are confused or weak may be restrained in a chair or wheelchair by a jacket restraint to prevent them from sliding down in the wheelchair and to prevent them from attempting to walk if they forget that they cannot walk by themselves.

3. description of skin integrity and skin care given
4. the time restraints were applied
5. the frequency of observation and removal of restraints (at least every 2 hours); range of motion exercise given
6. the time restraints were discontinued
7. how the patient tolerated restraints

Some alternatives to restraints include such diversions as music, crafts, magazines with pictures, and just moving the patient to a different area.

Purposes

to prevent the patient from injuring self or others
to immobilize the patient temporarily (as for a treatment)
to provide support for the patient

Types of Restraints

1. Posey waist restraint, soft belt model, limits movement; ties *under* bed or around chair
2. jacket restraint, limits movement but provides support; used in bed or chair
3. cloth wrist restraint, used to prevent patient from injuring self by pulling out IV's, and so on
4. leg restraint, seldom used except under supervision
5. leather restraints, used in cases of severe hyperactivity and confusion; rarely used

Dangers of Restraints

1. may limit circulation
2. may cause skin breakdown
3. may contribute to such effects of immobility as: a) contractures; b) decubitus ulcers; c) hypostatic pneumonia; d) loss of muscle tone
4. may give staff members a false sense of security
5. may cause restrained patient to feel rage or to feel helpless

How to Avoid Restraint Dangers

1. check patient at regular intervals, removing and replacing restraints *one at a time* to look at the skin
2. keep skin under restraints clean and dry; apply lotion and massage
3. give range of motion exercises at least once on each shift; encourage active exercise when possible (i.e., walk with patients who can be ambulated)
4. relieve pressure on bony prominences
5. turn patients at least every 2 hours

   Note. Just because a patient is restrained does not mean that he or she needs less observation. The long cloth ties of restraints have built-in risks. Also, there always seems to be a "helpful" patient around who unties the restrained patient. *A restrained patient is vulnerable.*

☐ MECHANICAL AIDS TO AMBULATION

Wheelchairs

The infirmity of the patient should determine the type of wheelchair to be used. Some wheelchairs come with adjustable back rests, head rests, and leg and arm rests. Detachable swinging footrests may be either removed or swung out of the way to get closer to furniture or equipment. Hands that are

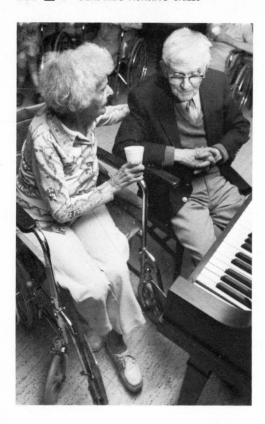

Figure 13–9 ☐ Wheelchairs are used for comfort and convenience. The older adult using a wheelchair can still be active and enjoy herself or himself. (Courtesy of Ring Nursing Homes.)

weak or affected by arthritis can wheel a chair easier if knobs are provided on wheels. These projections transfer the work of the fingers to the palms of the hands. The brake should always be on when a patient is being moved in or out of a wheelchair. Patients may tip geri-chairs over unless they are properly supervised. If the patient is able to walk, he or she should be ambulated for a few steps every 2 hours. No one should ever be left unattended in a geri-chair.

Wheelchair cushions are available from hospital supply firms; they help decrease the chances of pressure sores developing. Gel cushions filled with emulsions that shift with a patient's weight help to equalize pressure. A wheelchair should be kept clean and in good repair.

Walker

A walker is a light-weight metal frame with hand grips and safety-tipped legs. Some walkers have two front wheels. The patient lifts or wheels the walker in front as he or she walks. Various carrier bags for walkers that are useful for holding small items are available.

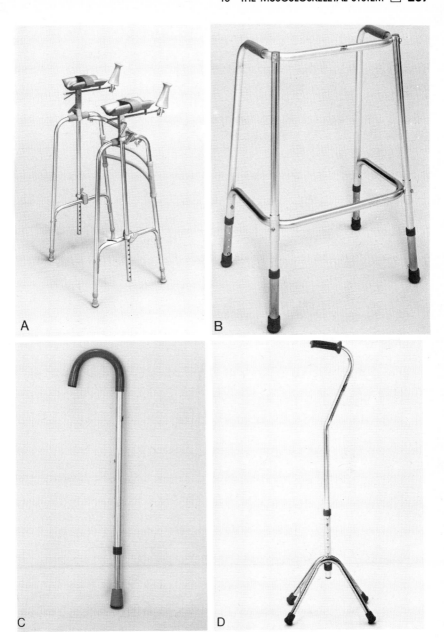

Figure 13–10 □ Various types of canes and walkers are used by older adults for support and confidence in walking.

Canes

Canes may be wood, metal, or plastic. A one-point cane has a curved handle and is used on the strong side of the body. There are also tripod and quad canes that stand alone. All canes should have safety tips to prevent slipping. Patients should be measured by a physical therapist for canes and crutches. Often a safety belt is used by the one teaching a patient to walk (whether with cane, walker, or independently).

Braces

Braces are supports for a part of the body with a musculoskeletal problem. They may immobilize, support, or protect and are prescribed by a physician. Remember:
- braces should be cleaned and repaired when necessary
- check the condition of straps; look for missing or loose screws
- after removing the brace for bathing, check skin for any reddened areas

Prostheses

A prosthesis replaces a missing part of the body. For example, an artificial breast is used for a patient who has had a mastectomy. A patient who has had an amputation will be fitted with a prosthesis and trained in its use. The length of time a patient needs to master the art of wearing a prosthesis varies with his or her condition and motivation. The main purpose of an artificial leg is to help the patient maintain mobility.

☐ RANGE OF MOTION (ROM) EXERCISES

"Use it or lose it!"

Flexibility and muscle tone are soon lost without exercise. Range of motion exercises should be carried out on all patients confined to bed at least once each day unless specifically contraindicated by the physician. For many, it may be their only exercise.

These exercises are done to prevent contractures, improve circulation, maintain joint mobility, and in general induce a feeling of well being. The exercises must be planned to use the muscles necessary to maintain joint mobility. The structure of a joint limits its movement; for example, hinge joints do not rotate but move in one direction only. Ideally, each joint should be put through its full range of movement daily. This is why patients should be encouraged to do as much of their own care as possible. Activity helps keep the joints flexible and the muscles toned. Besides, the independence is good psychologically.

But what if the range of motion exercises cannot be done actively by the patient? Then the nurse, or whoever is giving the beside care, should give

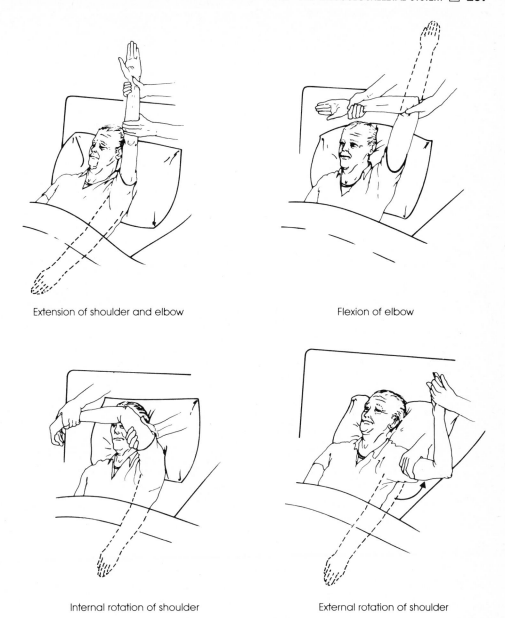

Extension of shoulder and elbow

Flexion of elbow

Internal rotation of shoulder

External rotation of shoulder

Figure 13–11 ☐ Examples of passive range of motion exercises.

ROM passively. A good time to carry out ROM exercises is during the bed bath. Enlist the cooperation of patients by telling them why ROM exercises are essential and just what will be done.

Exercising should not be done when the patient is tired or in pain.

☐ MOIST HEAT APPLICATIONS

Moist heat is a comfort measure designed to relieve joint pain, encourage circulation to the part, and reduce stiffness. The use of heat is always a possible risk, so great care must be given to the applications.

A warm tub bath or shower relieves the stiffness so apparent early in the morning. Warm soaks may be given to an affected extremity for 15 to 20 minutes at a temperature not exceeding 110°F. The nurse should be aware of the written policy regarding this procedure in the individual agency in which she or he practices.

Chapter 13 ☐ Review Questions

MULTIPLE CHOICE

1. Involuntary muscles
   A. accumulate lactic acid as waste
   B. work automatically
   C. are made up of striated muscle fibers
   D. are attached to bones
2. Joints are also called
   A. articulations
   B. cancellous
   C. hyoid
   D. fibrous
3. Adhesions that form between cartilages cause
   A. bleeding
   B. pallor
   C. overgrowth of bone
   D. impaired function
4. Degenerative joint disease
   A. is an inflammatory process
   B. is a result of wear and tear on the movable joints
   C. can be prevented by taking vitamins
   D. is more common in the nonmovable joints
5. Rheumatoid arthritis
   A. is most common in men
   B. is a symptom of muscle atrophy in the elderly
   C. is a chronic systemic disease
   D. is cured by vigorous exercise
6. Osteoporosis
   A. is most common in elderly, white women
   B. is cured by increased calcium intake
   C. cannot be prevented or slowed
   D. is another term for osteoarthritis

DISCUSSION QUESTIONS

1. Mr. Gardner, 82, is recovering from the repair of a fractured hip. His recovery is impaired because he is afraid of falling and injuring himself again. He resists going to physical therapy, complains about getting out of bed for any reason, and is being labeled as "uncooperative" by the nursing staff. How would you encourage Mr. Gardner to cooperate? What teaching does he need? What initial assessments would the nurse make before getting him out of bed?

2. Mrs. Rizzo, 75, is admitted from a nursing home for an open reduction of a fractured right ulnar. She is in a cast from her elbow to her fingers. What are some measures the nurse should take for the physical care of Mrs. Rizzo? For her emotional care?

3. You are assigned to take care of an elderly gentleman described by another worker as being confused and suspicious and "needs to be restrained all the time." What are some alternatives you might consider besides constant restraints? If restraints are indeed necessary, what are some safety factors to be considered? How will you document the restraining of this patient?

4. Mrs. Lord wants to take her 89-year-old mother into her home. She tells you that her mother is in fairly good health but has very poor vision and is, in general, frail. She asks you to suggest some ways in which she can eliminate safety hazards in her home and develop a safe, comfortable environment for her mother. How will you respond to her question?

☐ REFERENCES

Anaisson, A., et al.: Muscle function in 75-year-old men and women. A longitudinal study. Scand J Rehabil Med, (Suppl) 14(9):92–102, 1983.

Arthritis advice. Nurs Homes, 31(6):22–23, 1982.

Arthritis quackery: big business, big trouble. Your Life Health, 97(12):16–18, 1982.

Banwell, B.G.: Exercise and mobility in arthritis. Nurs Clin North Am, 19(4):605–616, 1984.

Boutaugh, M.: Arthritis—myths and realities. Occup Health Nurs, 32(7):346–349, 381–385, 1984.

Cunningham, L.S., et al.: Epidemiology of musculoskeletal impairments and associated disability. Am J Public Health, 74(6):574–579, 1984.

Evans, J.H.: Joint inflexibility: its relationship to psychological rigidity. Rehab Nurs, 9(4):26–29, 1984.

Googe, M.C.: Review of selected patient, family, and staff resources: the Arthritis foundation. Orthop Nurs, 3(5):43, 1984.

Hawley, D.J.: Non-traditional treatments of arthritis. Nurs Clin North Am, 19(4):663–672, 1984.

Holn, K., et al.: Perspectives on exercise and aging. Heart Lung, 13(5):519–523, 1984.

Johnson, J.A., et al.: Non-pharmacologic pain management in arthritis. Nurs Clin North Am, 19(4):583–591, 1984.

Kern, F.: Physical therapy and geriatrics: current issues and concepts. Phys Health Occup Ther Geriatr, 3(2):1–4, 1983.

Lewis, C.B.: Musculoskeletal changes with age. Clin Manage Phys Ther, 4(5):12–15, 1984.

Neuberger, G.B.: The role of the nurse with arthritis patients on drug therapy. Nurs Clin North Am, 19(4):593–604, 1984.

Simpson, C.F.: Adult arthritis: heat, cold, or both? Am J Nurs, 83(2):270–273, 1983.

Walker, J.M., et al.: Active mobility of the extremities in older subjects. Phys Ther, 64(6):919–923, 1984.

Wingate, M.B.: Geriatric gynecology. Primary Care, 9(1):53–63, 1982.

Objectives

After completing this chapter, the student should be able to

- [ ] describe briefly the anatomy and physiology of the circulatory system
- [ ] identify the age-related changes in the circulatory system
- [ ] describe three age-related circulatory disorders
- [ ] explain how to assist patients and family members to adjust to the effects of vascular disease
- [ ] explain the significance of accurate vital signs
- [ ] list the common risks of anticoagulant therapy and the related nursing responsibilities
- [ ] explain digitalis toxicity

Vocabulary

aneurysm
apical
arteriosclerosis
atherosclerosis
edema
hypertension
varicose

242

CHAPTER **14**

The Circulatory System

Chapter Outline

☐ *Anatomy Review*

☐ FUNCTIONS

The blood is a vital fluid that distributes oxygen and food to all parts of the body while removing carbon dioxide, a waste product. It is kept moving by the continuous pumping action of the heart.

The blood also helps fight infection through the action (phagocytosis) of the white blood cells, and by its circulation, it helps to maintain our body temperature. For example, if we are too warm, the capillaries of the skin expand, more blood flows through them, and the increased blood volume allows for a greater heat exchange. This results in a lower body temperature.

When there is external trauma to a blood vessel, we observe another characteristic of blood. It clots. Normally, blood is a liquid that flows smoothly through our blood vessels. But if a vessel is damaged, blood cells called platelets plug it up and then start releasing substances that produce a clot. Eventually this forms a scab.

Clots also form inside a blood vessel when its inner smooth lining becomes rough through trauma or deposits. This process is called arteriosclerosis or atherosclerosis.

☐ STRUCTURES

Blood Vessels. Arteries, veins, and capillaries are the three types of blood vessels. Arteries carry blood *from* the heart toward capillaries in the body's tissues. Veins carry blood away from capillaries *toward* the heart. A capillary is the body's smallest blood vessel and it is just wide enough for a red blood cell to pass through. Capillaries are microscopic in size. In a schematic drawing they appear as a web of fine tubules that branch out from arteries and unite with venules (small veins). Thus the vessels form a closed system by which the blood circulates throughout the body.

The wall of an artery is tough and heavy; it must withstand a lot of pressure. The largest artery is the aorta. A vein is much thinner because the pressure of the blood within it is less. The largest vein is the vena cava.

Heart. The heart is a powerful, cone-shaped, hollow muscle. This tireless, fist-sized organ beats over 100,000 times a day to supply blood to over 100,000 miles of blood vessels in the body.

Inside the heart is a septum (partition) that divides it in half. The four chambers of the heart are the right and left atria and right and left ventricles. There also are valves that make sure the blood flows in the right direction. The tricuspid (three-pointed) valve is between the right atrium and the right ventricle; the mitral valve is between the left atrium and the left ventricle. Semilunar valves monitor the blood flowing from the ventricles to the arteries.

Each side of the heart has its own job. The right side takes blood that is loaded with carbon dioxide, a waste product, and pumps it *to* the lungs. There, the carbon dioxide is removed and oxygen is added. Then the left side of the heart receives the blood *from* the lungs and sends it throughout the body.

□ *Age-Related Changes*

□ ARTERIOSCLEROSIS

The most common type of vascular change that occurs in the aged is the development of arteriosclerosis, a condition marked by the loss of elasticity and associated thickening of the walls of the blood vessels, particularly the arteries. One type of arteriosclerosis is atherosclerosis. In this situation, plaque, deposits of fat and some calcium, builds up inside the arterial walls. It is unclear why this occurs. Contributing factors are hyperlipidemia, cigarette smoking, obesity, physical inactivity, high-fat diet, stress of disease, hereditary tendencies, and the aging process.

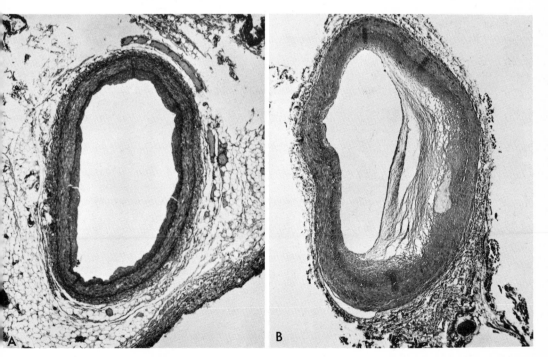

Figure 14–1 □ These photomicrographs show *(A)* a normal artery and *(B)* a diseased artery in which the channel is partially closed by atherosclerosis. (From Jacob, Francone, and Lossow, p. 393; courtesy of David M. Spain, M. D.)

The effects of arteriosclerosis are diverse. Systemically, it may result in an insufficient supply of blood to the cells of certain organs with the consequence that the cells die. Vital organs that can be affected are the brain, the heart, and the kidneys.

A local effect can also cause clotting problems. A healthy blood vessel collapses when it is cut, thereby encouraging clotting. Thickened arteries cannot collapse readily, so bleeding continues. That is why hemorrhage is a real threat to the elderly surgical patient. Perversely, the deposition of plaque on the blood vessel lining encourages clots to form and this is dangerous. These clots can occlude an artery, causing severe pain, necrosis, and ultimately, death.

□ VASCULAR DEGENERATION

Good health practices can prevent, or at least alleviate, the problems of vascular degeneration. For example, nicotine is a vasoconstrictor. Smoking contributes to vascular degeneration and should be discouraged in the interest of good health.

Neglected foot infections and varicose ulcers are commonly seen on the routine hospital admission of elderly patients. Although heredity plays a part in the development of varicose veins, obesity and poor posture (standing for long hours without a change of position or elevating the legs) increase the destructive process. Leg ulcers frequently occur in the elderly who have diabetes, and these lesions require prompt medical treatment. Nutritional adjustments, medications, warm compresses, and rest are utilized to bring relief.

□ REDUCED CARDIAC OUTPUT

In the elderly, each heartbeat puts out less blood volume than in younger persons. Reduced cardiac output and low maximum heart rate limit the amount of blood that flows to the various parts of the body. This explains why elderly people tire more easily than younger people. However, prudent exercise can increase endurance in the aged. Walking is the best exercise.

□ *Age-Related Disorders*

□ HYPERTENSION

Many elderly persons have high blood pressure due to the vasoconstriction associated with the aging process. The definition of hypertension given by the World Health Organization and by many life insurance companies is as follows: "Hypertension is a persistent elevation of the systolic blood pressure above 140 mm.Hg and of the diastolic pressure above 90 mm.Hg." *Blood pressure in elderly persons may be considerably higher and not be considered abnormal.* This points up the necessity for accurate readings and collection of data in order to form a baseline for comparison.

The nurse should take the patient's pressure in standing, sitting, and lying positions. Documentation about stress, anxiety, and activity prior to the blood pressure reading contributes to the data base.

Elderly persons who have diagnosed hypertension will be taught to reduce sodium intake, to reduce weight (if necessary), and to incorporate rest periods into their daily schedule.

□ HEART SIZE

The size of the heart does not change in the elderly as a rule. An enlarged heart indicates some heart disease; it is not a normal change due to aging. The resting heart rate does not change much with age either. But maximum heart rate decreases with age. For example, a 20 year old can, through exercise, increase his or her heart rate to more than 200 beats per minute. The average exercising 80 year old has a maximum heart rate of 120 to 130 beats per minute.

□ CONGESTIVE HEART FAILURE

Congestive heart failure (CHF) is characterized by diminished cardiac output. Food and oxygen no longer reach vital organs as needed. If the blood supply to the kidney is insufficient, sodium is not properly filtered. Patients will retain water, evidenced by the puffy, edematous legs of these people. The blood coming from veins and capillaries toward the heart backs up and congestion ensues. This contributes to dependent edema.

Acute care of the congestive heart failure patient is described in medical-surgical nursing texts. For long-term care or for the CHF patient at home, the following measures contribute to control of the disease:

1. emphasize the importance of taking medications exactly as ordered
2. confirm that the patient understands and follows the low sodium diet
3. check weight daily at the same time and in the same clothing to detect fluid retention
4. reduce stimulation in the environment
5. monitor visitors; avoid fatigue by pacing activities
6. stress recognition of danger signs of recurrent disease, e.g., shortness of breath; coughing; swelling of feet, legs, and ankles; and weight gain (Any of these symptoms should be immediately communicated to the physician.)

The nurse can educate and motivate the patient to follow a therapeutic program by being encouraging and reassuring in a relaxed, unhurried manner.

□ PULMONARY EDEMA

An outflow of serous fluid into the pulmonary interstitial tissues and air sacs is called pulmonary edema. This disorder is associated with congestive heart failure.

The patient appears dyspneic, cyanotic, and anxious. Pulse is rapid and cough is continual, resulting in *hemoptysis* (spitting up of blood). This is clearly an emergency situation because the patient can drown in his or her own secretions ("dry land drowning").

☐ AMPUTATIONS

When vascular problems do not respond to conservative treatment, an elderly patient may be faced with amputation. The shock is severe and demands not only the patient's physical care but also supportive emotional care. The nurse's attitude needs to be positive because the patient fears that if he or she has lost one foot (or leg) it will be only a matter of time before he or she loses the other. Postoperatively, independence and self-care should be encouraged as well as specific exercises designed to strengthen muscles and prevent flexion contractures.

☐ ANEURYSMS

Aneurysms usually occur in patients who have marked arteriosclerosis. Therefore, they are frequently seen in geriatric patients. An aneurysm is a ballooning out of the wall of an artery. The symptoms are severe pain, profound weakness, and shock. In this acute condition, surgery is the usual treatment.

☐ *Nursing Interventions*

☐ SOAKS

Warm soaks to the extremities are used to increase circulation, encourage healing, relax tissue, and inhibit infection. After soaking, medication may be applied. Soaks are a useful therapy, but they must be used with caution when the patient is elderly. *Many aged patients have peripheral circulatory problems and are vulnerable to heat injury.* They may not sense that the soak is too hot until damage has been done.

It is not practical to give a definite temperature and length of time for soaks. These judgments depend on the condition of the patient, the quality of the skin on the part to be soaked, and the size of the area to be soaked. Generally, most soaks involve putting an extremity into a prescribed solution for a given period of time. If there is an open wound, a sterile foot tub is obtained and dressings are applied as needed after the soak.

When a warm compress is ordered *to be applied continually*, the nurse uses an electric heating device designed to keep wet dressings warm at a constant temperature for an extended period of time. The usual safety precautions that apply to electrical devices are employed: checking wiring and plugs, avoiding the use of safety pins around the heating element, and, above all, emphasizing the *responsibility* of the patient to report any discomfort or over-heating.

☐ FOOT CARE

The geriatric patient often has foot problems that may be related to peripheral vascular disease. Good foot care can result in the patient's increased mobility. At the very least, it can prevent complications in patients who have diabetes and circulatory problems that affect the extremities.

Purposes

to improve circulation of the lower extremities
to prevent infection
to provide comfort
to promote cleanliness

Equipment

| basin | mild soap | nail clippers |
| soft cloth and towel | lotion | emery board |

Sequence

1. soak feet in lukewarm water
2. check skin surfaces for signs of infection, blisters, peeling, lesions
3. wash with mild soap, soft cloth
4. rinse
5. dry thoroughly and gently with soft towel, especially between the toes
6. trim nails with toenail clippers; smooth with emery board; *if nails are thick and long, a podiatrist should be employed*
7. apply lotion or cream before putting on clean socks or stockings

A daily foot soak and a daily change of socks and stockings that fit well are important. Self-care with OTC liquids that dissolve corns and calluses should be discouraged. They can be destructive to sensitive tissues. The elderly should also avoid using razor blades and pointed scissors for their foot care. Shoes should be well-constructed to give support and should be well-fitted for comfort.

☐ TAKING VITAL SIGNS

Vital signs, sometimes called cardinal symptoms, are those that can be measured. They are taken to help monitor a patient's condition. Strictly speaking, blood pressure and pulse (its rate and character) are the vital signs that belong with the circulatory system. However, procedures for taking respirations and temperature will be included in this section because these data are often obtained at the same time.

When an artery expands and contracts, the throbbing (pulse) that can be felt in an artery near the surface of the body is the blood being forced through the vessel by the beating of the heart. We usually time the pulse by locating the radial artery at the wrist. At times we take an apical pulse by counting the heartbeats with a stethoscope. (Other arteries where the pulse can be felt include the carotid, temporal, brachial, femoral, and popliteal arteries.)

Sequence for Taking Pulse (Radial)

1. identify patient; explain procedure
2. position patient's arm comfortably across his or her chest
3. place your first three or four fingers on the palm side of the patient's wrist close to the thumb (do not use *your* thumb; it has a pulse of its own)
4. time the pulse for 30 seconds if the beat is regular; if it is irregular, take the pulse for 1 full minute
5. note the character of the pulse, whether strong, weak, regular, irregular, bounding, and so on
6. document on graphic sheet as per institution's policy

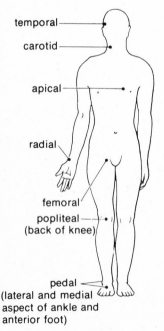

temporal
carotid
apical
radial
femoral
popliteal
(back of knee)
pedal
(lateral and medial
aspect of ankle and
anterior foot)

Figure 14–2 □ Common points at which the pulse is taken. (From Rambo and Wood, p. 416.)

GRAPHIC CHART

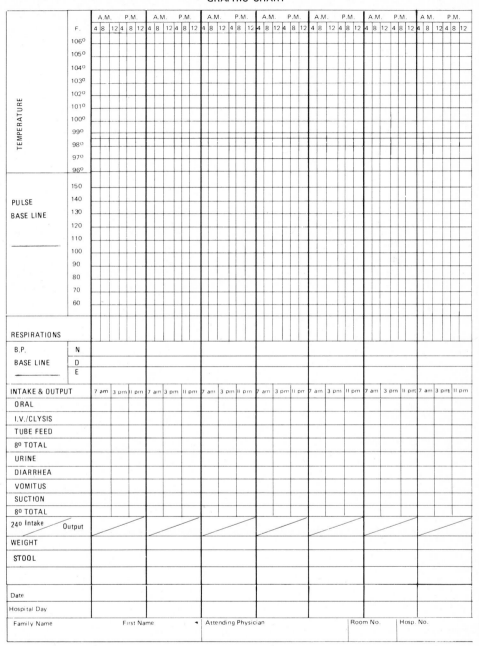

Figure 14–3 ☐ Graphic sheet used for documentation of temperature, pulse, and blood pressure.

Sequence for Taking Pulse (Apical)

1. using a stethoscope, listen for heartbeat to left of sternum
2. count heartbeat for 1 full minute by second hand of watch
3. document appropriately on a graphic sheet

Descriptions of any irregularity must be reported and documented. For example, tachycardia, bradycardia, and irregular pulse rhythm are significant and should be reported.

Respirations

Respirations should be counted when the patient is unaware of the procedure. This can be done at the time the pulse is being taken, when the patient has his or her arm across the chest. If someone knows his or her breathing rate is being timed, he or she may subconsciously alter it. The rate and character of respirations is noted to show either the progress or the change in a patient's condition.

One inhalation and one exhalation is counted as a respiration. A normal adult rate is about 16 per minute. Respirations are also described as shallow, labored, or difficult. If they fall into any of these categories, the patient's color should also be observed and the findings documented and reported.

Sequence for Taking Respirations

1. while taking pulse with patient's arm across chest, prepare to count respirations
2. observe each rise and fall of the chest and count as one respiration
3. time for 1 full minute
4. document as per hospital policy, recording rate, depth, and any unusual characteristics

Blood Pressure

Blood pressure is the force that the blood exerts against the walls of the arteries as it is being pumped through the body by the heart. The equipment used to measure it is a stethoscope and a blood pressure cuff (sphygmomanometer). There are two types of cuffs: a *mercury* sphygmomanometer has numbers on the glass column that contain the mercury, and the *aneroid* type has numbers on a dial that are read as the blood pressure is heard.

The reading obtained when the first sound is read measures the pressure of the blood at the height of the contraction phase of the heartbeat, which is called the *systole*. The reading at the last sound heard is a register of the blood pressure at the resting phase of the heart, called the *diastole*.

Arteries that have lost elasticity cause pressure to be high. Other factors responsible for high blood pressure are exercise, stimulants, and excitement.

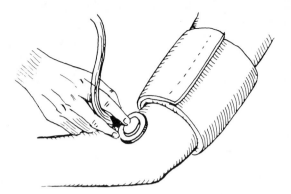

Figure 14–4 □ Blood pressure cuff. Stethoscope is placed in the antecubital space. (From Rambo and Wood, p. 430.)

Average adult pressure is 120 for systolic pressure and 80 for diastolic pressure (120/80), although these figures rise with age. A pressure of (150/90) might be considered normal for a person 70 years old. Generally, systolic pressures over 150 are considered high and diastolic pressures over 90 are also considered high. Low blood pressure in healthy adults is rarely significant (90 to 105 systolic). To take blood pressures,

1. identify patient; explain procedure
2. position patient's arm at the level of the heart
3. wrap cuff around patient's bare arm
4. locate brachial artery by palpation; place stethoscope over artery
5. inflate cuff while listening to pulsations
6. inflate cuff 20 points above that at which the pulse is no longer heard
7. slowly deflate cuff reading the *first* figure heard; the reading at this point is the systolic pressure
8. continue deflating cuff until *no* sound is heard; the reading at this point is diastolic pressure
9. document as per hospital policy; report abnormal readings immediately

   Note. Unless you use your own stethoscope remember to clean off the earpieces of the available stethoscope with an alcohol wipe.

Temperatures

Body temperature is the balance between the body's heat production and heat loss. Heat is generated by the metabolism of food. Exercise, external application of heat, and infection also cause an increase in body temperature. Heat is normally lost through perspiration and respiration. Hemorrhage and starvation also cause loss of body heat.

Two types of thermometers are used for registering body temperature— one based on the Fahrenheit scale and one based on the centigrade (or Celsius) scale. The Fahrenheit thermometer is most commonly used in health care facilities in the United States. Body temperature is most often taken by placing a thermometer under the tongue for 3 minutes, but in certain circumstances it can be taken by placing the thermometer in the rectum for 3 minutes or in the axilla for 10 minutes.

Some health facilities use electronic thermometers. The thermometer probe is covered with a disposable plastic probe cover and is inserted into the patient's mouth or rectum. The temperature is read on a small screen.

Note. It is important to wipe these devices with alcohol wipes between uses.

Normal oral adult body temperature is 98.6°F; the rectal temperature reading is usually 1° higher and an axillary temperature is usually 1° lower than an oral temperature. Elderly persons generally have slightly lower temperature. Early morning temperatures may seem to be very low (96°F). Slight elevations, therefore, may be significant. Baseline temperatures are important guidelines in geriatric nursing. Moreover, the geriatric nurse should be aware that all vital signs need to be checked accurately with careful attention given to changes.

Oral temperature must not be taken on

1. unconscious or confused patients
2. patients who have had oral surgery
3. certain patients on oxygen therapy
4. *any* patient with a condition for which the nurse deems it inadvisable to take the temperature orally.

Oral Temperatures

1. identify patient; explain procedure
2. check thermometer for possible defects (mercury that does not shake down, illegible markings, cracks, and so forth)

To convert centigrade to Fahrenheit, multiply by 9/5 and add 32. To change Fahrenheit to centigrade, subtract 32 and multiply by 5/9.

Examples of Equivalents

Centigrade	Fahrenheit
37.0	98.6
37.5	99.5
38.0	100.4
38.5	101.3
39.0	102.2
40.0	104.0
41.0	105.8

---

3. shake thermometer until mercury registers 96°F or below
4. place under patient's tongue; tell patient *not* to bite down; tell patient to keep in place in *closed* mouth for 3 minutes
5. remove thermometer, read; record reading

6. clean and care for thermometer as per facility's policy
7. document temperature reading; report abnormalities immediately
   Rectal Temperatures
1. identify patient, explain procedure, screen patient
2. lubricate end of rectal thermometer (after previous steps 2 and 3)
3. place patient in lateral position
4. insert thermometer 1 ½ inches and *hold* it for 3 minutes
5. remove thermometer after 3 minutes; wipe clean; read and record
6. care for thermometer as per facility's policy
7. document reading, report temperature of over 100°F immediately
   Note. Rectal temperatures are contraindicated in cases of rectal surgery or rectal inflammations.
   Axillary Temperatures
   If both oral and rectal temperature measurements are contraindicated for any reason, an axillary temperature may be taken
1. identify patient, explain procedure
2. dry axilla; repeat steps 2 and 3 of *Oral Temperatures*
3. place thermometer in axilla for 10 minutes; *hold thermometer* if patient is unable to cooperate
4. read and record as per facility's policy

□ ELASTICIZED STOCKINGS

Common peripheral circulatory problems cause edema and swelling in the lower extremities. Even after an attack of phlebitis has been cured, the damage to the valves in the vein may be such that they can no longer prevent backflow. This results in chronic venostasis, swelling, edema, and, eventually, leg ulcers. Elasticized stockings are useful in the conservative management of this condition. These stockings help to prevent backflow of blood in the lower extremities. They must be correctly fitted so as to exert uniformly decreasing pressure from the foot upward. The stockings may be ordered in two lengths; foot to below the knee and foot to thigh.

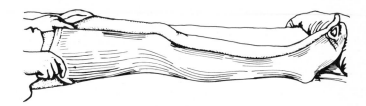

Figure 14–5 □ Elastic stockings help prevent backflow of blood in the lower extremities. The stockings are removed several times a day to check the skin color. The toes can be checked more frequently through the opening. (From Dugas, p. 583.)

These stockings should be changed daily. If the patient is confined to bed, the feet and legs should be bathed at least daily and the stockings removed and *reapplied* twice a day.

Sequence

1. identify and screen patient; explain procedure
2. check to be sure legs and feet are clean and dry. If there is an ulceration, be sure that the dressing is dry and intact
3. lightly powder the foot to decrease friction
4. roll stocking; stretch and ease over toes, gradually unrolling as foot and leg are covered
5. check toes for motion and sensitivity after stockings are on

☐ ELASTICIZED BANDAGES

Ace or tensor bandages are made of woven elastic and covered with another fiber. They are used to support or immobilize an extremity, to apply pressure to a part of the body, to hold a bulky dressing in place, or if the patient has a skin reaction to tape of any kind.

An Ace bandage should be applied firmly enough to keep it in place but not so tightly that it interferes with circulation. When used on an extremity, the arm or leg should be observed at regular intervals for color, motion, and sensitivity.

Elasticized bandages come in a wide variety of widths and lengths. They are used only by a physician's order.

☐ STUMP BANDAGING, STUMP CARE

As with all surgery, postoperative orders vary with the individual. Generally, early ambulation is encouraged. Casts are often used and patients may be able to use a prosthesis after 24 hours. An elderly patient needs special care because he or she may be dazed by the surgery and may not appear to know what type of surgery was performed even though he or she knew before the operation. Postoperative care includes

1. observation for shock and hemorrhage (tourniquet to be kept at bedside stand)
2. use of stump sock to help shrink and shape stump to prosthesis
3. use of elasticized bandage with or without stump sock
4. encouraging patient to turn from side to side and to assume prone position if possible to help prevent flexion contractures
5. elevating lower part of bed rather than elevating stump on pillow. The stump should *not* be held up in a flexed position as this might cause a permanent flexion deformity.

□ NURSING CARE DURING DRUG THERAPY

Anticoagulant Therapy

An anticoagulant is a medication that delays the clotting time of the blood and prevents further clot formation. Anticoagulant therapy is prescribed for patients with thrombophlebitis, recurrent clot formation, congestive heart failure, and hip fractures that may immobilize an elderly patient for a long time.

This therapy is not without risk and some physicians feel that the risks outweigh the gains. The primary complication is bleeding from or into any part of the body. Some examples are bruises caused by trauma to tissues, bleeding from minor cuts such as shaving nicks, bleeding from the nose, bleeding from the gums, bleeding from IV sites, bleeding from the urinary or gastrointestinal tracts, and hematoma at the injection sites.

Anticoagulants

Heparin sodium derivatives	*Coumarin derivatives*
(parenterally administered)	*(administered orally)*
Heprinar	Dicumarol
Lipo-Hepin	Coumadin
Panheprin	

Nursing Responsibilities

1. *warn patient not to take any other medication without the physician's knowledge*
2. tell patient to inform other health care professionals (dentists, podiatrists) that he or she is on anticoagulants
3. advise wearing of Medic-alert bracelet
4. emphasize the importance of the prescribed laboratory tests (prothrombin time, clotting time)
5. inspect the skin for bruises
6. report any bleeding from nose, mouth, or gums
7. observe urine for any signs of blood

Note. Anticoagulants used along with the following drugs have an enhanced effect: anabolic agents, clofibrate, phenylbutazone, and salicylates.

Also, when administering anticoagulants the nurse should verify the most recent laboratory values first.

Other Circulatory Drugs (Cardiotonics, Allied Glycosides)

Digitalis preparations are among the most widely used and most dependable drugs in the treatment of congestive heart failure. Some examples are

Digoxin	Digitoxin
Lanoxin	Crystodigin
	Purodigin

Digitalis preparations have two functions: slowing of the heart rate and strengthening the force of myocardial contraction.

When digitalis has improved myocardial contraction, circulatory functioning is restored.

Digitalis toxicity is a potential problem for all persons receiving the drug. Therefore, the nurse must recognize these major symptoms:

1. nausea, vomiting, diarrhea, anorexia
2. headache, fatigue, lethargy, restlessness, irritability
3. arrhythmias: bradycardia, tachycardia
4. double vision, blurred vision
5. gynecomastia in men

In all drug administration, it is essential to read labels carefully. Digitalis is prepared under several names and with widely varying strengths and dosages. Both patient and caregiver must be instructed to have digitalis medications checked by the physician on a regular basis in order to avoid unnecessary drug taking.

Note. The apical pulse is always taken for 1 full minute before any digitalis preparation is administered. If the rate is below 60 or above 100 the medication is withheld and the physician informed.

Chapter 14 ☐ Review Questions

MULTIPLE CHOICE

1. The blood, a vital fluid, removes wastes. An example of a waste product is
   A. oxygen
   B. carbon dioxide
   C. lipoproteins
   C. triglycerides
2. Another term for arteriosclerosis is
   A. atelectasis
   B. athetosis
   C. atherosclerosis
   D. astereognosis
3. A radial pulse is taken
   A. behind the knee
   B. over the heart
   C. at the temple
   D. at the wrist
4. The patient with congestive heart failure should immediately report
   A. shortness of breath
   B. drowsiness
   C. pruritus
   D. anxiety
5. Elderly patients receiving soaks are vulnerable to
   A. jaundice

    B. dyspnea

    C. heat injury

    D. diaphoresis

6. An elderly person's blood pressure is typically

    A. higher than a younger person's

    B. lower than a younger person's

    C. the same as it was in his or her youth

    D. difficult to determine

7. Elastic stockings are used to

    A. maintain alignment after a fracture

    B. keep the feet warm

    C. prevent pooling of blood in the legs

    D. prevent skin damage

DISCUSSION QUESTIONS

1. Outline a plan for a discharged congestive heart failure patient. Describe teaching for the patient and the caregiver.
2. Describe the action of digitalis preparations and identify the signs of digitalis toxicity.
3. Develop a check list that illustrates nursing responsibilities for the administration of anticoagulants.

□ REFERENCES

Boruch, I.M.: Heart rate response of elder women to non weight bearing ambulation with a walker. Phys Ther, 63(11):1782–1787, 1983.

Fogarty, T.J., et al.: A new approach to transliminal angioplasty. CVP, 12(2):14–16, 20, 22–24, 1984.

Galli, M.: Promoting self care in hypertensive clients through patient education. Home Health Nurs, 2(2):43–45, 1984.

Johnson, P.T.: Black hypertension: a transcultural case study using the Neuman model of nursing care. Issues Health Women, 4(2/3):191–210, 1983.

Haviland, S., and Garlinghouse, C.: Nursing foot clinics fulfill a great need. Geriatr Nurs, 6:338, 1985.

MacMurray, R.J.: Know your blood pressure and live longer. Your Life Health, 97(4):9–11, 1982.

McCauley, K., et al.: Your detailed guide to drugs for congestive heart failure. Nursing (Horsham), 14(5):46–50, 1984.

McCauley, K., et al.: Congestive heart failure: a step by step guide to better nursing management. Nurs Life, 4(3)(Suppl.):33–40, 1984.

Plunkett, L.W., et al.: Mild hypertension: the continuing dilemma of treatment. Family Community Health, 7(11):38–46, 1984.

Rahimtoola, S.H.: Options for the failing heart ... digitalis reexamined. Emergency Med, 16(15):46–50, 1984.

Wallis, C.: The fatty diet under attack. Time, 124(26):58, 1984.

Weber, K., et al.: Advances in the evaluation and management of chronic cardiac failure. Chest, 85(2):253–259, 1984.

Yen, P.K.: Fat, cholesterol and a healthy older heart. Geriatr Nurs, 5(6):254, 257, 1984.

Zeigler, M.G.: Mild hypertension: concentrate of treatment without drugs. Consultant, 24(1): 320–321, 1984.

Objectives

After completing this chapter, the student should be able to

- [ ] describe briefly the anatomy and physiology of the genitourinary system
- [ ] list the age-related changes and the age-related disorders of the genitourinary system
- [ ] assist with a pelvic examination
- [ ] institute measures that help induce voiding
- [ ] identify important factors of bladder training
- [ ] describe procedures related to the genitourinary system, e.g., catheterization, Foley catheter care, and douching

Vocabulary

dyspareunia
Escherichia coli
nocturia
polyuria
prepuce
pyuria
turgor

CHAPTER

The Genitourinary System

Chapter Outline

☐ Anatomy Review

☐ STRUCTURES AND FUNCTIONS

Kidneys. The kidneys, two bean-shaped organs that lie just below the diaphragm on the posterior abdominal wall on either side of the spine and behind the peritoneum, are very important organs of excretion. Blood reaches the kidneys by way of the renal arteries and wastes are strained from the blood as it passes through the kidneys.

Nephrons. Nephrons are the kidneys' filtering units and there are millions of them screening out substances not needed by the body. Nephrons accept certain substances from the blood, and these substances are reabsorbed into the body. They also regulate water and electrolyte balance. The body has tremendous reserves; we can lose vast amounts of nephrons to age and disease and still live. In fact, we can lose a kidney, one half of the filtering "team," and live normally.

Urine. Urine is the end product of the primary functions of the nephrons. It consists of filtered waste substances, excess salts, and water (Table 15–1). Certain conditions of the urine mean that disease is present. For example, sugar in the urine (*glycosuria*) can indicate diabetes mellitus. Pus in the urine (*pyuria*) indicates an infection in the urinary system. Copious, dilute urine (*polyuria*) is a symptom of diabetes insipidus.

Bladder. The bladder is a hollow muscular organ that acts as a storage vessel for urine. A bladder may hold 1000 ml. of urine, but the urge to void is felt at 200 to 400 ml.

Ureters. The body has two ureters. They are tubes, each about 25 cm. (10 inches) long, that extend from the renal pelvis (the kidney interior) to the bladder. Urine is passed from the kidneys into the ureters and then propelled by peristalsis down the ureters until it pools in the bladder.

Table 15–1 ☐ **Values of Components Found in Normal Urine of a Healthy Person**

Routine Urinalysis	Normal Value
Appearance	Clear, straw color
Specific gravity	1.010 to 1.025
pH	4.5 to 7.5
Erythrocytes—RBCs	Occasional cell
Leukocytes—WBCs	Less than 4 per high power field
Casts	0
Crystals	Most are not significant
Acetone—ketone bodies	0
Glucose	0
Protein—albumin	0

From Rambo, B.J.: Adaptation Nursing. Philadelphia, W. B. Saunders Company, 1984, p. 171.

Urethra. The urethra is also a tube, but thicker than the ureter. It extends from the bladder to the exterior. In the male, the urethra is about 8 inches long because it runs through the penis. In the female, it is about 1½ inches long. Urine does not drip right through the bladder and urethra to the outside because a sphincter controls the meatus, which is the opening at the end of the urethra through which urine passes out of the body. The bladder relaxes and expands as the urine begins to fill it. As it fills to a certain level, contractions are triggered that force the fluid to exert pressure against the base of the urethra and the sphincter muscle. This we interpret as the desire to urinate.

□ Age-Related Changes

Loss of Nephrons. With aging, the kidneys function less efficiently. The number of nephrons decreases. A newborn has about a million nephrons in each kidney. A 75-year-old has about half that number. The nephron, which filters the blood, also regulates the acid base balance in blood plasma. This is important to know when giving medications to the elderly because of the lesser number of nephrons in the older person's body. Thus, an elderly patient may exhibit an undesirable reaction to an average adult dosage of a drug.

Arteriosclerotic Changes. Arteriosclerosis may affect the blood vessels that supply blood to the urinary system. The reduction in the amount of blood going to the kidneys lowers their ability to resist infection and to recover from trauma.

Reduced Muscle Tone of Genitourinary Organs. The bladder, ureters, and urethra become less elastic with age and have poorer muscle tone. The capacity of the bladder often diminishes by half, and the urge to urinate does not occur until that capacity is nearly reached. As a consequence, many elderly are troubled by frequency, urgency, and nocturia. In an institutional setting where an elderly patient is on medication and is confined to bed, incontinence often develops.

Prostatic Enlargement. In elderly males a common problem is enlargement of the prostate gland that surrounds the urethra. Symptoms of benign prostatic hypertrophy are nocturia, difficulty in starting to urinate, and narrowing of the stream (because of the obstruction). The treatment is surgical intervention for prostatectomy.

□ Age-Related Disorders

Calculi. Residual urine is often associated with the development of calculi. If an elderly patient is immobilized, for example, with a fractured hip, the chance of developing calculi increases. Although the cause of stone formation is not completely understood, we do know that with failure to excrete certain substances (uric acid, calcium phosphate) stones may form.

Glomerulonephritis. Glomerulonephritis is present in many aged patients who do not have any obvious symptoms. It frequently is not discovered until there is a noticeable elevation of blood pressure or swelling of the extremities. Stroke can trigger glomerulonephritis. Beginning symptoms are polyuria, nocturia, and frequency. In severe cases the body becomes "waterlogged" with fluid collecting in the chest cavity, the abdominal cavity (ascites), and the sac that encloses the heart. If the condition is unchecked, the patient slips into uremia.

Urinary Tract Infections. Escherichia coli is a bacterium that is a normal inhabitant of the human intestinal tract. It is frequently a cause of infections in the urinary tract. Hospital employees who do not practice good personal hygiene may carry this organism on their hands and so infect either themselves or their patients. Other bacteria can cause such infections. Obviously, the elderly patient who is confined to bed or has an indwelling Foley catheter is especially vulnerable. Ambulatory elderly patients may develop urinary tract infections if they do not use proper hygienic measures after urinating or after a bowel movement. Nurses should see that these patients wash their hands before meals and after using the bathroom. Nurses themselves must do the same and, in addition, they must wash their hands after handling drainage tubing or bags and before giving direct patient care. Good nursing care includes encouraging fluids, observing and reporting temperature elevations and foul smelling urine, and giving special care to the external urinary meatus of any patient with an indwelling Foley catheter by washing the genitals when giving the daily bath.

Pyelonephritis is a serious urinary tract infection often seen concurrently with another infection. For example, a patient who has an oral infection may develop a kidney infection. Any one of many pathogenic bacteria may cause pyelonephritis.

If the passage of urine from the kidney to the bladder is slowed down for any reason, an infection such as pyelonephritis can ensue. Particular attention must be paid to a patient who has an obstruction anywhere in the urinary tract or who has urinary stasis because the microorganisms migrate upward. Likely candidates are those who are immobilized for a long period of time. Meticulous catheter care of the patients who have indwelling (Foley) catheters and handwashing after touching *any* such patient with a catheter are essential. *Health care personnel must wash hands when going from patient to patient because the microorganisms that thrive in the drainage bags are extremely resistant to antibiotics.*

Cystitis is an inflammation of the urinary bladder. Pathogens migrate from the kidneys downward or from the urethra up to the bladder. There are numerous other causes: enlarged prostate, urethral stricture, kidney infection, and, in women, improper perineal hygiene. Also, as mentioned earlier, the bladder loses muscle tone over the years. In fact, some bladders actually develop diverticuli; i.e., they become floppy with pockets that trap urine. When this residual urine becomes infected, cystitis results. Whereas an elderly person may put off seeking medical help for many infirmities, they usually consult a physician for cystitis because of the painful urination that accompanies this infection.

Women have a much higher incidence of cystitis than men because of their short urethra and the location of the meatus, which is easily contaminated by the organisms that are natural to the rectum. Cystitis is painful. It is characterized by frequency, burning upon urination, and elevated temperature. Antibiotics, increased fluids, and rest are measures to treat cystitis. In females, the importance of avoiding contamination and of wiping from the front to the back after voiding and defecating must be emphasized.

Vaginitis. Atrophy of the female reproductive tract progresses slowly but steadily after menopause, and atrophic vaginitis causes considerable distress for some elderly females. Three problems plague the shrinking vagina: thinning of the epithelium, decrease in estrogen production, and lack of acidity of the vaginal secretions. Irritation or pruritis because of decline in secretions may also be present. Left untreated, adhesions, infection, and dyspareunia (painful intercourse) can result.

Cancer. Cancer is the second major disorder of the aged. The genitourinary sites in women are

vulva	leukoplakia (thickened white patches) often is the first sign; precancerous lesion
vagina	seldom a primary site; usually is involved secondarily
cervix	more common in women of menopausal age than in elderly women
uterus	endometrial cancer is common; endometrial polyps can be precancerous
ovaries	high incidence in aged women
bladder	seen in elderly women but more common in aged men
breast	a significant cause of cancer deaths in elderly women

Prophylaxis is emphasized: the Papanicolaou (Pap) smear, physical examination of the pelvic organs, and prompt investigation of any bleeding from the body's orifices are means of identifying and controlling cancer. The nurse can also encourage the elderly woman to learn how to do a breast self-examination and to do it monthly.

Genitourinary cancer sites in men are

bladder	common cancer in the elderly, but significantly higher incidence in males; painless bleeding usually the first sign; linked to smoking
prostate	benign prostatic hypertrophy affects virtually all elderly males. The prostate can be examined by a physician during an annual checkup. Since urinary difficulty occurs mainly in men over 60, a physician's examination is necessary to determine whether the problem is benign prostatic hypertrophy or cancer of the prostate.

□ Nursing Interventions

Genitourinary problems are distressing, embarrassing, and annoying. Unfortunately, they are often regarded philosophically and are accepted as "to be expected" because of advancing years. The danger is that what some people are passing off as caused by old age may be early warning signs of infection or malignancy.

Elderly men have difficulty in accepting significant symptoms and they may misinterpret medical advice. Any threat to masculinity is intolerable—at any age. The nurse's attitude can generate trust and motivation. Shame and fear make patients delay the investigation of symptoms. Education of the genitourinary patient, particularly by stressing the seven danger signs of cancer, can help prevent the tragic outcome of neglect that so often shows up in physicians' offices and in hospitals.

□ ASSISTING WITH THE PELVIC EXAMINATION

Nurses can gain their patients' confidence and cooperation by giving a simple explanation of what is to be done and why. The nurse should bear in mind that the elderly patient may have limited movement in the joints, especially the hips. The lithotomy position may be uncomfortable. However, with the proper reassurance, draping, and adequate lighting the vaginal area can be visualized. The nurse can help the patient relax by *staying* at her side and holding her hand during the examination.

Purposes

to prepare the patient for a pelvic examination
to take care of any specimens obtained

Equipment

bath blanket	sterile glove	materials that may be
speculum	small hand towel	needed for taking
lubricant	small pillow	specimens

Sequence

1. identify patient; introduce self; explain procedure; have patient void; cleanse perineal area
2. assist patient onto examining table; position on table: legs in stirrups, pillow under head
3. drape with bath blanket after patient has hips brought down to end of table
4. reassure patient; adjust light for physician
5. if Papanicolaou smear is to be taken, have swabs, glass slide, and fixative ready for physician
6. be sure specimen is properly labeled
7. dry perineal area with hand towel (there may be some traces of lubricant left from the speculum)
8. remove both legs simultaneously from stirrups
9. encourage elderly patient to sit for a few minutes before getting off examining table
10. help patient with putting on gown or assist with dressing if needed

□ MEASURES TO INDUCE VOIDING

The nurse should be familiar with many separate ways of helping the patient who has difficulty voiding. Inability to pass urine is uncomfortable and anxiety producing. The nurse's "bag of tricks" should include the following:

1. offer fluids, particularly warm drinks
2. have the patient blow bubbles through a straw in a glass of water (blowing relaxes the urethra)
3. let the patient listen to running water
4. place patient's hands in a basin of water
5. give patient a sitz bath (with physician's or supervisor's permission)
6. try to place the female patient in a sitting position—this position is the preferred position for females
7. if the male patient's condition permits, have him stand at the bedside
8. give a *warm* bedpan
9. place the patient on a bedpan and pour warm water over the genitalia
10. apply gentle downward pressure on the lower abdomen
11. have patient bend forward and rock gently
12. put spirits of peppermint *on* a cotton ball *in* a paper medicine cup *in* the bedpan (why this works is unclear—it may be that the vapors from the spirits of peppermint are warm and that this relaxes the sphincter muscle)

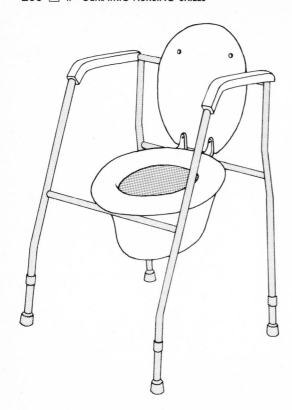

The bedside commode encourages bowel and bladder functioning. It is a better choice than a bedpan, if the person can get out of bed to use it. In the home, if the patient cannot walk to the bathroom (e.g., the bathroom is on another floor), various kinds of commodes are available. A small amount of water added to the commode before use facilitates cleaning it after use.

The most important move of all when trying to induce voiding is to help the patient relax. Providing privacy and time helps, as does a lessening of emotional tension. *Frequently, all that is needed is to leave the patient alone for a few moments.*

☐ PROVIDING THE BEDPAN AND URINAL

Bedpans, urinals, and commodes are used to provide for a patient's elimination and to aid in measuring output. Patients who cannot ambulate, should be given the opportunity to use a bedpan or urinal before starting any treatments and before leaving the room for trips to x-ray and physical therapy. Use of the bathroom or commode is preferable. For the patient who cannot move from the bed, however, the nurse should offer the bedpan before each meal, when the patient awakens in the morning, and at bedtime.

Purposes

to give and remove a bedpan and urinal
to measure and record output
to collect a specimen

Equipment

bedpan or urinal	towel	basin of water
cover	toilet tissue	room deodorizer
soap		

Sequence

1. identify patient; introduce self; screen patient; elevate bed to level of comfort
2. run hot water over rim of pan if necessary to warm it
3. if possible, have the patient help by digging his or her heels into the bed and pushing up on his or her elbows while the nurse places a hand under the lower back and slides bedpan or urinal into place
4. for a helpless patient, roll patient on to side with the aid of another person; position pan against buttocks and roll patient back on pan; *then* elevate bed after patient is positioned correctly
5. leave patient with call signal and toilet tissue at hand
6. remove bedpan as it was given, remembering to use bedpan cover
7. roll helpless patient on side, wrap tissue around hand and wipe from pubic area to anus; use wet cloth if necessary; inspect the perineum carefully to check for redness or excoriation
8. do not discard contents of any bedpan until you are sure contents do not have to be measured *or* that a specimen does not have to be taken
9. collect specimens as per hospital policy, being careful not to let toilet tissue get into bedpan
10. offer basin of water, soap, and towel to patient or wash the patient's hands if he or she is unable to do so.
11. Clean and replace equipment and wash your hands.

A way to clean an incontinent patient is to have the patient sit on the bedpan and pour a quantity of warm water over the perineal area. This helps prevent skin problems and contributes to a feeling of cleanliness.

Very thin patients should have the bedpan padded with a folded towel as a comfort measure. When there is a problem in sitting on a bedpan either because of dressings, contractures, or casts, a fracture pan should be offered.

The nurse should remember that it can be very embarrassing for people to have to use a bedpan. And, although it would be ideal for male patients to

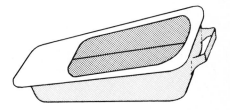

Fracture pan. The fracture pan is useful for the person confined to bed who has very limited mobility.

be given bedpans and urinals by male attendants, it is not always possible. A cheerful, matter-of-fact attitude demonstrates a sincere interest in the patient's well-being and lessens self-consciousness.

☐ INCONTINENCE

Urinary incontinence (involuntary voiding) is as distressing to patients as it is to nurses. Stress incontinence is the involuntary escape of urine that occurs with straining, such as heavy lifting, sneezing, coughing, or laughing. The literature review suggests that the prevalence of urinary incontinence is greater in women (Simons, 1985). There is also strong indication that there is a lack of interest on the part of health care providers in the problem of incontinence (Simons, 1985).

The fact that urinary incontinence occurs most often in women is thought to be due to their shorter urethras. The incontinence may occur as early as middle age in otherwise well women. It appears to be more prevalent in women who have had a number of pregnancies.

Urinary incontinence sometimes occurs temporarily after an operation. It can also result from diseases of the nerves and muscles of the bladder. There may be a complete inability to control the flow of urine and, as a result, a constant dribbling occurs.

Bladder Training

The first step in a bladder retraining program is an assessment of bladder function and urinary output (Table 15–2). The nurse will have to document the amount of voiding in a 24-hour period, the number of voidings, and the amount voided each time. Retraining can be achieved by following a regular schedule. At first, the interval between trips to the bathroom or times when the urinal or bedpan is offered is short. The interval is gradually lengthened, and within a few days the patient will usually begin to feel the stimulus to urinate. At first, an hour is usually as long as the patient can retain urine. This period, however, can be lengthened gradually to 2 then to 3 or 4 hours.

When the patient is fully prepared to undertake a program for developing urinary continence, certain general rules for bladder training may be followed:
1. encourage daily fluid intake of approximately 2000 to 2500 ml. per day
2. record voidings in order to establish a pattern; involve the patient in record keeping, if possible
3. encourage voiding shortly after taking fluids
4. take patient to bathroom every 2 to 3 hours (or offer urinal or bedpan), especially first thing in the morning and periodically after meals
5. teach patient perineal exercises (Kegel exercises), that is, how to contract muscles as though trying to stop urinating followed by relaxing them; done 10 to 15 times daily, these exercises help tone muscles that are involved in voiding

Table 15–2 □ Assessment of Bladder Function and Urinary Output

Factors to Assess	Normal Behaviors	Maladaptive Behaviors
Characteristics of urinary output	_____ ml./24 hr.	Less than 25–30 ml./hr. Oliguria, anuria Less than 100 ml./voiding
Components	Clear, yellow to amber Normal urinalysis	Contains glucose, blood, protein, acetone, sediment Other: _____
Control	Continent, controls sphincter Can stop and start stream	Loss of control, dribbling Retention of urine
Sensation	Voids easily No discomfort	Pain on voiding, bladder spasms, urgency, burning, frequency, or bladder distention
Altered means	Voids normally	Use of catheter, cystostomy catheter, ureterostomy tube, or urinary diversion

From Rambo, B.J.: Adaptation Nursing. Philadelphia, W. B. Saunders Company, 1984, p. 171.

6. keep the incontinent patient clean, dry, and comfortable when incontinence has occurred
7. observe skin frequently for rashes
8. use tact and understanding; offer emotional support; encourage and praise successes

The nurse must carefully evaluate the patient before undertaking a program of bladder training. If total continence is not possible, the goal should be adjusted to meet the patient's needs. Perhaps daytime continence would be a more realistic goal.

If continence is not possible and a medical evaluation of the problem has been made, then protective undergarments should be used. Again, careful attention to hygiene and a supportive attitude on the part of the nurse are essential to preserve the dignity and self esteem of the patient.

External Appliances

External appliances for collecting urine are available for male patients. A rubber bag that slips over the penis and is fastened to a belt and also secured to the patient's leg may be worn inconspicuously under clothing.

Incontinent females wear protective panties or perineal pads. There is no external urinary device for females. In the last 3 to 4 years, manufacturers have developed many new disposable materials for incontinence use. They are advertised both in media for health care workers and directly to the public. There are advantages and disadvantages to disposable products versus reusable (washable) garments and pads. Some aspects to consider are price, convenience, effectiveness, effect on skin condition, comfort, ease of use, and esthetics. Some adults who have compared disposable to reusable products rate the disposable poorly because they create noise when the person moves, causing embarrassment.

The Incontinent Person at Home

Incontinence at home is just as traumatic and embarrassing as incontinence in a hospital or nursing home. At no time should the patient at home believe that incontinence must be accepted because of aging. If there is no medical reason why incontinence exists, then bladder retraining should be implemented.

The best way to deal with incontinence is to prevent accidents. If, in spite of preventive measures, accidents do occur, the caregiver should deal with the problem quickly and nonjudgmentally.

- Offer the bedpan, urinal, or use of the commode regularly and frequently for the bed-confined person.
- Do not focus attention on the incontinence in a way that is demeaning, i.e., using diapers or placing an absorbent pad directly underneath the patient. It can be traumatic to the self esteem of the elderly person for it to be obvious that she or he is incontinent. An absorbent pad can be slipped into a pillowcase that is the same color as the linen on the bed or into a cover that looks like a chair cushion. This reduces attention to the problem and allows the person to maintain dignity.
- Purchase knit underpants with replaceable high-absorbency pads (Dignity, available through Humanicare International Inc., 5 Joanna Court, East Brunswick, N.J. 08816). Another alternative is checking with local surgical supply stores and pharmacies that stock various products.
- Incontinence in the elderly home patient ranges from occasional stress incontinence to total dependence on the family for personal care. For the patient who is alert and aware, the nurse can explain the causes of incontinence and options for control, allowing the patient to choose his or her own plan of care. An incontinent person in the home can be a strain on the whole family, and the nurse needs to help the family in selecting the best options for control.

Note. Patients and caregivers may be taught the Credé method of emptying the bladder after bladder training. Either patient or caregiver makes a fist and presses down directly over the bladder and down toward the pubic bone with a kneading motion.

☐ OBTAINING A URINE SPECIMEN

At one time all specimens for a urine culture were obtained by catheterization. Within the last few years, however, *clean catch specimens* have been found acceptable for this laboratory test. The nurse should first determine whether "midstream" and "clean catch" are used synonymously. Then she or he should find out if the container must be sterile (many agencies use "clean", not sterile, containers). Once there is a clear understanding of terms, the nurse may proceed to collect the specimen.

There are many elderly patients who are capable of carrying out this procedure without the assistance of the nurse. Simply review the instructions to be sure the patient understands what is expected of him or her.

Equipment

sterile disposable "clean
  catch" pack
OR sterile collection container

antiseptic swabs
clean gloves
sterile bedpan or urinal (optional)

Sequence

1. identify patient; introduce self; explain procedure; screen patient
2. inspect perineal area to be sure external meatus is clean
3. wearing clean gloves, wash off external meatus area with antiseptic swabs (keep labia of female patient separated)
4. if the patient is confined to bed, place a female on a bedpan and have her void a small amount into the pan; now, holding the sterile container at the meatus, let the urine fall directly into it (Some agencies have patient void into a *sterile* bedpan and then collect the specimen; check policy of health care facility); offer a urinal to a male patient; instruct him to void a small amount into the urinal and then to void directly into the sterile specimen container
5. provide whatever aftercare is necessary
6. label specimen; record procedure; take or send specimen to laboratory

□ RECORDING INTAKE AND OUTPUT

About two thirds of the body's weight is water. It is important that the amount of fluid taken in by the body compensates for the amount of fluid used and excreted by the body. This is what fluid balance means.

The elderly adult needs about 2500 ml. (about 2½ quarts) of oral fluids daily, and the nurse should encourage adequate fluid intake. *Some elderly people restrict their fluids for fear of incontinence or because they hope to avoid frequency and nocturia.*

The body tolerates losing body weight better than losing body fluids. Fluids leave the body in urine, feces, respiration, perspiration, wound drainage, and vomitus. A hospitalized patient may lose more fluid than is normal because of severe vomiting, diarrhea, and fever.

An elderly patient will react to dehydration in the following ways: loss of skin turgor, dry mouth, elevated urea levels in the blood, and confusion. Inadequate fluids can also result in infections and constipation. Conversely, overhydration can pose a threat to the aged adult because of decreased renal and cardiovascular functioning with resulting collection of fluid in the tissues.

There are medical reasons for the physician to order the intake and output of the patient to be measured. It is helpful in making a diagnosis, in evaluating the condition of a patient, and in monitoring the action of drugs.

Patients who are edematous may be on diuretics. Nursing considerations here (besides recording of intake and output) are daily weight-taking and replacement of lost electrolytes. Electrolytes are salts in the blood, mainly potassium, sodium, calcium, and bicarbonate. Diuretics are used to eliminate sodium, which is the cause of fluid retention. To some extent, potassium is also eliminated. Potassium may be replaced by medications or by eating foods that are rich in potassium, namely, bananas, raisins, orange juice, cabbage, and celery.

Intake and output records must be accurate. For example, if a 120 ml. glass of juice is on the patient's tray and he or she drinks only half of it, 60 ml. is recorded. Intake fluids recorded are

fluids administered parenterally
water, juices, soft drinks, milk
tea, coffee
soups
jello
ice cream
dietary supplemental drinks (Ensure, Sustecal, and so on)

Output recorded includes urine, feces, perspiration (slight, moderate, profuse), any vomitus, wound drainage, and suction drainage.

Most agencies have the intake and output sheet taped to the patient's door or to the bedside stand. Entries must be prompt, accurate, and neat.

Purposes

to find out how much fluid has been gained or lost from the body
to determine whether the patient is dehydrated
to learn the results of fluid restriction
to keep an accurate record of fluids taken and excreted

Equipment

fluid balance record on patient's chart
intake and output sheet   calibrated graduate

	MERCY HOSPITAL Springfield, Mass.			
	INTAKE AND OUTPUT CHART			

Water, cup 210 cc Cooked cereal, fruit juices, pudding,
Coffee, tea 210 cc custard, sherbet, Italian ice 120 cc
Soups, broths 180 cc Ice cream, Popsicles 90 cc
Gelatin 150 cc Creamers 15 cc
Milk 120 or 240 cc

NOTE: 1. Oral intake is recorded _after_ drinking.

2. I.V. fluids are recorded when started _and_ finished. At shift change, nurse must record both the amount left in bottle and the _amount absorbed._

Date / /			INTAKE PARENTERAL				OUTPUT (Specify Amount and Describe)					
			I.V. To Go		cc	Irriga-tions				Drainage		
Time	Oral	Tube	Amount	Type	Amount Absorbed		Urine	Vomitus	Stool	Hemo-vac	Suction Chest–GI	Duodenal Bile, Wound
A.M. 12												
1												
2												
3												
4												
5												
6												
7												
Total 11–7			Amount Remaining in Bottle ▶									
A.M. 8												
9												
10												
11												
12												
1												
2												
3												
Total 7–3			Amount Remaining in Bottle ▶									
16-Hr. Total												
P.M. 4												
5												
6												
7												
8												
9												
10												
11												
Total 3–11			Amount Remaining in Bottle ▶									
24-Hr. Total												

Fluid balance record. (Courtesy of Mercy Hospital, Springfield, Massachusetts.)

Sequence

1. identify patient; explain procedure
2. encourage patient participation if feasible
3. record all liquids taken at meals and between meals
4. record all fluids administered parenterally
5. measure specimens voided into urinal or bedpan in a calibrated graduate
6. record Foley catheter drainage at the end of each shift
7. estimate wound drainage as scant, moderate, profuse; record
8. estimate perspiration if significant; record
9. be sure bedside input and output sheet is transferred to fluid balance record

Common Fluids Measured in ml. when Recording Intake

container	
4-ounce Dixie cup	120 ml.
juice glass	100 ml.
½ pint carton of milk	240 ml.
drinking glass	200 ml.
coffee cup	150 ml.
serving of Jello, custard, junket	150 ml.
1 Dixie cup ice cream	90 ml.
small soup bowl	100 ml.

Notes. The previous listing is just a sample. Most health care agencies have intake equivalents posted in the diet kitchen on the unit or on the intake and output sheet itself, or both.

Intake should be recorded each time the nurse takes a tray, glass, or pitcher away from the patient. Otherwise, it will be forgotten.

☐ CATHETERIZATION

Catheterization is the act of inserting a catheter (tube) into the urinary bladder to empty it of urine. The procedure is done for many reasons. For example, when surgery is to be done, an indwelling catheter may be ordered preoperatively to keep the bladder reduced in size. This allows the surgeon more room and allows for hourly urine measurement. Postoperatively, catheterization may be ordered when the patient is unable to void and all other measures to induce voiding fail. The procedure is also used to measure residual urine and to obtain specimens for some laboratory examinations. Frequently, indwelling catheters are placed in incontinent patients to keep them dry.

A Foley indwelling catheter has a separate valve that allows for the inflation of a 5-ml., 10-ml., or 30-ml. balloon on the end of the catheter. When inflated, the balloon acts as an anchor to hold the catheter in the bladder. This catheter comes in sizes 14, 16, 18, 20, and 22.

A French catheter is a plain tube with no balloon and comes in sizes 10 Fr., 12 Fr., 14 Fr., 16 Fr., and 18 Fr.

Equipment

sterile disposable catheterization kit
bath blanket
container for soiled equipment

goose neck lamp
extra pillows
tape

Sequence

1. identify patient; introduce self; explain procedure; screen patient
2. clean patient as necessary before beginning procedure if patient is incontinent
3. place patient in dorsal recumbent position and drape appropriately with bath blanket; pillows may be used under legs as a comfort measure. Many institutionalized elderly women are too contracted to be catheterized in

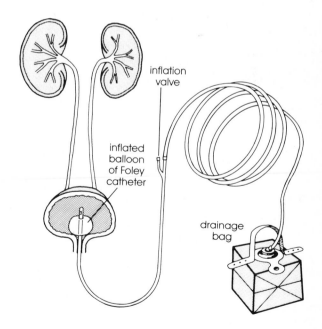

Kidneys, ureters, bladder, and inflated Foley catheter with drainage tube and drainage bag.

inflation valve

inflated balloon of Foley catheter

drainage bag

the traditional position. The nurse may use a side lying position to allow for patient comfort. However, since it is more difficult to visualize the meatus, an assistant will have to hold a flashlight or position an extra light for the nurse who is gloved and doing the catheterization.

4. adjust light until perineal area is clearly seen
5. place protective underpad under hips, plastic side down
6. open catheterization kit near the work area, being sure to maintain a sterile field
7. put on sterile gloves
8. place drape from the kit on patient (sterile towels may be substituted)
9. lubricate tip of catheter liberally and keep catheter on sterile field
10. open container of cleansing solution and pour solution over all rayon balls in the kit *but one*
11. use *dry* rayon ball to protect fingers and separate labia; cleanse area using forceps to hold the moistened rayon balls (warn patient, "it's cold and wet")
12. discard all rayon balls and forceps in appropriate container—*not* on sterile field
13. tell patient to breathe deeply while you insert the catheter 2 to 3 inches for female patient and 6 to 8 inches for male patient
14. hold catheter while urine is draining into container or into drainage bag (obtain specimen at this time if ordered)
15. allow no more than 500 ml. to empty out of the bladder; if there is more urine in the bladder, simply clamp off the catheter and observe the patient for 20 minutes before proceeding with emptying the bladder
16. when urine stops flowing, if French catheter is used, pinch the catheter and withdraw it slowly
17. if Foley catheter is used, reinflate the balloon using a prefilled syringe
18. tape drainage tubing to leg, being careful not to kink tubing
19. leave patient clean, dry, and comfortable
20. record time of procedure, observations of urine, how patient tolerated procedure

Note. If a male patient is to be catheterized, steps 1 to 10, *omitting 3*, are the same. The foreskin of an uncircumcised male is drawn back as the penis is cleansed. The penis is then raised nearly perpendicular to the body and the catheter inserted. The foreskin is then reduced and the procedure as just outlined is followed.

Additional Information. Never catheterize a patient without an assistant or observer. Always be sure the lighting is adequate. The nurse must prepare to adapt all procedures to the individual patient. Catheterization is one of the more complicated procedures and demands practice and review in order to maintain sterile aseptic technique.

☐ URINARY MEATUS CARE OF PATIENT WITH INDWELLING FOLEY CATHETER

Urinary meatus care is given during the patient's bath. After the perineal area of the male or female patient has been thoroughly cleansed, proceed in the following way:

1. female patient—with labia well separated, apply antiseptic swab or bacteriocidal ointment to urinary meatus and around the indwelling Foley catheter
2. circumcised male—apply antiseptic swabs or bacteriocidal ointment to urinary meatus around Foley catheter
3. uncircumcised male—retract foreskin, apply swabs or ointment as above, then draw foreskin back over penis

☐ FOLEY CATHETER IRRIGATION

Catheter irrigation is usually done to remove clots, to fight infection by instilling medication, or to make sure the catheter is patent. There are some physicians who feel that an excellent way to keep a catheter patent and draining well is to encourage fluid intake. The major risk with the procedure of irrigating catheters is that of infection. Proper handling of the irrigation equipment and of the catheter, drainage tubing, and catheter is the use of sterile technique. Both ends of the drainage tubing must be kept sterile when it is disconnected because organisms travel up the tubing into the bladder after the tubing is reconnected.

Irrigation equipment available may be sterile disposable equipment that is for one use only or sterile syringe and sterile basin obtained from central supply. Whatever choice the nurse has, it is crucial to follow sterile technique.

It is essential for nurses to wash their hands before and after giving a catheter irrigation. Handwashing by patients is to be encouraged and provided for.

Purposes

to maintain a patent Foley catheter for urinary drainage
to promote patient comfort

Equipment

sterile disposable irrigation kit
OR bulb or Asepto syringe
  and sterile basin

sterile catheter plug
OR dry sterile dressing

protective underpad   emesis basin (clean)
Alcowipe   sterile irrigating solution

Sequence

1. identify patient; introduce self; explain procedure; screen patient
2. pour sterile irrigating solution into sterile basin
3. fold covers back far enough to just expose the catheter connected to the drainage tubing
4. place protective underpad under patient's hips; place emesis basin on bed
5. disconnect catheter; plug or cover tubing, to preserve sterility
6. fill syringe with prescribed amount of solution
7. instill solution slowly into catheter
8. permit solution to drain into emesis basin by way of gravity
9. repeat as ordered
10. wipe catheter end with alcohol and reconnect to drainage tubing
11. record the kind of solution and the amount used; describe the returns and how the patient tolerated the procedure.

Note. Many elderly patients have been told that this is a painful procedure. Although it is true that in some surgical cases a bladder irrigation may produce bladder spasms, the patient should be reassured that every precaution will be taken to relieve distress and maintain comfort.

□ VAGINAL IRRIGATION (DOUCHE)

A douche is irrigation of the vagina; that is, an amount of fluid is instilled into the vagina and allowed to drain out via gravity. Physicians order douches preoperatively when certain types of surgery are scheduled. Sometimes douches are used to instill medication or to promote cleanliness when there is an abnormal discharge. A deodorizing douche may be ordered for a patient with a vesicovaginal fistula (abnormal passageway from the bladder to the vagina).

Routine home douching is discouraged as this can alter the natural flora of the vagina and cause dryness, irritation, and bacterial growth that may contribute to infection.

Equipment

warm irrigating solution and   bedpan
  irrigating container with   protective underpad

curved irrigating nozzle
OR sterile disposable douche kit

clean gloves
bath blanket

Sequence

1. identify patient; introduce self; explain procedure; screen patient
2. have patient get in dorsal recumbent position; drape patient with bath blanket
3. pour solution into container
4. place patient on bedpan with protective underpad under hips
5. put on gloves
6. allow some solution to wash over perineum slowly to cleanse vulva and to accustom patient to temperature of solution
7. gently introduce curved irrigating tip into vagina, rotate slowly to cleanse all folds of vagina while solution flows in; control flow so it is not running too fast
8. when container is empty, dry perineum but keep patient on protective underpad as some solution may remain in vagina for a while

Chapter 15 □ Review Questions

MATCHING

_____ 1. glomerulus

_____ 2. calculi

_____ 3. ascites

_____ 4. vaginitis

_____ 5. speculum

_____ 6. incontinence

_____ 7. Kegel exercise

_____ 8. nephron

A. excess fluid collects in tissues

B. filtering unit

C. small structure within kidney made up of blood vessels

D. uric acid, calcium phosphate

E. potassium

F. used in pelvic examination

G. decline in estrogen production

H. fluid in abdomen

_____ 9. edema   I. involuntary loss of feces, urine

_____ 10. electrolyte   J. strengthens perineal muscles

DISCUSSION QUESTIONS

1. Rose Andrews, 79, was recently operated on for repair of an inguinal hernia. She lives alone and is in fairly good health. Shortly before discharge, she confides in the nurse that she has been troubled with stress incontinence. Develop a plan to help this lady deal with her problem.
2. List some specific measures for a bladder training program that could be implemented in a home situation and in a long-term-care situation.
3. Describe some unique bladder problems common to elderly women. Identify solutions to these problems.
4. Identify some dangers of dehydration to the older adult.

□ REFERENCES

A look at urinary stress incontinence. Emer Med, 16(5):79–82, 1984.

Autry, D., et al.: The voiding record, an aid in decreasing incontinence. Geriatr Nurs, 5(11): 22–25, 1984.

Badlani, G., et al.: Urinary tract dysfunction: how to evaluate elderly patient. Consultant, 24(6):181–182, 184–185, 188–189, 1984.

Bates, P.: Three post-op perils of prostate surgery. RN, 47(2):40–43, 1984.

Bradshaw, T.W.: Making male catheterization easier for both of you. RN, 46(12):43–45, 1983.

Brodoff, A.S.: A new look at cystitis in women. Patient Care, 18(4):16–21, 25, 1984.

Brink, C., et al.: A continence clinic for the aged. Gerontol Nurs, 9(12):651–655, 1983.

Clark, N., et al.: Prostatectomy: a quick guide to answering your patients' unspoken questions . . . patient teaching aid. Nursing (Horsham) (Can Ed), 14(4):48–51, 1984.

Engram, B.W.: Do's and don'ts of urologic nursing. Ten easy ways to improve your urologic nursing care. Nursing (Horsham) (Can Ed), 13(10):49, 1983.

Fuller, E.: Infections to watch for in the elderly. Patient Care, 18(8):132–135, 137–138, 1984.

Gramse, C.A.: Indwelling catheter care: a run through. Nursing (Horsham) (Can Ed), 14(10): 26–27, 1984.

Hart, M., et al.: Do increased fluids decrease urinary stone formation? Geriatr Nurs, 5(6):245–248, 1984.

Hay, J.: Incontinence pants: one system. Nurs Mirror, 158:28–30, 1984.

Kennedy, A.: Promoting continence . . . catheters in the community. Comm Out, 51, 53, 55, Feb., 1984.

King, M.: Aids for incontinence. Nurs Mirror, 158:30–36, 1984.

Lawler, P.E.: Benign prostatic hyperplasia: knowing pathophysiology aids assessment. AORN J, 40(5):745–748, 750, 1984.

McConnell, J.: Preventing urinary tract infection . . . nursing measures alone reduced UTI in a nursing home. Geriatr Nurs, 5(8):361–362, 1984.

Nahata, M.C., et al.: Effect of chlorophyllin on urinary odor in incontinent geriatric patients. Drug Intell Clin Pharm, 17(10):732–734, 1983.

Plantimoli, L.V.: When the patient has a Foley. RN, 47(3):42–43, 1984.

Robbins, S.: Incontinence in the elderly mentally infirm. Nurs Times, 80(14)(Suppl):25, 27, 1984.

Rooney, V.: Incontinence in the elderly in the community. Nurs Times, *80*(14)(Suppl):13–14, 1984.

Schnelle, J.F., et al.: Management of geriatric incontinence in nursing homes. J Appl Behav Anal, *16*(2):235–41, 1983.

Simons, J.: Does incontinence affect your client's self-concept? Gerontol Nurs, *11*(6):40, 1985.

Tallis, R.: Incontinence in the elderly: preventing the disability. Nurs Times, *80*(48) (Suppl): 9–12, 1984.

Objectives

After completing this chapter, the student should be able to

☐ describe briefly the anatomy and physiology of the nervous system
☐ list age-related changes in the nervous system
☐ describe age-related disorders of the nervous system
☐ explain how sensory deficits can cause accidents
☐ explain what is meant by risk factors in cerebrovascular accidents
☐ list warning signals of stroke
☐ list some nursing measures critical to care of the stroke patient

Vocabulary

aphasia
autonomic
cognitive
comatose
hemiplegia
ischemic
palpation
percussion
postural hypotension
prophylaxis
spatial
vertigo

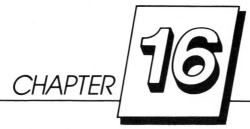

CHAPTER 16

The Nervous System

Chapter Outline

☐ *Anatomy Review*

The brain and the spinal cord are the chief components of the nervous system, which is a vast communication network made up of nerve cells called *neurons*. The nervous system helps to regulate the functions and movements of the body.

All nerve tissue is extremely delicate. That is why the brain and the spinal cord are carefully protected by fluid, membranes, and bones.

☐ STRUCTURES AND FUNCTIONS OF THE SPINAL CORD AND NERVES

Neurons. The neuron is an odd type of cell. Most of our cells reproduce; cells of the skin, bone, and blood are replaced when they wear out. But when neurons, the cells of the nervous system, die, they cannot be replaced. A neuron is made up of a cell body and two types of extension—*dendrites* (one or more of them), which conduct nerve impulses to the neuron's cell body, and an *axon*, which conducts nerve impulses away from the cell body. The axons are also referred to as nerve fibers.

Signals entering and leaving the body are passed via nerve fibers to the brain, which, with its billions of neurons, analyzes the signals and transmits their meaning through other neurons, thereby giving direction to muscles.

There are two types of nerves: *sensory nerves* that go from sense organs to the brain and *motor nerves* that go from the brain and spinal cord to the muscles. Some messages are conscious (voluntary) and some are involuntary. There are also reflex actions.

In a reflex action, the nerve impulses travel a special route called a reflex arc. For example, if you touch something hot, the impulse on the skin of your finger races along a sensory nerve to the spinal cord. There it generates another impulse that activates the muscle of your arm and you immediately pull your hand away. It is actually a shortcut whereby the muscles move before the brain knows why. Reflex actions protect the body from harm.

Special motor nerves make up the autonomic nervous system; they control the activities of our internal organs such as the heart, lungs, stomach, and intestines.

This is the way nerves carry messages: A stimulus, such as a pin, cotton ball, or ice cube, touches a nerve ending in the skin of the hand. This sets up an impulse (reaction) in the dendrite. The impulse speeds along the dendrite until it reaches the cell body. It then penetrates the cell body and exits through its axon away from the cell body to the dendrite of another neuron. Eventually it ends up in the brain. The brain interprets the impulse to be pain, a tickle, or perhaps a feeling of cold.

Spinal Cord. The spinal cord is a rope of nerve tissue about 16 inches long that is threaded through the protective bony arches of the vertebral foramina. It extends from the medulla (a part of the brain) through the vertebrae downward approximately four fifths of the length of the spinal column.

Cranial Nerves. Twelve pairs of nerves branch off the brainstem and pass through the base of the skull into the brain. Thirty-one other pairs of nerves branch off the spinal cord at regular intervals between the vertebrae and reach all the organs of the body.

Nerves that reach upward from the spinal cord to the brain pass through the medulla oblongata (in the brainstem) where those from the left side of the body cross to the right side of the brain and vice versa. This is why the left side of the brain controls the right side of the body and the right side of the brain controls the left side of the body.

□ STRUCTURES AND FUNCTIONS OF THE BRAIN

The brain may be compared to a master computer that analyzes information and transmits orders to all parts of the body. It is made up of several components, each with its own functions.

Cerebrum. This is the largest part of the brain. It is composed of two hemispheres of convoluted (wrinkled) nerve tissue. The outer layer is called the cortex and is made up of "gray matter." The cerebrum helps with understanding, problem solving, memory, and thinking.

Cerebellum. The cerebellum is smaller than the cerebrum. It also is made up of two hemispheres. It is located at the back of the head. It coordinates our muscular activity.

Brainstem. The brainstem connects the cerebrum with the spinal cord. Within the brainstem are the diencephalon, midbrain, pons, and medulla oblongata.

Diencephalon. This part of the brainstem contains the thalamus and the hypothalamus.

Midbrain. This is a short part of the brainstem just below the thalamus and above the pons. It sends signals on to the cerebrum along with the pons.

Pons. The pons passes signals from the cerebrum to the cerebellum.

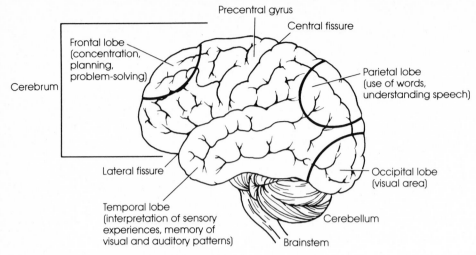

Figure 16–1 ☐ Major structures of the brain.

Medulla Oblongata. This is the lower portion of the brainstem. It is a bulbous enlargement of the spinal cord that accepts and transmits nerve impulses, which control breathing, digestive processes, and the circulation of the blood.

Four important concepts you should learn about this complex system of the body are:

- All conscious activities (seeing, hearing, thinking, and so on) are controlled by the cerebrum.
- Involuntary muscles such as those of the heart are controlled by the medulla oblongata.
- Voluntary muscles are controlled by the cerebellum, although this control is automatic.
- The spinal cord is the place where the nerve branches that reach out to all the organs of the body originate.

☐ Age-Related Changes

☐ NEURONAL LOSS

There is a slow, gradual loss of neurons as people age. Neurons are lost by the thousands starting at age 25. Because of the large number we begin with, most of us function rather well despite the loss.

☐ ATHEROSCLEROSIS

In this country, almost everyone has some degree of atherosclerosis. This is probably due to a combination of genetic and environmental factors. A 75-year-old has blood flow to the brain that is about 80 per cent of that of a 30-year-old. In advanced stages of atherosclerosis, however, plaque (a deposit of fatty material on the lining of the blood vessels) narrows the lumen of vessels and gradually occludes them. This serious impairment of blood flow to the brain can result in dizziness and stroke.

☐ BEHAVIORAL CHANGES

Neuronal loss and atherosclerosis contribute to such behavioral changes as difficulty in remembering recent events, slowing of reaction responses, and difficulty in mastering motor skills. Older people who have trouble getting about or who are worried about what seems to be increasing helplessness are likely to be irritable. These reactions must be handled calmly, quietly, and constructively by the nurse. If an elderly person is not rushed, or is not confused by being moved into a new environment or by being subjected to a new routine, he or she usually can adapt to inevitable changes. Nurses must realize that most elderly persons *are* a bit slower mentally and physically than when they were younger. It may take longer for them to understand what is said and to accomplish a given direction. The key is to try to avoid pressure situations.

☐ ACCIDENT PRONENESS

Progressive changes in vision and hearing, plus advancing neuromuscular changes, make the elderly vulnerable to accidents. Falls are extremely common at home and in health care facilities. Postural hypotension, medication the patient is taking, momentary confusion, and furniture that is not in its usual place are a few of the causes of these falls. Simple preventive measures are needed. The environment at home and in the hospital must be made as hazard-free as possible. Routine safety precautions include:

adequate lighting
no scatter rugs or slippery floor surfaces
bedrails at night
clearly labeled medications
handrails in bathtubs and on stairways
electrical equipment in good working order (no frayed or worn cords)

A younger person recovers quickly from injuries incurred by a fall. An elderly person is likely not only to have more serious consequences but also to take a longer time convalescing.

☐ Age-Related Disorders

☐ CEREBROVASCULAR DISEASE

There are several types of cerebrovascular disease. The main types are cerebral infarction, transient ischemic attacks, intracranial hemorrhage, and hypertension.

Cerebral Infarction. Cerebral infarction, also called stroke, shock, or CVA, means that there is vascular disease that involves either a vein or an artery. The problem is caused either by a hemorrhage from a torn vessel or by an obstruction of the lumen of the vessel.

Cerebral Thrombosis. Cerebral thrombosis is the most common cause of CVA's in the elderly. There is usually a previous history of arteriosclerosis. Some early warning signs may be vertigo, headache, lightheadedness, sudden falls without loss of consciousness ("drop attacks"), blurred vision, memory loss, and behavioral changes.

Transient Ischemic Attacks. Transient ischemic attacks (TIA's) are temporary dysfunctions of the central nervous system. Atherosclerotic vessels impair the circulation of the blood to a part of the brain and the patient experiences vertigo, loss of vision in one eye, aphasia, or confusion. The entire episode may last a few minutes or several hours. Treatment is either anticoagulant therapy or reconstructive surgery of the blood vessel (endarterectomy). The person who has transient ischemic attacks has an increased chance of having a cerebral vascular accident.

Smoking has a vasoconstrictive action and the action of certain drugs, namely antihypertensives and diuretics, can also cause poor cerebral circulation.

People with hypertension and arteriosclerosis are candidates for *intracranial* or *intracerebral hemorrhage*. The pressure builds up in the defective artery and the artery eventually ruptures and bleeds into the surrounding tissues. A clot forms and causes pressure on the site of the brain where the hemorrhage took place. Sometimes there are early warning signals, but often the attack is sudden. Symptoms vary widely, from severe headache, vertigo, and loss of consciousness to mental confusion, aphasia, nausea, and a feeling of weakness.

The initial effect of cerebral vascular accident is paralysis of one or both sides of the body. A right-sided paralysis (hemiplegia) indicates that the left side of the brain is involved. Occasionally the hemorrhage is slight, nerve damage temporary, and the paralysis not too serious.

Stroke patients have a characteristic appearance. Speech is indistinct, there is no muscle control on the affected side, and there may be no bowel or bladder control. These men and women suffer some mental confusion and are emotionally labile, i.e., they may laugh and cry inappropriately.

☐ HYPERTENSION

Hypertension, which is accompanied by inelasticity of blood vessels, is a significant cause of CVA's in the elderly. Any sign of epistaxis, disorientation, confusion, or poor memory should be investigated. A fine balance between blood pressure that is high enough to allow good circulation without being so low as to cause complications must be reached. Rest, sodium restriction, weight reduction (if indicated), and drug therapy can improve the condition of the hypertensive geriatric patient by helping to lower the blood pressure.

☐ TUMORS

Most brain tumors occur in younger adults. Unfortunately, the few brain tumors that do occur in the aged adult are often not diagnosed for a long time because the symptoms are so easily attributed to the aging process. Forgetfulness, personality changes, headaches, visual disturbances, and poor coordination are what we have grown to expect from the elderly. Most of the time the symptoms are attributed to arteriosclerosis; on other occasions "senility" is blamed.

Metastatic disease is prevalent in the elderly. A test that is done frequently on elderly patients is a brain scan. It is a painless procedure involving an intravenous injection of a substance that is picked up by lesions. These lesions are recorded by a scanner. What frightens the patients is that they must remain perfectly still when this is being done and usually the head is immobilized. The scanner passes over the patient's head and seems very threatening. If the patient is prepared for this and reassured, the experience is not anxiety provoking.

☐ TREMORS

Tremor is occasionally observed in the elderly. A fine trembling of the jaw (distinguished from drug-induced *tardive dyskinesia*) or of the hand that increases when the person is hurried or under stress is sometimes referred to as "senile tremor." It is distinguished from the tremor of Parkinson's disease in that it is more rapid and is not medically significant.

☐ PARKINSON'S DISEASE

Parkinson's disease, or paralysis agitans, is a degenerative disease of the nervous system. It involves a slow destruction of nerve cells. The symptoms are muscle weakness, tremor of the head and hands, shuffling gait, masklike facial expression, and slow, wooden speech.

☐ Nursing Interventions

☐ ASSISTING WITH THE NEUROLOGIC EXAMINATION

A patient who is suspected of having a disease of the nervous system will be examined by a neurologist, that is, a physician who specializes in the field of nervous system deficits. A complete neurologic examination may be done at intervals, since it can be exhausting for the patient. After testing reflexes, gait, and special senses, the examiner will then order one or more of the diagnostic tests that are required to determine the cause of dysfunction. Refer to a medical-surgical nursing text for discussion of these highly specialized diagnostic examinations.

The nurse's responsibility with assisting at the neurologic examination is to have the necessary equipment and materials ready for the physician and to prepare and reassure the patient. The patient should be clean, should have had an opportunity to void, and should have been given an explanation about the examination in keeping with his or her state of alertness at the moment.

Equipment

percussion hammer	colored yarn	applicators
straight pin	flashlight	substance with aro-
safety pin	pocket watch	matic, nonpungent
cotton ball or soft	substances with sweet and	odor (such as onion,
fine brush	salty tastes (sugar, salt,	coffee, or tobacco)
tuning forks	vinegar)	

Sequence for Testing Cranial Nerve Functions

1. olfactory: one nostril is closed; substance with a characteristic odor is held beneath the other nostril to test sense of smell; repeated with first nostril
2. optic: patient wears glasses if customary; color sense is tested with yarn; cover one eye and test for visual field by moving finger from behind head toward line of vision and note when patient first sees the finger; repeat

3.,4., and 6. oculomotor, trochlear, and abducent:
   a. patient is in semidarkened room; light is shone into eyes one at a time to see reaction
   b. patient holds head still and follows moving finger of examiner
5. trigeminal: test done with cotton or pinprick, or both, to check superficial sensations of face; heat and cold reaction also tested; corneal reflex tested with cotton strand (blinking)
7. facial: examiner places salty and sweet substances on tongue, asks for patient's reaction

8. acoustic: examiner tests hearing using pocket watch and various tuning forks
9. and 10. glossopharyngeal and vagus: examiner tests for gag reflex with applicators
11. spinal accessory: patient rotates head, shrugs shoulders
12. hypoglossal: testing of movements of tongue

Other Tests

In addition to testing the cranial nerves, a neurologic examination includes testing for

Speech. The examiner will ask the patient to identify ordinary objects (key, dollar bill, and so on), to follow simple commands ("raise your right hand"), and perhaps even to read.

Muscle Status. Muscles are measured to check for symmetry of contraction. The use of palpation and a percussion hammer help to demonstrate muscle tone.

Gait. Gait observation involves having the patient walk forward, backward, and then with eyes closed.

Coordination. To test coordination, the examiner may have the patient pour a glass of water from a pitcher or close his or her eyes and try to touch his or her nose with a finger.

Reflexes. An example of reflex testing is the classic patellar reflex test in which the patellar tendon is hit with a percussion hammer. Another reflex is the plantar reflex, which is tested by stroking the sole of the foot to see if the toes flex or extend.

Sensitivity. This may be determined by pinching, squeezing, or pricking the patient's skin to observe for reactions to pain. It can also include having the patient close his or her eyes and then tell the examiner which finger or toe is being held by the examiner. A strand of cotton may be used to touch the skin lightly to see if the patient can feel it.

□ NEUROLOGIC ASSESSMENT

When working with patients who have a disease of the brain or spinal cord, you may be required to take "neuro signs." This means that the physician will order observations of neurologic signs on a periodic basis.

Neurologic signs include orientation, bodily movements, pupillary reaction, speech, vital signs, and affect.

Orientation. Does the patient know who he or she is? Where he or she is? What day it is?

Bodily Movements. Is the patient lethargic? Stuporous? Comatose? Does the patient voluntarily move his or her arms and legs? Is the patient's muscle tone strong? Weak? Is his or her grip strong?

		NEUROLOGICAL ASSESSMENT SHEET												
DATE ➤━━➤														
TIME ➤━━➤		AM PM	AM PM	AM PM	AM PM	AM PM	AM PM	AM PM	AM PM	AM PM	AM PM	AM PM	AM PM	AM PM
L.O.C.														
ORIENTATION	NAME													
	PLACE													
	DAY													
MOVEMENTS	GRIP													
	Ⓛ ARM													
	R ARM													
	Ⓛ LEG													
	R LEG													
PUPIL SIZE	R													
	Ⓛ													
SPEECH	CLEAR													
	RAMBLING													
	INCOHERENT													
	APHASIC													
VITALS	B. P.													
	PULSE													
	RESP.													
	TEMP.													
MISC.														
NURSE'S SIGNATURE														

ABBREVIATIONS	ORIENTATION	MISCELLANEOUS	PUPIL CHART	
Q – QUIET	MOVEMENTS	ABBREVIATIONS	2 ● 5 ● 8 ●	RB – REACT BRISKLY
D – DROWSY	I EXCELLENT	＝ EQUAL		R – REACT
A – ALERT	II GOOD	> STRONGER	3 ● 6 ●	RS – REACT SLOWLY
C – CONFUSED	III AVERAGE	< WEAKER		F – FIXED
SS – SLIGHTLY SLURRED	IV BELOW AVERAGE		4 ● 7 ●	

Figure 16–2 ☐ Neurological assessment sheet. (Courtesy of Mercy Hospital, Springfield, Massachusetts.)

Pupillary Reaction. Do the patient's pupils constrict when a light is shone into the eyes? How long do they take to constrict? How much do they constrict? (Beam light on closed eye and then watch constriction of pupil when eye is opened; repeat for the other eye and compare pupillary reaction of second eye with first).

Speech. Can the patient speak? Is his or her speech clear? Is the patient confused? Aphasic? Can he or she identify ordinary objects or follow simple directions?

Vital Signs. What are the patient's temperature, pulse, respirations, and blood pressure?

Affect. Does the patient appear depressed? Hostile? Tense or anxious? Or does he or she appear normal, with appropriate comments and responses?

□ NURSING THE STROKE PATIENT

The two most common neurologic problems of the central nervous system in the aged adult are transient ischemic attacks (TIA's) and cerebrovascular disease (Paulsen, 1983). Stroke or cerebrovascular accident (CVA) killed 159,000 Americans in 1982. Each year there are 500,000 victims. Hypertension, a risk factor of stroke, afflicts 37,900,000 Americans. The economic costs of this massive health problem in 1985 are estimated to exceed a staggering 72.1 billion dollars (American Heart Association, 1985)!

Risk Factors

There are some risk factors in cerebrovascular accidents that cannot be changed: sex and race. The risk of stroke is less in females. Females who smoke probably increase this risk, however. Black Americans have a significantly higher incidence of stroke.

Risk factors that can be changed are hypertension, elevated red blood cell count, heart disease, and diabetes. Medical management of these disorders and patient compliance decrease the risk of stroke.

Warning Signs

There are four warning signals of stroke:
- sudden temporary weakness, numbness or tingling of face and extremities on one side of the body
- slurred speech or temporary loss of speech
- any visual disorder, particularly in one eye; double vision
- sudden falls; unexplained dizziness

A stroke occurs when oxygen-rich blood is cut off on its way to the brain. The person afflicted may lose consciousness. The face is flushed and respirations are labored and noisy. The pulse is slow and blood pressure is elevated. The patient may become comatose and the thrust of medical care is aggressive treatment in order to stabilize the patient. The early stages are critical.

Immediate Care

The CVA patient is usually unconscious on admission. Nursing measures include proper positioning to maintain an open airway and to prevent aspiration. A lateral position on the unaffected side is the position of choice. Suctioning may be necessary, and in critical situations a mechanical airway or tracheostomy may be required. Oxygen will be used.

Careful monitoring of vital signs is essential since a danger sign is lowered pulse and respiration rate.

When consciousness returns, frequent turning, coughing, and deep breathing are vital nursing measures. Prolonged immobility leads to hypostatic pneumonia, urinary retention, renal calculi formation, and fecal impaction. Meticulous skin care is needed in order to prevent decubitus ulcers.

General Care

After the immediate nursing needs are met, efforts must be made to prevent flexion deformities by positioning and body alignment. Foot drop, external rotation of the hip, adduction of the affected shoulder, and contractures of the affected hand must be prevented through positioning and exercises.

The following are general measures you should be familiar with when planning the nursing care of the convalescent CVA patient.

1. prevent hypostatic pneumonia by changing the patient's position every 2 hours; encourage coughing and deep breathing if the patient is responsive
2. prevent contractures and other deformities by using hand rolls, trochanter rolls, range of motion exercises, footboards, and so on
3. encourage good nutrition and hydration; note input and output
4. maintain good skin condition by keeping the bed linen clean and dry, changing the patient's position frequently, and giving back rubs with position changes
5. encourage the patient's participation in whatever Activities of Daily Living he or she is capable of even if it is in a very small way; example—let the patient handle a piece of toast while being fed breakfast
6. get the patient out of bed and out of the room as soon as this is permitted to expose him or her to the stimuli of other sights and sounds
7. allow the family to participate in the patient's care by feeding him or her, wheeling the wheelchair, caring for the patient's hair, and so on
8. follow the plans of the physical therapist, speech therapist, and occupational therapist to ensure reinforcement of therapy

The amount of brain damage governs the degree of impairment. Brain damage affects opposite sides of the body. For example, right-brain damage affects the ability of the patient to deal with spatial-perceptual situations. There are deficits in judgment of distance, size, position, rate of movement, form, and the relation of parts to the whole. The nurse must remember that although speech is unimpaired, other abilities may be affected. Right-brain damage, which produces left hemiplegia (paralyzed left side), may be manifested by such disabilities as inability to steer a wheelchair through a doorway without bumping the frame; buttons may not be fastened correctly. There may be difficulties with simple, self-care activities.

The patient with left hemiplegia appears impulsive; he or she is often a poor judge of his or her own abilities. This person will benefit from being encouraged to slow down and check carefully each step of the task he or she is trying to accomplish.

Attention to environment is important. Minimize clutter and avoid rapid movement around the patient. A well-lighted room is helpful.

Left-brain injury produces right hemiplegia. Typically, the patient will have speech and language deficits. This means that there will be difficulties in both speaking and understanding. However, alternative means of communication should be used. For example, gestures and pantomime to demonstrate questions and answers are often used. Speech and language problems of the stroke patient (aphasia) often produce frustration, disappointment, and confusion. It is not necessary to shout at the aphasic patient who has no hearing deficit. He or she might be more able to understand when spoken to in short, simple phrases accompanied by appropriate gestures. Support and encouragement of any indication of progress is essential for the patient's improvement.

Recovery and Rehabilitation

Generally speaking, the patient should start relearning activities of daily living as soon as possible. The rationale is that if this is done the patient will maintain strength in the unaffected extremity and trunk muscles, will be more alert, and will have a more hopeful attitude. There is also the chance that some improvement in strength in the affected side will occur.

Depending on the condition of the patient, it may be necessary to increase activities very gradually. Aged patients with CVA may need much longer rehabilitation efforts than would be the case in younger individuals. In either situation, frequent rest periods should be provided between activities so that the work is not too strenuous.

Some beginning activities of daily living to be encouraged are rolling over in bed, changing position, lifting hips onto bedpan, feeding, and partial bathing.

The efforts of the multidisciplinary rehabilitation team and the consideration of alternative settings and levels of care are critical factors in the restoration and preservation of function in the elderly. Stroke has both high frequency of occurrence and strong positive association with advancing age. Stroke survival has always been one of the classic conditions amenable to structured and detailed medical rehabilitation.

Stroke rehabilitation requires specific and complete neurologic diagnosis. For example, assessments must be made of the degree of motor weakness, sensory deficits, cognitive dysfunction, and speech problems.

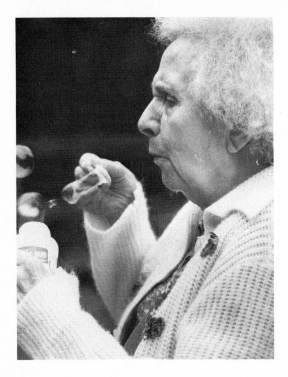

Figure 16–3 ☐ Rehabilitation of the stroke patient. Activities of daily living and self-care are resumed as soon as possible for the stroke patient. Depending on the extent of the stroke, basic abilities such as rolling over in bed, changing position, feeding, and bathing may return slowly. This woman is blowing bubbles as part of a rehabilitation program to exercise facial muscles and arm.

The Setting

Stroke patients used to spend several weeks in the hospital, receive rehabilitation there, and then go either home or to a long-term-care facility. Now, because of escalating hospital costs, utilization review, and changing attitudes in regulating agencies and third party payors, stroke patients move on as soon as they are medically stable.

Some alternatives are hospital-based and free-standing medical rehabilitation (both relatively intensive), skilled nursing facilities in extended-care facilities that offer similar rehabilitation services on a less intensive basis, innovative programs in home care, and day care with varying amounts of rehabilitation services available (Gresham, 1982).

Since the degree of neurologic return that occurs is hard to predict, it is essential that *no* preventable complications be allowed to develop. For example, a patient eventually gains enough motor power to walk but cannot do so because joint flexion contractures were allowed to develop. Nursing management of the stroke patient includes the following techniques if rehabilitation is to take place:

- proper positioning and turning
- range of motion program
- knowledgeable approaches to bowel and bladder management

Prophylaxis

The single therapeutic measure most likely to prevent vascular disease is control of hypertension. Even elderly patients deserve control of their blood pressure (Busse, 1982). Cessation of smoking, a prudent life style, and a prudent diet are the best ways for a person to prevent vascular disease.

Further Nursing Measures for Patients with Cerebrovascular Disease

The following are some general measures for the care of the aged person with cerebrovascular disease:
1. be sure that the aged patient with cerebrovascular disease gets enough rest and sleep
2. avoid overstimulation
3. supervise the patient's nutritional intake, fluid intake, elimination, and personal hygiene in order to prevent vitamin deficiencies, constipation, and urinary tract infections
4. avoid embarrassing the patient by remarking about his or her confusion or memory loss
5. reinforce reality (use clocks, calendars, patient's name)
6. see that the patient's environment is safe; that furniture is in the same place he or she is accustomed to; that handrails are where needed; that he or she is suitably clothed when going out
7. pay attention to the patient as an individual; comment about the weather, the seasons, his or her appearance; this lets the patient know you care and also reinforces security

□ NURSING MEASURES FOR THE PATIENT WITH PARKINSON'S DISEASE (PARALYSIS AGITANS)

Patients with parkinsonism may not be seen by the nurse until they have endured the disease for years. When they are hospitalized, it is often due to a secondary infection; they may have increased stiffness and weakness. There is no cure. Medication, surgery, and physical therapy are the three methods of treatment. Effective nursing care focuses on controlling rigidity and preventing contractures.

Nursing Care

1. keep the skin scrupulously clean, using lotion on dry areas
2. encourage frequent oral hygiene where there is drooling
3. provide a nutritionally adequate diet; encourage fluids; assist with feeding if needed, but allow the patient to do as much for himself or herself as possible; see that patterns of elimination are established

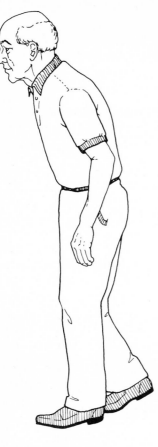

Figure 16–4 □ A person with Parkinson's disease shows a typical stooped, rigid posture. Active and passive exercise is encouraged to reduce rigidity.

4. encourage active and passive exercise such as walking, movement of arms, squeezing sponges or balls, and range of motion for patients confined to bed
5. see that the patient gets enough rest and sleep; reduce stress
6. observe, report, and document changes in patient's condition; example— report any temperature elevation since this could be the beginning of an infection
7. encourage the family; be an interested listener to those who live with this long-term disability

Note. The patient with Parkinson's disease may be alert and aware even though the masklike face shows no emotional reaction, either positive or negative.

Chapter 16 □ Review Questions

MULTIPLE CHOICE

1. The major structures of the nervous system are
   A. neurons and dendrites
   B. axons and neurons
   C. sensory nerves and dendrites
   D. brain and spinal cord
2. Autonomic nerves control
   A. sense organs
   B. internal organs
   C. peripheral nervous system
   D. central nervous system
3. The part of the brain that helps us to understand, solve problems, and re-member is the
   A. cerebrum
   B. cerebellum
   C. medulla
   D. pons
4. As we age, we all have
   A. behavioral changes
   B. neuronal loss
   C. tremor
   D. hypotension
5. An early warning sign of CVA is
   A. irritability
   B. hyperpyrexia
   C. sudden dizziness or weakness
   D. anorexia

MATCHING

_____	1. hemiplegia	A. early warning sign of stroke
_____	2. vertigo	B. emotion
_____	3. hypostatic	C. dizziness
_____	4. symmetry	D. temporary deficiency of blood
_____	5. ischemic	E. decreased blood flow, circulation

_____ 6. affect   F. problem solving

_____ 7. numbness, tingling in face,   G. evenness
extremity

_____ 8. reinforces reality   H. half the body is paralyzed

_____ 9. dendrite   I. calendars

_____ 10. cerebrum   J. extension of neuron

DISCUSSION QUESTIONS

1. Develop a 5 minute presentation to give to a group of older adults in your community. Include statistics, risk factors, and practical suggestions regarding diet and life style to prevent strokes.
2. Mr. C, a 72 year old black male, has learned upon a routine physical examination that he has hypertension. How will you, as his nurse, tell him what the significance of this finding is? What kind of information will you incorporate into your teaching?

⌐ REFERENCES

Busse, E.: Cardiovascular disease and psychopathology in the elderly. Psychiatr Clin North Am, 5(1):159, 1982.

Caine, S.: Parkinson's disease—helping the patient with a movement disorder. Can Nurs, 80(11):35–37, 1984.

Chase, M., et al.: Nursing management of a patient with a subarachnoid hemorrhage. J Neurosurg Nurs, 16(1):23–9, 1984.

Duthie, J.: The nervous system: structure and function. Nursing (Oxford), 2(15):431–432, 434, 1983.

Gresham, G.: Rehabilitation of the geriatric patient. Primary Care Geriatric Patient. Primary Care Geriatric Medicine, 9(1):240–243, 1982.

Hart, G.: Strokes causing left vs right hemiplegia: different effects and nursing implications. Geriatr Nurs, 4(1):39–43, 1983.

Hartshorn, J.C.: Aneurysm! Keeping your patient alive until surgery. RN 47(1):30–33, 74, 1984.

American Heart Association: Heart Facts, 1985.

Hickey, J.V., et al.: Effective discharge planning and the neurosurgical nurse. J Neurosurg Nurs, 16(2):101–106, 1984.

Hendrickson, S.: Psychological care of the patient with a neurological dysfunction. J Neurosurg Nurs, 16(4):202–207, 1984.

Holt, P.: Parkinson's disease. Nursing (Oxford), 2(15):448–450, 1983.

Ilson, J., et al.: Current concepts in Parkinson's disease. Hosp Med, 19(11):33–34, 36–37, 42–43, 1983.

Iveson-Iveson, J.: Parkinson's disease . . . innovative treatment in the 18th century. Nurs Mirror, 30(22):158, 1984.

Lindsey, M.: Developing an understanding of Parkinson's disease. Nurs Times, 79(10):24–26, 1983.

Mancell, E.L., et al.: Therapy of neurologic disorders in the elderly . . . parkinsonism and ischemic cerebrovascular disease. Hosp Prac, 19(10):106E, 106, 106L–M, 1984.

Mawson, D.: Organic psychiatric disorders: the assessment of patients. Nurs Times, 79(23):29–31, 1983.

Paulsen, G.W.: Disorders of the central nervous system in the aged. Med Clin North Am, 67(2):354–355, 1983.

Rainer, J.K., Sr., et al.: Evaluation of the comatose patient. J Neurosurg Nurs, 15(5):283–286, 1983.

Roberts, B.L., et al.: Improving balance: therapy of movement . . . elderly receiving vestibular stimulation . . . rocking in a rocking chair. J Gerontol Nurs, 9(3):150–156, 1983.

Shreeve, C.: Why another anti-Parkinson's drug? . . . selegiline hydrochloride. Nurs Mirror, 158(9):38–40, 1984.

Stewart, R.M.: Extrapyramidal syndromes: update on managing parkinsonisn and tardive dyskinesia. Consultant, 26(6):51–55, 59, 64–65, 1983.

Turning off the "on-off" syndrome in parkinsonism . . . fluctuating clinical response to levodopa. Emergency Med, 16(18):60–61, 64, 1984.

Objectives

After completing this chapter, the student should be able to

☐ describe differences between exocrine and endocrine glands
☐ list age-related changes in the endocrine system
☐ list age-related disorders of the endocrine system
☐ define and differentiate between the two major types of diabetes
☐ describe some factors associated with identifying the elderly diabetic
☐ list and explain common treatment modalities for diabetes
☐ identify two major complications of diabetes
☐ explain the differences between oral hypoglycemics and insulin
☐ list significant factors in patient education

Vocabulary

acidosis
beta cells
diurnal
glucagon
hypoglycemia
ketosis
kilogram
polyphagia
polyuria
reagent
retinopathy

CHAPTER

The Endocrine System

Chapter Outline

□ *Anatomy Review*

A gland is a structure that produces and secretes certain chemical substances that are necessary for the functioning of the body's organs. There are two kinds of glands: exocrine and endocrine.

Exocrine glands have ducts (tiny tubes) through which their secretions pass directly to the area of the body that needs them. Some examples of exocrine glands are lacrimal glands, salivary glands, mammary glands (in females only), intestinal glands, sebaceous glands, and bulbourethral glands.

Endocrine glands, on the other hand, are ductless; their secretions are discharged directly into the blood or lymph. The major endocrine glands are the adrenals, gonads (ovaries in the female and testes in the male), pancreas, parathyroid, pituitary, and thyroid.

Two other endocrine glands are the *thymus*, which secretes one hormone that promotes cellular reproduction and growth and another that affects lym-

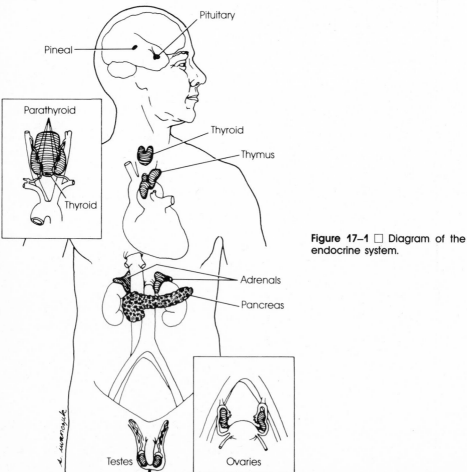

Figure 17–1 □ Diagram of the endocrine system.

phatic tissue and immune mechanisms, and the *pineal gland*, which secretes a hormone that acts on the hypothalamus and pituitary glands. In addition, there are other ductless glands whose functions are relatively minor or not clear.

The pancreas is both an exocrine and an endocrine gland. It channels pancreatic fluid into the digestive tract, and its islets of Langerhans secrete the hormone insulin directly into the bloodstream.

Endocrine glands, together with the nervous system, govern the body's systems, but the endocrine glands also govern each other. The best example of this is the pituitary, the master gland of the body. The pituitary hangs by a stem from the base of the diencephalon and fits into the sphenoid bone at the base of the skull just above the roof of the mouth. It secretes a variety of hormones, including those that influence growth; sexual development; some gonad, thyroid, and adrenal functioning; milk production after childbirth; and some kidney functioning.

□ *Age-Related Changes*

Aging causes changes in endocrine glands that are subtle and still being studied. This text will limit its discussion to changes to pituitary gland, adrenal glands and pancreas. Disorders caused by over- or undersecretion of the glands are reviewed in Table 17–1.

□ PITUITARY GLAND

There is a decrease in weight and blood supply to the pituitary gland. Nevertheless, the concentration of pituitary hormones seems to be unaltered (Campbell, 1985). It is unclear, however, what the effects of stress are, especially if prolonged, on the elderly individual.

□ ADRENAL GLANDS

There is an increase in connective tissue and pigmentation of the adrenals. The aging adrenal glands are also characteristically affected by a loss of lipids (substances made up of fatty, waxy compounds) and an increase in the dilatation of blood vessels. The plasma levels of the glucocorticoids as well as their diurnal (occurring during the daytime or period of light) rhythms seem similar to those of younger adults. A major consideration, however, is that the multiple chronic illnesses that elders are prone to can affect diurnal patterns and confuse the distinction between changes due to aging and changes due to disease.

□ PANCREAS

Controversy surrounds distinguishing normal aging changes in the pancreas from those of diabetes mellitus. The obvious structural changes occur

Table 17–1 ☐ The Major Endocrine Glands

Gland	Location	Clinical Information
Adrenals	One above each kidney (actually 2 glands—a. cortex and a. medulla)	Hypercorticalism: Cushing's syndrome (moon face; "buffalo" hump on back; obese trunk; spindly legs) Hypocorticalism: Addison's disease (increase in pigmentation of skin, weight loss, hypotension) Tumors of a. medulla: can cause hypertension, hypoglycemia, diaphoresis, emotional instability
Gonads: Testes in male	Scrotum	Secrete testosterone, a hormone essential for male sexual characteristics
Ovaries in female	Flank the uterus in pelvis	Secrete estrogens and progesterone, hormones that govern ovulation and female sexual development
Pancreas	Behind the stomach	Double duty gland: exocrine because it secretes digestive juice and endocrine because it secretes the hormone insulin via islets of Langerhans; hyposecretion of the islets of Langerhans causes diabetes mellitus
Parathyroid	Attached to and behind the thyroid	Hyperparathyroidism: destruction of bone; pathologic fractures; kidney stones Hypoparathyroidism: patient feels tingling in extremities; muscle spasms; seizures; treat by regulating calcium and phosphorus
Pituitary	Base of brain	Hyperpituitarism: frequently caused by tumors; may result in acromegaly, giantism, Cushing's disease Hypopituitarism: dwarfism; reproductive problems
Thyroid	In neck	Goiter: enlarged thyroid; may be due to lack of iodine in diet, inflammation, or hyper- or hypofunction of thyroid Thyroiditis: inflammation of thyroid caused by bacteria or virus Tumors: usually benign in younger patients Hyperthyroidism: Graves' disease, caused by overproduction of thyroid hormone; patient has exophthalmos, weight loss, enlarged thyroid, nervousness Hypothyroidism: caused by lack of thyroid gland; in women over 60, myxedema is common, causing weight gain, dry skin and hair, sluggishness; cretinism in children with stunted growth, mental retardation

with obstruction of ducts and degeneration of alveoli. The certainty is that glucose tolerance declines progressively with age. Elderly persons have less muscle mass and more adiposity. This may provide less tissue in which to store carbohydrates.

☐ Age-Related Disorders: Diabetes Mellitus

The major endocrine system disorder of concern in the elderly is diabetes mellitus. This is a disease characterized by *hyperglycemia, insulin deficiency, and premature degenerative changes in the nervous and circulatory systems.* Research now indicates that diabetes may be a pattern for aging.

There is an unmistakable similarity between the development of atherosclerosis in the elderly and in diabetics. The most common cause of death in both diabetics and nondiabetics is atherosclerotic cardiovascular disease. The difference is that atherosclerotic cardiovascular disease develops prematurely in the diabetic.

Briefly, diabetes is a chronic metabolic disease marked by a deficiency in the production or utilization of the pancreatic hormone *insulin.*

There is a decrease in the use of glucose by cells and the blood sugar rises (hyperglycemia). When blood sugar reaches a certain elevation, the kidneys excrete the excess and glucose appears in the urine. The elevated sugar level upsets normal kidney function and causes more water and electrolytes to be excreted. Excessive urine output (polyuria) causes the person affected to become dehydrated and extremely thirsty (polydipsia).

One result of abnormal fat metabolism is an increase in ketones, the by-products of fat metabolism. Excess ketones may be excreted in the urine (ketonuria), but they can reach levels whereby they are not all safely excreted, and this condition is called acidosis. A person with acidosis can progress into diabetic coma and die.

Diabetes mellitus may be growth-onset (Type I, juvenile diabetes) or maturity-onset (Type II, beginning in adulthood). Since Type I diabetics usually lack insulin, they need to take it because insulin decreases blood sugar levels. Maturity-onset diabetics have some insulin circulating in their blood and often respond well to oral hypoglycemic drugs and diet therapy. They may also be receiving relatively small amounts of insulin.

Insulin, a protein, is a hormone secreted by the islets of Langerhans, which are the endocrine portion of the pancreas. In the islets, there are two types of cells: alpha cells, which secrete glucagon, and beta cells, which secrete insulin.

Insulin causes a decrease in blood sugar levels because it apparently aids the movement of glucose through cell membranes; this in turn causes the sugar molecules to leave the blood and go into the cells. When blood glucose levels elevate, insulin is secreted and released into the bloodstream. When blood glucose levels fall, insulin is not secreted.

☐ THE ELDERLY DIABETIC

Diabetes is a disorder of metabolism marked by hyperglycemia and glycosuria. It is caused by inadequate production of or utilization of insulin. It is probably the most common metabolic disease among older adults.

At least 20 per cent of adults over the age of 65 have diabetes. There are many reasons: people are living longer, obesity is a contributing factor (and it is becoming more prevalent), and methods of detecting diabetes are more frequently being used.

Points to Remember when Teaching the Diabetic Patient

1. Know your subject (diabetes) and your technique (insulin injection) thoroughly
2. Use words the patient understands
3. Instruct on the basis that the patient knows nothing about diabetes and insulin injection
4. Ask questions of the patient to see how much he or she is learning
5. Choose a quiet time and private place for instruction
6. Do not flood the patient with too many facts at once
7. Use cassettes, booklets, and visual aids that can be used by the patient when the instruction period is over
8. Instruct a family member at the same time

As the body ages, the ability to handle glucose decreases. The diagnosis of diabetes on the basis of glucose intolerance, however, is difficult. Fasting glucose levels rise slightly with age, and elevated concentrations must be found repeatedly before the elderly person is considered diabetic. Positive diagnosis is on the basis of repeatedly elevated 2-hour postprandial (after meals) glucose levels or when diabetic complications, such as neuropathy or retinopathy, are associated with elevated glucose levels (Steffl, 1984).

Since the elderly diabetic may have an elevated renal threshold and yet test negative for glycosuria with urine testing, the physician may recommend capillary blood glucose monitoring.

Of course, capillary blood glucose monitoring is used for Type I diabetics only, i.e., those who are insulin dependent or who are taking oral hypoglycemic agents. Type II diabetes is referred to as non–insulin-dependent diabetes mellitus (NIDDM). NIDDM frequently will resolve itself if patients (usually elderly women) reduce their weight to appropriate levels.

Identification of the Elderly Diabetic

About 50 per cent of all elders may have abnormal results on the standard oral glucose tolerance test (OGTT) (Marchesseault, 1985). The frequency of the abnormal results can be related to the tendency of the elderly to have higher blood glucose levels and to the fact that interpretation of tests is usually based on the norms of younger persons.

The standard symptoms that nurses have been taught to recognize (polydipsia, polyuria, and polyphagia) may not be present. Instead, there may be other physical problems that not only coexist with the diabetes but also require more immediate attention. Some examples are stroke, glaucoma, digestive disturbances, and infections. Diagnosis is difficult because some disorders mask obvious symptoms; for example, polyuria can be caused by diuretics, medications commonly taken by elderly men and women.

Renal threshold increases with age, and glycosuria may not occur until blood sugar levels reach 300 mg. per cent or more. It is generally agreed among physicians that the recommended criteria for diagnosis of diabetes in the elderly is based on measurements of blood or plasma glucose on a fasting basis and/or after oral glucose administration.

☐ COMPLICATIONS

Initially, diabetes seems to be less severe in elders than in younger adults. However, it must be remembered that older people have multiple health problems and all the body's systems are losing reserve.

Vascular disorders are responsible for 75 per cent of the deaths in diabetes (Marchesseault, 1985). In addition, circulatory problems and ocular (diabetic retinopathy), neurologic, renal, and infectious problems are often encountered.

Diabetics also have been shown to have a higher incidence of cerebral atherosclerosis than nondiabetics. Again, age rather than duration of disease seems to be the important factor (Schrier, 1982).

Diabetic Hyperosmolar Coma

A major complication of diabetes in the older adult is hyperosmolar coma. The chief symptom is an unusually high blood sugar. Blood sugar levels may range from 750 to 2000 milligrams per 100 milliliters (Written 750–2000 mg./100 ml.) Glucose draws water from the cells. When this occurs in the brain, the result is stupor and then coma. Hyperosmolar coma may be precipitated by a heart attack. Although it is infrequent in the elderly, it is very serious and is associated with a high mortality rate (Ernst, 1983).

☐ NURSING IMPLICATIONS

The goal of the geriatric nurse is to aid older adults in managing their lifestyle so as to control diabetes and, insofar as is possible, to limit the effect of the disease on the body.

Medication may be unnecessary. In fact, insulin and oral hypoglycemic agents can increase the risk of hypoglycemia. Satisfactory control can be achieved through regular exercise, dietary management, and maintenance of healthy skin.

Since elderly persons have elevated renal thresholds, many long-term-care facilities have eliminated routine urine testing in their non–insulin-dependent diabetics. However, some physicians require their elderly Type II diabetics to routinely test urine. It is important that the first voided specimen of urine, which has been stored in the bladder for hours, be discarded. The urine voided half an hour later is a more accurate indication of glucose in the bloodstream and excreted by the kidneys in the last 30 minutes.

☐ TREATMENT

Therapy includes diet, weight control, exercise, and medication as needed. It is important to remember that in Type II diabetes, therapy should be directed toward preventing vascular disease by reducing hyperglycemia since the major clinical manifestations are the result of atherosclerotic disease. Research has shown that the higher the blood sugar and the longer it is high, the more changes occur in the vascular system.

Diet and Weight Control

Obesity is common among patients with Type II diabetes and the most important aspect of dietary treatment of maturity-onset diabetes is reduction of weight until ideal weight (or even slightly below ideal weight) is reached (Marchesseault, 1983). Normal body weight decreases with aging. However, a higher proportion of women remain obese after age 65 than do men (Natow and Heslin, 1980). For some individuals, weight loss should be a goal. Symptoms associated with degenerative joint disease and hypertension, as well as diabetes, can be substantially alleviated by weight reduction.

In many elderly diabetics, a modification of diet is all that is needed. High carbohydrate, high fiber diets have been found to both improve glucose metabolism and decrease the hyperlipidemia so often seen in Type II diabetes (Scherer, 1985). A moderate regimen using the American Dietetics Association exchange diet program is appropriate.

After the physician has established the needed energy and nutrient requirements, the amounts are divided into *exchanges*. The exchanges group foods according to their carbohydrate, protein, and fat content. There are six exchange food groups: milk, vegetables, fruit, bread (includes cereal and starchy vegetables), meat, and fat. All exchanges within one group contain about the same number of calories. An individual is allowed to eat a specified number of food exchanges from each group every day. The term *exchange* may be confusing to some persons who believe that they can exchange a food in one group for a food in another group (Schrier, 1982). This is why it is essential for the nurse to emphasize that exchanges are made only *within* an individual food group, not among the various groups.

As important as dietary regulation is, most physicians do not impose rigid requirements on their elderly diabetic patients, *provided* there are no severe complications and the hyperglycemia is asymptomatic. Often the decision is made just to observe these patients periodically.

Exercise

Physical activity or exercise is as important as diet or medication. Exercise helps to maintain strength and muscle tone, improves joint mobility, encourages circulation, and aids digestion and elimination. Exercise also improves insulin effectiveness and mental attitude.

Exercise *is* possible for frail elders. Walking or non–weight-bearing exercise such as bicycle exercise or swimming are alternatives. Even rocking chairs are highly recommended. The activity of rocking increases cardiac output (the amount of blood pumped by the heart per minute), promotes respiration, and discourages lung congestion. It stimulates muscle tone and not least important maintains the feeling of relatedness.

Medication

Oral Hypoglycemics. Sulfonylurea drugs are the oral hypoglycemics used to lower the blood glucose in patients with non–insulin-dependent diabetes mellitus (Type II) whose hypoglycemia cannot be controlled on diet alone. They are also used as an adjunct to insulin therapy in the stabilization of insulin-dependent maturity-onset diabetes resulting in a reduction of insulin requirement and a lesser chance of hypoglycemic reactions.

These drugs appear to lower blood glucose acutely by stimulating insulin release from the pancreas. Oral hypoglycemics will *not* lower blood glucose in the patient who lacks pancreatic function and are only effective in those with some insulin production.

Examples of oral hypoglycemic drugs are Dymelor, Diabinese, Tolinase, and Orinase. Orinase is a short-acting compound with a 3- to 8-hour duration of action. Dymelor and Tolinase are intermediate in duration of action, 24 to 36 hours.

Insulin. If the patient with Type II diabetes remains hyperglycemic despite orally administered drugs and diet therapy, the logical answer is the use of insulin.

Insulin has been available since 1921, when it was first prepared for injection by Drs. Banting and Best. Earlier, the outcome of diabetes was fatal. The first insulin was similar to the regular insulin presently in use. Today there are several different kinds, which allows for adaptation to individual lifestyles and metabolisms.

Insulin is prepared in a solution containing 100 units per ml. It can be measured in any kind of hypodermic syringe, but for accuracy and ease of administration, a U100 insulin syringe is recommended. The person who is insulin dependent need only buy U100 insulin of whatever kind he or she needs along with U100 syringes from the several convenient types available.

Human insulin, made by altering the genes of a bacterium, was synthesized in 1978. It is similar in metabolism as well as in hypoglycemic effect to pork insulin. A major advantage of recombinant human insulin (sold under the name Humulin) is that it can ensure an adequate supply of insulin to patients. A disadvantage, for now, is that it is more costly than conventional insulin.

The nurse will have to evaluate carefully the patient's, or family member's, ability to understand the usage of the drug, which is potentially hazardous. Consideration should be given to community assistance in the form of visiting nurses, homemaker home health aides, and public health nurses to ensure proper supervision. Insulin may be drawn up into several syringes to give the patient a week's supply if he or she has difficulty seeing or measur-

---

Patients' Guidelines for Taking Oral Hypoglycemic Agents

1. Remember to take your pills from ½ to 1 hour before meals unless your doctor directs otherwise. This will give the pills time to be absorbed in your system before food enters your bloodstream and raises the amount of glucose in the blood.
2. Get your doctor's approval before you switch from one pill to another. One tablet of one drug will not always give the same results as one tablet of another drug, even though they have the same amount of milligrams that are equal in strength. Let your doctor determine the correct amount of milligrams for you. Each drug has a maximum amount that is considered effective. Taking more than this amount may increase the number of side effects.
3. Report all side effects to your doctor. Diarrhea, nausea, and loss of appetite may be due to the drug causing an irritation in the stomach. Skin rashes seem to occur most often with chlorpropamide (Diabinese).
4. Know the symptoms of hypoglycemia, low blood sugar caused from the stimulation of too much insulin: *confusion, headache, hunger, nervousness,* and *pale, moist skin.* Keep a concentrated source of sugar, such as a candy bar, on hand to curtail this reaction.
5. Beware of reactions with other drugs. Always check with your doctor or pharmacist before you combine a new medicine with your treatment for diabetes. If you drink alcohol while on these drugs, you may experience an unpleasant reaction such as flushing, nausea, and rapid heartbeat. The oral hypoglycemic agent prevents the alcohol from being broken down in the body.
6. Other drugs, such as steroids (prednisone), estrogens, diuretics, Dilantin, Inderal, and the decongestants that are found in many cough and cold medications, may interact with oral agents or interfere with diabetic control.
7. Over-the-counter remedies for colds, sore throats, and congestion contain syrups that will increase sugar intake.

---

ing. *The fact that the patient is older does not mean that he or she cannot be successfully maintained.* In fact, many physicians report that compliance is better in older adults than in younger diabetics.

The nurse should know the kind of insulin the patient is taking, the time it begins its action, when peak action is reached, and when effectiveness declines.

Regular insulin is quick acting, which means the effect begins in 30 minutes to 1 hour. It reaches peak action in 2 to 4 hours and lasts 6 to 8 hours. Intermediate insulins are NPN, Globin Zinc, and Lente. These insulins have a 1- to 1½-hour onset, reach peak in 6 to 8 hours, and last from 12 to 16 hours. The long-acting insulins are Protamine zinc (PZI) and Ultralente, which have as their onset of action a 4- to 6-hour span, peak in 14 to 20 hours, and last 36 hours. About one third of elderly diabetics require insulin.

Monitoring

Urine Testing. Routine testing of urine of nursing home patients has been criticized as a meaningless task since their higher renal threshold means that they are unlikely to spill sugar in their urine. However, the nurse may be asked to teach a patient to test his or her urine for sugar and acetone. There are a number of tests available, all of them relatively easy to do. There are two basic types:

1. A tablet is dropped into the urine specimen for a specified period of time after which the color of the urine is compared with a color chart.
2. A testing tape (a strip of treated paper) is held in a specimen of urine for a specified period of time and its color is then compared with a color chart.

Blood Glucose Tests. In some instances, the physician will recommend that the patient monitor blood glucose at home. There are several devices available. The Glucometer is an easy to read testing apparatus.

The patient pricks a finger (a lancet or automatic finger puncturing device like the Autolet can be used), places a drop of blood on a reagent strip, inserts the strip into the Glucometer, and reads the test results. The advantage of self testing is that it minimizes laboratory testing and costs. (It also encourages independence and control in self management of diabetes.)

Most insurance companies cover a major part of the cost of these devices.

Patient Education

When teaching patients urine testing and self medication the nurse must emphasize the importance of record keeping. There are several resources where printed materials both for educational purposes and to aid in record keeping are available at no cost. The American Diabetes Association, 600 Fifth Avenue, New York, NY, 10020, and the Eli Lilly Company, Indianapolis, IN, 46285, are two such resources. The patient can request a self-monitoring record and a dictionary of terms relating to diabetes, as well as information on diet and health practices.

The nurse will recommend avoidance of sweets, limitation of animal fats and fried foods, and a sensible intake of low-fat dairy products. A variety of fruits and vegetables and whole-grain cereals and breads together with physical activity will ensure a healthful diet.

Habits and lifestyles are hard to change: a person's motivation must be strong to change them. Compliance with dietary restrictions is best if the diet is a modification of previous eating habits. The nurse must know the patient, his or her patterns of living, educational background, and limitations. A detailed explanation of carbohydrate metabolism will probably not be as beneficial as emphasis on dietary intake, shopping patterns, and patient likes and dislikes. There should be special attention paid to establishing a regular meal time and planning for snacks that are a part of the total dietary plan. The patient must understand what will happen if meals are skipped or improper food is eaten.

The hazards of infection should be stressed. Prompt medical attention to signs and symptoms of infection can prevent the development of major diseases. Virtually all elderly diabetics have some degree of atherosclerosis. The problems of peripheral vascular disease are intensified by this deterioration of circulation. The dependent extremities are especially vulnerable. This is why foot care is so important. In addition to daily washing of feet with mild soap and lukewarm water, checking for any sign of skin disorder, and massaging with lanolin or petroleum jelly, the following foot tips for the diabetic should be taught:

- *never* cut corns or calluses with a razor blade or knife.
- *never* wear elastic garters or hose that are not properly measured.
- *never* apply extreme hot or cold to your feet.
- *never* wear cut-out shoes or sandals.
- *never* apply strong antiseptics or chemicals to your feet.
- *do* use anti-fungal powder between toes daily.
- *do* wear shoes and socks whenever you can.
- *do* visit your podiatrist regularly.
- *do* trim your nails (using a file or nail clipper) straight across.

Administering Insulin

The following are safety rules for the preparation of insulin injections:

1. verify the label on the insulin bottle along with the physician's order for the correct *type* of insulin, the correct concentration (U100), the expiration date, and the appearance of the insulin (clear, cloudy)
2. remove insulin from refrigerator a few hours before giving it; always prepare at room temperature
3. use U100 insulin syringe for U100 insulin
4. roll bottle between palms of hands until mixed; do not shake
5. some health agencies have two nurses check dosages; some have nurse and patient verify dosage (patient may draw up and administer insulin in selected cases).
6. double check patient's identity before giving insulin
7. never give insulin to patient who is to receive nothing by mouth (NPO) without checking with the physician
8. wipe off rubber stopper with alcohol
9. inject air into the vial equal to the number of units to be injected
10. withdraw insulin into syringe equal to number of units ordered

The insulin-dependent patient at home needs to be taught the following:

1. always have extra insulin at home
2. observe thorough handwashing
3. use only sterile equipment
4. always cleanse top of insulin bottle

Recognizing the Symptoms of Insulin Reaction and Acidosis

Nurses should be able to recognize the symptoms of insulin reaction (insulin shock) and acidosis (diabetic coma). They are both serious conditions and require prompt treatment.

Insulin Reaction (hypoglycemia)
(caused by too much insulin or
too little food, or by stress, vomiting, diarrhea, unusual activity)

Symptoms:
hunger
diaphoresis
dizziness
pale, moist skin
blurred vision
nervousness
tremor
convulsion
coma

Treatment:
fruit juice with added sugar,
hard candy, glucagon

Acidosis (hyperglycemia)
(caused by lack of insulin and
accumulation of ketone bodies
or by stress, illness, or injury)

Symptoms:
nausea, vomiting
drowsiness
confusion
characteristic sweet, fruity odor
to breath
rapid pulse
abdominal pain
restlessness
flushed face
coma

Treatment:
contact a physician, who will
order blood and urine tests.
When results are reported, a
rapid-acting insulin will be
ordered.

Note. Never attempt to give anything orally if the patient is unable to swallow. Contact a physician.

Diabetic patients often need counseling to help improve their control of blood glucose levels. Information about the diagnosis and control of diabetes is rapidly increasing and changing. New products are continuously being developed to help normalize blood glucose levels. Informed, responsible nurses have the opportunity to significantly affect the health and lives of their diabetic patients.

Chapter 17 ☐ Review Questions

MULTIPLE CHOICE

1. Endocrine glands are
   A. sebaceous glands
   B. ductless glands
   C. active in females only
   D. active in males only
2. A result of abnormal fat metabolism is
   A. an increase in ketones
   B. a decrease in ketones

    C. a decrease in beta cells

    D. an increase in alpha cells

3. Insulin is secreted by the endocrine portion of

    A. the pituitary

    B. the parathyroids

    C. the pancreas

    D. the gonads

4. An adrenal disturbance, hypercorticalism, is manifested by

    A. kidney stones

    B. dwarfism

    C. moon face, "buffalo" hump

    D. pathologic fractures

5. An important factor to consider when instructing the geriatric patient in management of diabetes is

    A. to assess the patient for sensory deficits

    B. to keep a record of his or her weekly blood pressure

    C. to take a height and weight periodically

    D. to recommend monthly glucose tolerance tests

6. A Type II diabetic is described as

    A. usually obese, requires insulin to control blood glucose

    B. normal in body weight; has frequent hypoglycemia

    C. usually non–insulin-dependent and is treated with oral agents, diet, exercise, self monitoring, and education

    D. having high blood glucose levels due to an increase in insulin receptors

7. A Type I diabetic patient is

    A. a non–insulin-dependent diabetic

    B. a maturity-onset diabetic

    C. ketosis resistant

    D. a juvenile-onset diabetic

8. Which of the following is a sulfonylurea hypoglycemic agent?

    A. insulin

    B. orinase

    C. sulfizin

    D. surfak

9. Insulin in current use should be stored

    A. at room temperature

    B. at any temperature

    C. at freezing temperatures

    D. in the refrigerator

10. The advantage of Humulin is that

    A. it ensures a supply of insulin

    B. it is less expensive than beef or pork insulin

    C. there are no known side effects

    D. it can be taken orally as well as by injection

MATCHING

_____ 1. diabinese   A. vision deteriorates

_____ 2. diabetic retinopathy   B. fainting

_____ 3. hyperglycemia   C. raises level of glucose

_____ 4. hypoglycemia   D. parathyroid disturbance

_____ 5. dwarfism   E. give orange juice

_____ 6. hypoparathyroidism   F. give insulin

_____ 7. Addison's disease   G. oral hypoglycemic

_____ 8. regulates hormones   H. adrenal disease

_____ 9. glucagon   I. pituitary disease

_____ 10. syncope   J. gonads

DISCUSSION QUESTIONS

1. Mrs. Webber is a 70-year-old diabetic who is scheduled for surgery to correct problems with varicose veins of her left leg. Develop a plan of care to help achieve the following:
   a. improved dietary habits
   b. meticulous foot care
   c. adequate exercise
   d. accurate testing of urine for sugar and acetone

2. If you were assigned a project that required you to teach an elderly couple how to manage the husband's diabetes, what are some of the factors of diabetes and diabetic management you would emphasize?

☐ REFERENCES

Campbell, R.K.: Diabetes mellitus update. J Practical Nurs, 35:59, 1985.

Covington, T., and Walker, J.: Current Geriatric Therapy. Philadelphia, W.B. Saunders, 1984, p. 342.

Diabetes Forecast, 1982.

Ernst, N.: The Aged Patient: A Sourcebook for the Allied Health Professional. Chicago, Year Book Medical Publishers, 1983, pp. 103–104.

Frankel, L., and Richard, B.: Be Alive as Long as You Live. Philadelphia, Lippincott, 1980, p. 219.

Huey, F.L.: What nursing homes are teaching us. Am J Nurs, 85(6):678–683, 1985.

Marchesseault, L.C.: Diabetes mellitus and the elderly. Nurs Clin North Am, 18(4):791, 792, 793, 796, 1983.

Natow, A., and Heslin, J.: Geriatric Nutrition. Boston, CBI Publishing, 1980, pp. 139–141.

Scherer, J.C.: Nurses' Drug Manual. Philadelphia, Lippincott, 1985, p. 996.

Schrier, R.W.: Clinical Internal Medicine in the Aged. Philadelphia, W.B. Saunders, 1982, pp. 235, 239, 243.

Steffl, B.: Handbook of Gerontological Nursing. New York, Van Nostrand Reinhold, 1984, pp. 241, 242.

Objectives

After completing this chapter, the student should be able to

☐ describe briefly the anatomy and physiology of the ear and eye
☐ explain how the aging process affects the sense organs
☐ perform ear and eye irrigations correctly
☐ instill ear, eye, and nose drops correctly
☐ list conditions that make the use of a hearing aid appropriate
☐ communicate effectively with hearing impaired and visually impaired adults
☐ suggest ways the nurse can assist the family of the hearing impaired and the visually impaired

Vocabulary

auditory
cerumen
conjunctiva
diplopia
hyperopia
lacrimal glands
otosclerosis
photophobia
presbycusis
presbyopia
prosthesis
ptosis
retina

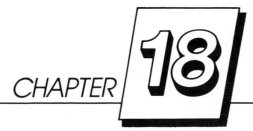

CHAPTER

The Special Sense Organs

☐ The Ear

☐ STRUCTURES AND FUNCTIONS

Outer Ear. This is the pinna, the visible part of the ear, and consists of cartilage covered by skin. It includes the external auditory canal, at the end of which is the tympanic membrane. Under normal circumstances the eardrum (tympanic membrane) vibrates with incoming sound waves.

Middle Ear. The middle ear contains air sacs and three small bones called ossicles. These tiny, linked but movable bones are the malleus (hammer), which is attached to the tympanic membrane, the incus (anvil), which is attached to both the malleus and the stapes (stirrup), which is the third bone. Sound waves from the air enter the external auditory canal, pass through the tympanic membrane, and cross the three bones to the inner ear.

Inner Ear. The inner ear (labyrinth) transmits sound to the brain. The cochlea, a complex, snail-like structure, is filled with a fluid that reacts to the vibrations of sound waves by rippling. The movement of the fluid activates the hair cells that make up the organ of Corti, where the hearing receptors are located. When these hair cells are stimulated, they send messages through the acoustic (eighth cranial) nerve to the brain's center for hearing.

☐ AGE-RELATED HEARING CHANGES

Conductive and Perceptive Deafness. With age, all of us lose some portion of our hearing. Two kinds of impairment are conductive deafness and

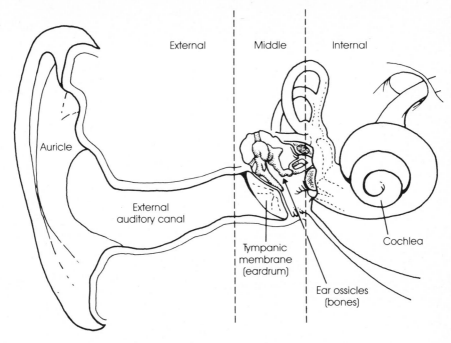

Figure 18–1 □ Anatomy of the ear.

perceptive deafness. Conductive deafness indicates that there is an obstruction in the path of sound waves in the middle ear. One cause of this condition is impacted cerumen (wax); another is otosclerosis, a disease of the bone that interferes with the conduction of sound.

Perceptive deafness is caused by a defect in the inner ear. The nerve endings just do not register sounds.

There are, of course, other reasons for hearing loss, such as injuries, illnesses that affect hearing, and long-term exposure to excessive noise.

Presbycusis (Degenerative Nerve Deafness). The type of deafness most frequently encountered in geriatric nursing is degenerative nerve deafness or eighth nerve deafness. Its medical name is presbycusis. Its early manifestation is an inability to hear high-frequency sounds. The condition is made worse by malnutrition, diabetes, circulatory disorders, and chronic systemic infections.

Presbycusis may lead to behavioral changes. The elderly patient may become irritable, depressed, and at times paranoid. He or she may withdraw and become isolated as he or she participates less and less in activities. It is difficult for this patient to use the telephone, a communication device we take for granted. It is estimated that one person in ten over the age of 65 has this problem.

Impacted Cerumen. The oil glands of the ear produce a wax called cerumen that, along with the hairs near the external opening, helps prevent foreign substances from entering the ear. Some individuals produce more cerumen than others and it can become hardened. A nurse or physician skilled in the procedure of removing earwax may be consulted. The patient should be cautioned, of course, against introducing anything into the ear to take out the wax because this only packs it more tightly against the eardrum. In addition, the eardrum could be punctured by using such objects as bobby pins, cotton tipped applicators, and so on.

☐ HEARING DEFICITS IN THE OLDER ADULT

Several physiologic changes occur in most elderly adults' hearing: the auditory nerve fiber degenerates, the eardrum thickens, and the production of cerumen declines. These changes occur to a certain degree in all older persons.

The effect of these physiologic changes is that normal speech sounds are more difficult to hear and the ability to hear tones within the range of normal conversation decreases.

The elderly client may have either conduction deafness or perception deafness. Conduction deafness is caused by some interference with the transmission of the physical sound waves. Perception deafness describes the ineffective registering of electrical signals by nerve endings. Both conduction and perception deafness may occur in the same patient.

Less common but equally important causes of hearing impairment are vascular problems and viral infections. Middle ear infections are uncommon in the elderly, and when they do occur they usually accompany such diseases as tumors or diabetes.

All persons who have a hearing deficit should receive written explanations and instructions to ensure accuracy. There are, however, other measures the nurse should be able to use when communicating with the hearing impaired:
- face the individual when talking
- talk into the least impaired ear
- use gestures, facial expressions
- when high frequency loss exists, talk slowly, distinctly, and in a low voice
- *never raise the voice or shout.*

The hard-of-hearing individual suffers social isolation. An elderly person with a hearing deficit may become emotional in his or her reaction to this additional loss. Anger, impatience, frustration, and suspicion are the common results of being unable to understand conversation. There is a feeling of insecurity in being unable to hear sounds of danger. The client may be self conscious and avoid social interaction deliberately. As a result, physical, emotional, and social health can be affected by hearing impairment.

☐ NURSING INTERVENTIONS

Helping with the Hearing Aid

Being hard of hearing is serious, but not hopeless. There are corrective measures. First of all, the hard of hearing should see an otologist, a physician who specializes in diseases of the ear. If medication or surgery is not the answer, a hearing aid may be recommended. The nurse should know that such a device must be individually fitted and that the patient must be taught how to use and care for it. The following hints are written for differing degrees and types of losses. They will alert caregivers to the problems that the hard-of-hearing older person may encounter with the hearing aid.

Initial Hearing Aid Use

1. A hearing aid should be used in quiet, familiar situations at first. It takes time for most persons to become adjusted to listening to amplified sounds. Gradually, the aid may be used in more difficult situations, such as when among large groups of people, in large rooms, and in noisy places such as restaurants. Success depends on the specific type and degree of loss a person has.
2. New hearing aid users should initiate use gradually. The skin that lines the ear canal is sensitive and, if irritated, takes time to heal.
3. A hearing aid has a volume control that has to be adjusted to different listening situations. Too little volume will cause other persons to have to speak louder than normal and too much volume will distort incoming sounds and over-amplify unwanted background sounds.
4. Anticipate that in everyday situations unexpected loud sounds can occur before the volume can be controlled. The user should not become alarmed when this happens.

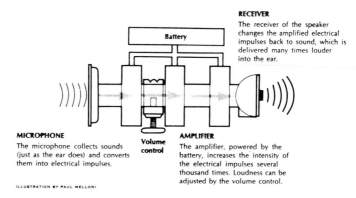

RECEIVER
The receiver of the speaker changes the amplified electrical impulses back to sound, which is delivered many times louder into the ear.

Battery

MICROPHONE
The microphone collects sounds (just as the ear does) and converts them into electrical impulses.

Volume control

AMPLIFIER
The amplifier, powered by the battery, increases the intensity of the electrical impulses several thousand times. Loudness can be adjusted by the volume control.

ILLUSTRATION BY PAUL MELLONI

Figure 18–2 ☐ Basic components of a hearing aid. (From Gardner, p. 94.)

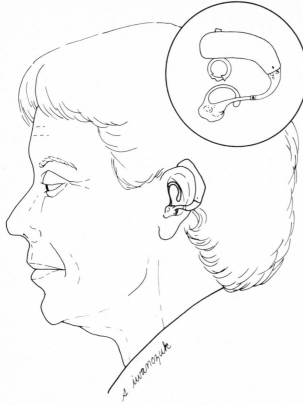

Figure 18–3 □ Hearing aids. The behind the ear (BTE) aid is the most popular hearing device. It hooks behind the ear. A plastic tube connects it to the ear mold in the ear canal.

5. Some aids have tone control. Depending on the kind of hearing loss a person has, tone controls can markedly affect the clarity of speech heard with the hearing aid.
6. It takes time and practice to adjust to a new hearing aid. Several trips to the hearing aid dealer may be necessary in order to insure a properly fitted earmold.

Part-Time Hearing Aid Use (for Persons with a Mild Degree of Hearing Loss)

1. It may be that amplification is needed in certain types of situations only.
2. Hearing aids may hinder, rather than help, the communication of a person with a mild loss in some cases, particularly in noisy situations.
3. If part-time hearing aid use has been recommended, there is no logical reason to wear it in situations for which it is not helpful.

Limitations of Hearing Aids. A hearing aid is a mechanical prosthesis. It does not give normal hearing. It makes sounds and words *louder*, but it cannot make them clearer than a person's ability to understand speech clearly.

Although hearing aids have been constructed to provide a range of pitches or frequencies, they do not cover all the pitches the human ear is capable of hearing. For understanding speech, however, the hearing aid is adequate.

Common Complaints of Hearing Aid Users. If the user feels his or her voice sounds different or loud, it might be because he or she is very close to the microphone of the hearing aid, which picks up the sound. Therefore, the user's voice will sound louder than the voice of a person several feet away. A person with hearing loss is not used to hearing his or her own voice so loud. The hearing aid is actually amplifying the user's own voice. Hearing one's own voice through a mechanical instrument is never the same as hearing it otherwise.

If the hearing aid seems to pick up more noise than speech, turning the volume down may help. Less volume will moderate the background noise and voices will be heard better. People tend to speak louder when in a noisy place.

A hearing aid that whistles may have a mechanical defect. It is possible to have sounds that come into the ear canal leak out and then feed back into the microphone, which causes a squeal. This problem may have to be investigated by the dealer. The earmold may be improperly fitted; this is the most common cause of whistles and squeals.

Sometimes a person complains that he or she can hear more but cannot understand what is being said. For some types of disorders, a person may have difficulty in being able to distinguish between vowel and consonantal elements of speech. The person will have to rely on visual clues as well as the hearing aid. It is always possible that the hearing aid is not working properly; if the user complains about not being able to hear, have the instrument checked.

If the wind whistles in the aid when the person is outside or is driving a car with the window open, placing a small bit of porous material over the microphone may help. This complaint is only on hearing aids worn on the head; a body model is shielded by clothing.

Clothing noise (clothing rubbing on a body model hearing aid) is not easily corrected; a harness that holds the aid may help.

If there is a feeling of "fullness" in the ear (common with new hearing aids), air may be trapped between the tips of the earmold and the drum membrane. The feeling usually passes in a few days.

Suggestions for Special Listening Situations

Hearing in Groups. It is extremely difficult to engage in group conversation when one is wearing a hearing aid. The criss-crossing of talk results in word scrambling. Keen concentration and attention is required. A beginning user should avoid group conversations. Later he or she can try groups but concentrate on one person at a time. The ability to concentrate in groups will develop in time.

Listening to Radio and TV. Announcers and commentators speak rapidly because of limited time allotments. The voices and sounds that are broadcast are mechanically reproduced and sometimes that results in poor quality. With practice, especially by paying attention to TV's visual clues, the person with a hearing aid can enjoy TV and also radio.

Using the Telephone. Many persons with even moderate to severe loss have little difficulty on the phone, especially if the telephone company has installed an amplifier. Those persons with poor ability to discriminate between speech sounds may have considerable difficulty.

The receiver should be held close to the microphone on the hearing aid. If the aid has a telephone pick-up switch, the switch should be flipped to "T" before the telephone is used. If a person is using a body hearing aid, he or she should hold the telephone upside down so the receiver is held close to the microphone on the body. The other end is help up to the mouth to speak into.

If hearing loss is not too severe in the unaided ear, it may be more practical to have the phone company install an amplifier that can be controlled for loudness by the speaker.

Care of the Hearing Aid

Earmolds. Keep the earmold clean. Check it every day to be sure wax is not accumulating in the canal tip. If the opening is plugged with wax, simply remove it with a toothpick or pin. Detach it and wash it with warm water and soap. Accumulations of wax on the outside can cause a poorly fitting mold and will result in feedback when the aid is turned on. *Do not* use alcohol to clean the mold as this has a tendency to cause cracks in the material.

Whistling or feedback is annoying. Be sure to check that the user knows how to put the earpiece in properly. The noises may be caused by a poorly fitting earpiece or by wax on the mold. Minor adjustments may have to be made by the dealer.

Earmolds need to be replaced periodically. Some types of materials will shrink over a period of time as they are exposed to the air. Persons' ears change in size (especially very young ears). But it is a mistake to think that there is no change in the size of the ear canal after maturity.

Tubing. The tubing that connects the hearing aid to the earmold will also need to be replaced periodically. It will dry out and have a tendency to crack. This is a very inexpensive part of the aid.

Batteries. If the hearing aid "goes dead" quickly, it is very likely the battery is no longer functioning. Replace it with a fresh one. Most hearing aids operate with mercury or silver oxide batteries. The voltage keeps a fairly stable level throughout its life but will burn out quickly.

Some new batteries are defective. If a user puts a fresh battery in a hearing aid and it "warbles," it may be caused by a defective battery. Faulty batteries will be replaced free of charge.

Store batteries in a cool, dry place away from the direct rays of the sun or heat from a radiator. Do not keep too many on hand. Though the shelf life of mercury and silver oxide batteries is good, batteries that are stored 6 months or more may lose a good deal of their voltage and usefulness. It is better to buy only a half a dozen at a time and ensure having fresh ones.

Avoid mixing old, worn-out batteries with a fresh supply. Since they "go out" rather quickly, always carry a spare for emergency use. Do not carry batteries loosely in a pocket. A plastic container protects better than a metal con tainer.

Keep contacts clean. Oxygen in the air may cause corrosion on the metal contacts in the hearing aid or on the surface of the batteries, resulting in an unpleasant "frying" noise. If this occurs, the rubber eraser on the end of a lead pencil may be used to polish the contacts.

Cleaning and Repairs. A hearing aid needs to be cleaned periodically, about once a year. If the aid is exposed to an excessive amount of dirt, it can be done oftener.

Precautions. Do not drop the hearing aid. It is delicate and although it will take a considerable amount of jarring, the less there is the longer will be the lifetime of the aid.

Do not get the instrument wet.

Turn off aid when not in use to preserve battery.

A hearing aid does not last indefinitely, nor does any mechanical device. The average length of time during which an aid will perform satisfactorily is from 4 to 6 years. Some people have them for 10 years. An aid can be changed for a new model, just like a car. Of course, a great deal depends on the care that is given to the aid, but every aid will wear out sooner or later. If costly repairs are needed, it may be time to replace the aid.

First Aid for Hearing Aids

If the hearing aid gives no sound at all:
Check the battery by trying a fresh one.
The battery may be upside down.
Check the earmold to be sure wax is not stopping up the opening.
Check the tubing to see that it is not cracked, warped, or bent.
If hearing aid has a telephone pick-up, be sure to check the switch; it may accidentally have been pushed to telephone.
With a body aid, try a spare cord; the old one may have cracked or broken.

If the sounds are weaker than usual:
Try the same things as above; especially try a new battery.
A hearing aid exposed to excessively cold weather will be weak; it will act normally as soon as the indoor temperature takes effect.

If there are scratchy noises and if operation is intermittent:
Clean battery and battery contact springs with a pencil eraser.
Try a spare cord if it is a body aid.
Move all switches back and forth; this may remove fine particles of lint or dust that can interfere with proper electrical contacts. Removing and inserting the cord plugs several times in the receiver may also correct the trouble.

If there are whistling noises:
All hearing aid users are familiar with the "whistling" problem. If the aid does not whistle when it is removed from the ear with the volume turned up, the instrument is not performing properly. Feedback can be caused by certain conditions existing inside the instrument. A leak between any connections from the aid to the earmold can cause feedback.

Irrigating the Ear and Instilling Medications

There is an important difference between ear irrigations and ear instillations. An irrigation is a solution that flows over a specific area. An instillation is the topical administration of a drug drop by drop to a specific site that will benefit by the action of the drug being instilled.

Ear irrigations are used to remove impacted cerumen, the protective secretion produced by glands in the ear. The production of cerumen may increase when the ear is infected by fungi or bacteria. Dark-haired people produce more cerumen than light-haired people.

If cerumen becomes hard and impacted it will impair hearing and may cause discomfort. Instilling hydrogen peroxide half an hour before the irrigation helps to soften the ear wax. In stubborn cases, drops of mineral oil should be instilled several days before irrigation.

Equipment

hydrogen peroxide	dropper
rubber bulb syringe or	curved basin
metal Pomeroy syringe	protective underpad
towel	prescribed solution

Sequence

1. identify and screen patient; explain procedure
2. ask patient to turn head to side with affected ear uppermost
3. pull the ear upward and backward in order to straighten the normally curved auditory canal
4. instill a few drops of hydrogen peroxide in the ear; tell patient to hold this position for 10 or 15 minutes and reassure patient that the bubbling and fizzing is the sound that hydrogen peroxide normally makes
5. return to patient to complete procedure; place curved basin under the ear to be irrigated; have patient hold this to catch return flow
6. drape patient with protective pad and towel
7. fill syringe with solution at tepid temperature (check doctor's order before beginning procedure for prescribed solution)
8. pull the outer ear upward and backward
9. direct the flow of solution toward the side of the auditory canal, *not* toward the center of the canal (to avoid pushing the impaction against the eardrum); administer solution slowly
10. watch for wax returns; stop irrigation when plug of cerumen is noted in returns
11. aftercare of patient as needed; watch for dizziness
12. record results and note how patient tolerated procedure

Abbreviations Used for Ear Treatments and Medications

A.D.	auris dextra	right ear
A.S.	auris sinistra	left ear
A.U.	aures utrae	both ears

Some texts suggest that a Water Pik may be used successfully at low pressure when giving an ear irrigation. If a foreign body is in the ear, *do not attempt ear irrigation*. It may cause the obstruction to swell and compound the problem. See a physician. Bugs that fly or crawl into the ear can be killed with oil instillation and then flushed out.

Ear irrigation should not be done if there is any discharge from the ear. Let the physician decide what to do in such cases.

□ *The Eye*

□ STRUCTURES AND FUNCTIONS

The eyeball is made up of three layers of tissues:

Sclera. This is the tough outer layer. It serves as a supporting framework for the two inner layers. Light enters through the transparent cornea in front of the eye and the aqueous humor (clear fluid) lies right behind the cornea.

Middle Layer. This is divided into three parts: the choroid, which contains blood vessels; the ciliary body, which contains the ciliary muscles that keep the lens in place; and the iris, the colored part of the eye.

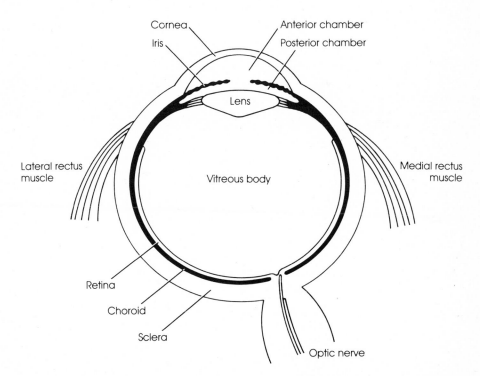

Figure 18–4 □ Anatomy of the eye.

Retina. This is the inner layer of the eyeball. It has light sensitive cells (rods and cones) and touches the choroid. Nerve fibers in front of the rods and cones mesh to form the optic nerve. The optic nerve (second cranial nerve) enters the eyeball slightly below the center of the back of the eye.

The eyeball is protected by the bony orbit in which it lies. Also contributing to protection are the eyelashes, lids, and brows.

Light rays are slightly bent toward each other as they meet the cornea. The iris regulates the amount of light that enters the eye because it is able to change the size of the pupil. The pupil contracts if too much light is beamed toward the eye, and it expands if light is dim. The rays bend even more as they pass through the curved lens. They meet at the focus, which *should* be on the retina. Light rays will be blurred if they meet in *front* of or in *back* of the retina. The eye is constructed so we can focus perfectly on near or far objects, but not simultaneously. Light enters the eye and changes a chemical in the retina, which permits us to see.

If an eyeball is too long, the lens brings the light rays into focus too far in front of the retina. Concave lenses are used to compensate for this nearsightedness.

Farsightedness occurs when the eyeball is too short and rays focus *behind* the retina. Glasses with convex lenses help sharpen vision.

☐ AGE-RELATED VISUAL CHANGES

Slowed Responses. The slowed responses to stimuli that are noticeable in so many elderly patients' reactions are also true of the eye. The slowness with which the eye reacts to dust specks and other foreign bodies makes it vulnerable to injury.

Reduced Secretions. The tear-producing lacrimal glands secrete less fluid, and therefore the eyes look dry and lack luster.

Diminished Visual Perception, Ulcers, Iritis. Visual perception diminishes for several reasons. There is a degeneration of the blood vessels that nourish the tissues; the pupil is smaller and less light gets to the retina. Ulcers of the cornea and inflammation of the iris (iritis) occur frequently, and just as frequently the elderly person puts off seeking treatment, attributing many of these changes to "old age."

Detached Retina. This condition is often found in the elderly since chronic disease, old age, and debility predispose to this problem, in which the retina separates from the choroid. Trauma can also cause this condition, as in the case of a severe shaking up, with or without bruises, and other injuries from accidents. A detached retina can be treated surgically, but the condition sometimes recurs. Strict attention to postoperative measures and positive health practices during convalescence help prevent recurrences.

Corneal Ulcers. These occur following fever, nutritional deficiencies, or a stroke. They can also be caused by irritation, as from eyelashes. Reduced muscle tone and loss of elasticity of the skin cause ectropion, the turning outward of the lower eyelid. Entropion irritation can cause corneal ulcers because the lashes can scratch the cornea. Ectropion exposes the conjunctiva in the lower lid and dries the natural secretions before they are able to lubricate the cornea.

Glaucoma. Glaucoma, a disease characterized by increased intraocular pressure, causes blindness in many elderly. Some early symptoms are headache, loss of peripheral vision, and seeing halos around lights. Glaucoma is never cured, although treatment relieves symptoms. Although physician's orders are specific, there are some general guidelines nurses should know when caring for patients with glaucoma. Increased intraocular pressure can result from stress, wearing tight clothing, upper respiratory infections, and excessive fluids. Activities to be encouraged are moderation in exercise and in using the eyes, avoiding constipation, and use of medications with the physician's authority *only*. The patient should wear a Medic-alert bracelet that identifies him or her as having glaucoma.

Cataracts. This condition, in which the lens becomes clouded, is very common among the elderly. About eight out of ten geriatric patients 80 and over have some loss of the transparency of the lens. The cause of senile cataracts is unknown. Fortunately, surgery for this problem is highly successful, restoring vision in 95 per cent of those patients who have uncomplicated cataracts.

Blindness. Blindness can occur when nephritis with high blood pressure is present in the geriatric patient. Diabetic retinopathy, caused by hemorrhaging of the small blood vessels that nourish the retina, causes blindness in young as well as old persons.

Presbyopia. Even if the aged adult is in excellent health with no eye pathology, there are unavoidable vision changes. The most common of these is presbyopia (far-sightedness), a condition caused by the decreasing elasticity of the lens, which results in a lack of accommodation for near vision. A prescription for reading glasses corrects this deficiency. This decreasing elasticity begins at about the age of 45.

Senile Macular Degeneration. Senile macular degeneration may result from a decrease in the vascular supply to the macula. The cause is unknown and there is no definitive treatment for this common retinal disorder. However, laser photocoagulation has proven effective in some cases.

☐ NURSING INTERVENTIONS

The nurse can be helpful by discouraging people from using glasses that are not specifically prescribed for them. It is common practice not only to borrow eyeglasses but also to use outdated eye medications or eye medications that are prescribed for someone else.

Another drawback to maintaining optimal eye care is the tendency to put off seeing a physician when there are unpleasant symptoms either with the fear that "if I go, he'll find something wrong," or with the thought that "maybe things will clear up in a few days."

Many people do not differentiate between an optician, an optometrist, and an ophthalmologist. An optician grinds and fits lenses; an optometrist is a licensed person who examines the eyes, prescribes, and adjusts lenses; and an ophthalmologist is a physician trained in diagnosing and treating diseases of the eye.

Care of the eyes and of eyesight includes good nutritional intake. For example, night blindness (absent or defective vision in the dark) may result from a vitamin A deficiency as well as from degenerative changes of the aging adult. Diet may not be able to cure eye diseases but a balanced diet may delay aging's unpleasant side effects by slowing lens opacity and possibly deterring many other degenerative processes.

Working with the Visually Handicapped*

1. Provide adequate lighting at all times, especially for reading, sewing, writing, and similar activities. Lighting is extremely important. A room that is well lit is better than a room that has only a table lamp or floor lamp. The reason is that it is hard for an elderly person to adapt from light to dark and vice versa. A lamp accentuates light in a small area with vast areas of darkness around it. It is hard to accommodate to this if you are over 65.
2. Avoid bright glare, e.g., highly polished floors, windows without curtains or shades.
3. Supply a nightlight in the bathroom, kitchen, or any other area where the individual is likely to go at night.
4. Elderly people should be discouraged from driving at night because of "night blindness."
5. Large-print newspapers, magazines, and books should be made available.
6. Take advantage of other useful aids that are available such as needle threaders and playing cards with enlarged figures and numbers.
7. Talking book records and machines can be obtained free from the Library of Congress.
8. Face the visually handicapped person when speaking to him or her.
9. It is easier for a visually impaired person to lipread if the speaker wears bright lipstick.
10. Do not cover your mouth, smoke, or chew gum when speaking to a visually handicapped person.
11. Provide a transistor radio for the visually handicapped person to carry from place to place.
12. Special dials for phones are available that enlarge the numbers and glow in the dark; provide if possible.
13. Do not move furniture or belongings around without explaining what you are doing and why.
14. Give simple but detailed instructions for anything you plan to do. Wheel-

*Courtesy of Holyoke Geriatric Convalescent Center, Holyoke, MA.

chair patients in particular need to be told about obstacles, warned that they will be pulled backwards, and so on, to diminish their fears.

15. Large clocks and large calendars are a must for orientation.
16. Do not use colors that blend. For example, avoid white dishes on a white table, beige light switches on beige walls, and so on.
17. Eyeglasses must be cleaned often and checked for scratched lenses, cracks, or faulty screws. Eyes should be checked regularly.

Working with the Blind Elderly*

1. Face the person directly when speaking to him or her.
2. Touch the person you are speaking to: a handshake will help place where you are. It is especially important to touch hallucinating patients when speaking to them. However, be sure to speak before touching a blind person.
3. Provide pockets on clothing.
4. Provide a transistor radio.
5. A rope or cord leading to the bathroom may be useful. Be careful that it does not create a hazard, however.
6. Do not move personal belongings or furniture around.
7. Remove the glass from clocks so the person can tell time by touch. Have him or her use a Braille wristwatch.
8. Provide a calendar with raised letters and numbers.
9. Arrange for free talking books from the Library of Congress.
10. Speak clearly, slowly, and distinctly. If the person is confused or has a short attention span, allow for this.
11. Check to see if the person's hearing is impaired also. You may have to move closer or talk directly into the ear.
12. Give the blind person simple but detailed instructions about all the things you plan to do. Remember that there are no nonverbal or visual clues to help the person understand. It is especially important to explain to the blind person what is happening in group meetings.
13. Do not leave an elderly blind person alone in the room for long periods of time. He or she may begin to hallucinate.
14. Do not change the daily schedule. Blind people often judge the time of day by the day's regular events; they do not have sunrise and sunset for reminders.
15. Use as many external clues as possible, e.g., clocks that chime, a noon whistle, intercom, radio, and so on.
16. Constantly use sensory stimulation through touch, sounds, and smells since visual stimulation is absent. Increase such stimulation if there are signs of apathy, withdrawal, depression, or a diagnosis of chronic brain syndrome.
17. The newly blinded individual should be told about his or her disability in a straightforward manner. It decreases the impact of the disability.

Courtesy of Holyoke Geriatric Convalescent Center, Holyoke, MA.

Instillation of Eye Medications

For instillation, the patient may be in bed or seated in a chair. Any solution or ointment instilled should be sterile and used for the individual patient only. Most eye drops have the dropper built into the bottle cap, but there may be times when the nurse will use a sterile eye dropper. As the drops are instilled, the nurse should be careful to drop the solution into the lower conjunctival sac (in the lower eyelid) to avoid traumatizing the sensitive cornea. The medication is recorded after the procedure by indicating the treated eye as follows:

O.D.	oculus dexter	right eye
O.S.	oculus sinister	left eye
O.U.	oculus uterque	both eyes

Equipment

medication
sterile eye dropper, if needed
sterile cotton balls or gauze squares

Sequence

1. identify patient; introduce self; explain procedure; screen patient
2. with cotton ball or gauze square cleanse the affected eye, wiping from the inner canthus (corner of the eye near the nose) to the outer canthus; if there is a discharge from the eye, or if it is encrusted with dried secretions, sterile normal saline may be used to cleanse the affected eye
3. with a dry wipe protecting the finger of the nurse, depress the eyelid, tell the patient to look upward, and drop the prescribed medication into the lower conjunctival sac to avoid traumatizing the sensitive cornea
4. caution the patient not to rub the eye; rather, suggest he or she close both eyes and move them around to help distribute the medication
5. record the time, amount of drug, patient's reaction, and which eye was treated

If an eye ointment is to be applied, follow the same basic procedure but apply a thin line of the ointment along the conjunctiva of the lower lid.

Naturally, the nurse will wash her or his hands thoroughly *before* giving eye medications; this includes handwashing after treating *each* eye if both eyes are medicated in order to avoid cross contamination. The nurse should again wash her or his hands *after* the procedure is concluded.

Eye Irrigation

Purposes

to cleanse the eyes
to treat for inflammation, and other conditions

Equipment

prescribed solution, tepid temperature

curved basin
towel

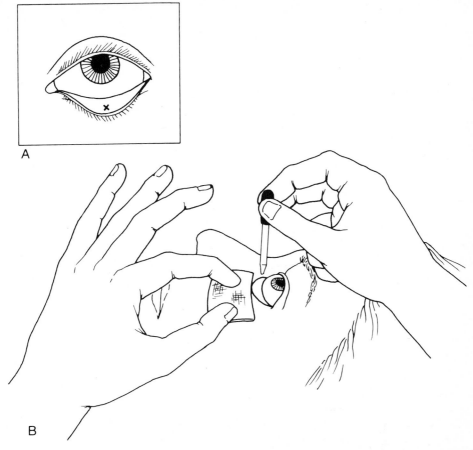

Figure 18–5 □ A, Eye drops are administered into the lower fornix (indicated by X). B, The nurse can steady the hand by resting it against the person's forehead.

rubber bulb syringe or eye dropper
  as ordered

waterproof protective pad
gauze squares

Sequence

1. identify patient; introduce self; explain procedure; screen patient
2. have patient tip head toward the *affected* side so solution flows from inner aspect of eye to outer (to avoid cross contamination)
3. place protective underpad and towel over shoulder, tuck up under head and neck so gown and sheets are not saturated
4. have patient hold curved basin at cheek on affected side to catch waste solution
5. depress lower conjunctival sac while holding upper lid open
6. gently introduce tepid solution from the inner canthus toward the outer canthus, being careful not to touch the eye, eyelid, or eyelashes with the tip of dropper or syringe; allow patient to blink from time to time

7. after prescribed length of time for treatment, have patient close eyes; blot dry
8. record as for instillation

Removal of a Foreign Body

Eyes are self-cleansing and the use of over-the-counter eye-cleansing preparations for the geriatric patient should be discouraged. Valuable time is lost with such self-medication. Many a physician has struggled to conceal frustration when faced with a health problem that could have been solved quickly and easily if only the patient turned up in the office sooner.

Occasionally the nurse will be asked to remove a foreign body from the eye. Of course, anything other than a small dirt particle or an eyelash should be referred to a physician.

Sequence
1. wash hands
2. grasp upper lid by the lashes and pull outward and downward; the eye will tear and may wash out the foreign body
3. evert upper lid on an applicator (Fig. 18–6)

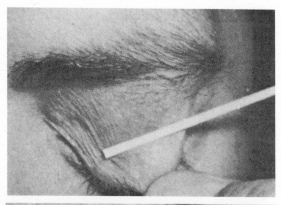

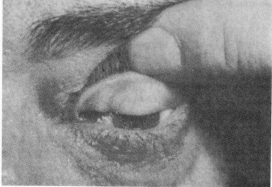

Figure 18–6 ☐ Technique for everting the eyelid in order to remove a foreign body. (From Carr, P. 53.)

4. holding the eyelid everted, slide the applicator out and discard
5. remove lash or cinder with new, moistened applicator

Compresses

Warm or cool compresses may be ordered. Compresses may be used with either clean (medical asepsis) technique or sterile (surgical asepsis) technique. For example, if medication (such as a sterile ointment) is ordered *before* the compress is given, the nurse will wear sterile gloves while carrying out the procedure.

Most physicians approve of sanitary napkins being used as the material for the compress. They absorb more fluid than gauze does and are easier to handle.

Care of the Eye Prosthesis

An enucleation, removal of an eye, is surgery performed in case of malignancy or severe eye trauma. A solid ball-shaped implant can be attached to the eye muscles. After healing is complete, a glass or plastic prosthesis can be fitted over the implant. This operation permits the prosthesis to move as the healthy eye focuses.

Most patients in this situation care for their own prosthesis, but occasionally the nurse assists.

Scrupulous cleanliness of the eye and of the socket is necessary to prevent infections and irrigations. The prosthesis should be gently cleansed with warm water and mild soap or saline. It should be stored in a suitable place. Generally, the eye is kept dry and stored on clean gauze.

Insertion of an Artificial Eye

1. wash hands before handling an artificial eye and before touching the socket
2. rinse prosthesis with saline or with water; sometimes the physician's order may require the socket to be rinsed also
3. hold the eye so that the pointed end is toward the nose
4. lift the upper lid and slide the eye under the lid
5. hold the eye in place, pull the lower lid down until it slides over the lower edge of the eye

Removal of an Artificial Eye

1. wash hands
2. depress the lower lid
3. cup hand under the eye
4. exert slight pressure under the eye; it will slip out

Artificial eyes are fragile and should be inserted and removed over a soft surface, e.g., a folded towel or pillow.

☐ *Taste and Smell*

Taste buds are located primarily on the surface of the tongue and in three places in the throat. Many substances taken into the mouth cause the taste buds to produce the sensation of taste. It is not clearly known how this happens.

The organ of smell is the nose. As we breathe, we inhale odorous gases that are mixed with the natural gases of the air. These gases touch a small cluster of epithelial cells that line the upper part of the inner surface of the nose. The cells then generate impulses that race along a pair of nerves to the cerebrum where the interpretation is an odor. Every gas we inhale does not set up the "smell" sensation. However, the more of an odorous gas that does contact these special cells, the stronger the odor.

The smell receptors, located high inside the nasal cavity, adapt to a scent quickly and the intensity of perception drops. That is why it is possible to enter a room, smell a strong odor, and after a while barely notice it.

Excessive mucus secretion can mask the sense of smell. If one has a cold, mucus coats the epithelial cells that pick up scent and inhibits gases from contacting them.

☐ AGE-RELATED CHANGES IN TASTE AND SMELL

Impaired smell among the elderly is common. It can actually be a safety hazard, as in the case of fire, escaping gas, or spoiled food.

The senses of smell and taste are linked. If something smells good we are inclined to taste it. The decline in appetite noticed in many geriatric patients is partly because of loss of smell and partly because there is a marked decrease in taste buds. By the age of 75, 65 per cent of the taste buds are lost.

Dietitians in nursing homes and hospitals and other health care workers seem to feel that elderly adults prefer bland food. They do not. They like highly seasoned food because it takes more sugar to get the right sweet taste and more of other seasonings to make foods palatable. It is true, of course, that many of the elderly are on bland diets because of medical or surgical problems, but those who are not should be allowed condiments.

The elderly like variety but the variety should include familiar foods because that is what their digestive tracts are used to. Long periods of time between meals should be avoided. Five or six small meals a day are preferable to three large meals.

☐ NURSING INTERVENTIONS

Nose Drop Instillation

Nose drops are drugs that are made up in solutions of normal saline. Oily solutions are never used because of the danger of aspiration pneumonia.

To administer nose drops, ask the patient to sit with his or her head and neck hyperextended. If the patient is confined to bed, the head may be tilted back over a pillow. The solutions should flow to the back of the nose. Before giving nose drops, the patient may gently blow both nostrils together to clear the nose.

The tip of the dropper is placed just inside the nose and the prescribed medication instilled. The patient should maintain the position for several minutes after the instillation. If the solution runs down the back of the throat, the patient will want to expectorate, so tissues should be provided. He or she should be encouraged not to blow the nose for half an hour after the instillation.

Chapter 18 ☐ Review Questions

MULTIPLE CHOICE

1. The middle ear is separated from the external auditory canal by
   A. the cochlea
   B. the organ of Corti
   C. the tympanic membrane
   D. the malleus
2. The type of deafness the geriatric nurse most frequently encounters is
   A. presbycusis
   B. conductive nerve deafness
   C. otosclerosis
   D. impacted cerumen
3. Impacted cerumen may be softened with:
   A. moistened cotton-tipped applicators
   B. Dobell's solution
   C. hydrogen peroxide
   D. sterile water
4. Light sensitive cells are:
   A. ciliary bodies
   B. rods and cones
   C. neurons
   D. electrons
5. Farsightedness occurs when:
   A. light rays focus too far in front of the retina
   B. light rays fail to be regulated by the iris
   C. light rays fail to be regulated by the choroid
   D. light rays focus too far behind the retina

MATCHING

_____ 1. Ménière's syndrome   A. outer layer of eyeball

_____ 2. tinnitus   B. right ear

_____ 3. glaucoma   C. clouding of lens

_____ 4. cataract   D. inner layer of eyeball

_____ 5. myringotomy   E. exposes conjunctiva in lower lid

_____ 6. auris dextra   F. incision of tympanic membrane

_____ 7. auris sinistra   G. ringing in ears

_____ 8. sclera   H. increased intraocular pressure

_____ 9. retina   I. left ear

_____ 10. ectropion   J. vertigo

DISCUSSION QUESTIONS

1. What community agencies are available in your locale to assist the older adult with the following:
   diabetic screening   foot care   nutrition counseling
   vision, hearing testing   dental problems
2. Prepare an outline for an inservice education program on the hearing impaired older adult. Include effect of aging process, emotional problems, aids for the family, tips for the nurse, and initial hearing aid use.

☐ REFERENCES

Childs, E.: Blind and deaf, but not daft as well. Nurs Mirror, 156(15):30–31, 1983.
Fairweather, W.: Care of adults with hearing loss. Nursing (Oxford), 1(28):1236–1238, 1981.
Gladstone, V. S.: Hearing loss in the elderly. Phys Occup Ther Geriatr, 2(2):5–20, 1982.
Hayter, J.: Modifying the environment to help older persons. Nurs Health Care, 4(5):265–926, 1983.
Jundra, L. F.: Cataract surgery before and after. Hosp Pract, 19(5):142A–B, 142G, 142J, 1984.
Kakritz, L. W.: Glaucoma: the silent thief: Pressure inside the eye can insidiously destroy sight. Your Life Health, 99(5):33, 1984.

Kaufman, J. H.: Eye surgery: improved techniques for age-related disorders. Consultant, 24(7):63–64, 69, 72–73, 1984.

Kopac, C. A.: Sensory loss in the aged; the role of the nurse and family. Nurs Clin North Am, 18(2):373–384, 1983.

Stag, C.: Resident for a day . . . experiencing blindness and physical restraint opened the staff's eyes. Geriatr Nurs, 5(6):239, 1984.

Smith, J. F.: The patient having cataract surgery. J Ophthalmic Nurs Technol, 3(3):124–126, 1984.

Wineburg, R.: Geriatric blindness: a neglected public health problem, Health Soc Work, 9(1):36–41, 1984.

Yen, P. K.: Taste, smell and appetite: they go together. Geriatr Nurs, 3:56–57, 1982.

Zachow, K. M.: Helen, can you hear me? J Gerontol Nurs, 10(8):18–22, 1984.

Answers to Review Questions

Answers to the Self-Check on Page 15

1. *True.* Life expectancy has been increased through modern medical advances. In 1900, life expectancy was 43 years. In 1920, it was 54 for men and 55 for women. In 1950, it was 66 for men and 72 for women. In 1978, it was 67 for men and 74 for women.
2. *False.* Aged individuals may need more *rest*, but they actually need less sleep. Five to seven hours a night is sufficient.
3. *True.* Very few of the total population of elderly persons are institutionalized. About 80 per cent live in their own homes. Another 14 or 15 per cent live with relatives.
4. *False.* When we speak about biologic aging we are talking about cellular life. Chronologic age means age in years. No two people age the same biologically, and different rates and degrees of aging can be found in the same age group. Also, one body system can deteriorate with age (the skin, for instance) while there is almost no change in the other systems.
5. *False.* Depression, which increases in incidence among the aged, is the most common problem that psychiatrists treat elderly people for. It is difficult to diagnose because the symptoms are often obscured by stereotypical behaviors—lack of vitality, sluggishness, brooding—which are thought to be an inevitable part of growing old.
6. *False.* Senile patients can become depressed. In fact, sometimes it is depression, not chronic brain syndrome (or organic brain syndrome), that provokes symptoms of senility.
7. *False.* Certain medical problems can be treated and thus improve the blood supply to the brain. Examples of such medical problems are congestive heart failure and dehydration with resulting electrolyte imbalance.
8. *True.* Short-term memory does decrease with age, but long-term memory is rarely impaired.
9. *False.* Elderly people tolerate pain quite well. It is not a good thing,

though, because some complaints that they shrug off as due to "old age" should be investigated before they develop into something serious. Peripheral pain sensations are reduced and this can be harmful as in cases of heating pad burns, scalding, and so on.

10. *False.* Many elderly people have a healthy interest in and need for sexual activity. Sexual information is necessary for the aged so that they can avoid feeling guilty about sexual feelings, and it is necessary for the younger members of society so that they will recognize that the sexual experiences of the aged are natural and good.

11. *True.* Reminiscing is important and can be therapeutic for elderly people. Memories are sometimes all older people have to remind them that they were once vital contributors to society.

12. *True.* By listening to older people, you can begin to appreciate many of the changes that take place in the elderly—impaired hearing, short-term memory loss, slowed reaction time, and others.

Chapter 1 ☐ Answers to Matching

1. g
2. i
3. b
4. h
5. e
6. a
7. j
8. c
9. d
10. f

Chapter 2 ☐ Answers to True/False

1. F
2. F
3. T
4. T
5. F
6. F
7. T
8. T
9. F
10. T

Chapter 3 ☐ Answers to Matching

1. e
2. d
3. b
4. g
5. c
6. a
7. f

Chapter 3 ☐ Answers to True/False

1. T
2. T
3. F
4. F
5. F
6. F
7. T
8. T
9. T
10. T

Chapter 4 ☐ Answers to Matching

1. e
2. h
3. i
4. a
5. g
6. j
7. f
8. b
9. c
10. d

Chapter 5 ☐ Answers to Multiple Choice

1. b
2. d

3. c
4. c
5. d
6. c
7. b
8. b
9. d
10. b

Chapter 5 ☐ Answers to True/False

1. T
2. F
3. T
4. F
5. F
6. T
7. T
8. T
9. T
10. F

Chapter 6 ☐ Answers to Multiple Choice

1. a
2. b
3. d
4. d
5. b

Chapter 6 ☐ Answers to True/False

1. T
2. T
3. T
4. F
5. F

Chapter 7 ☐ Answers to Multiple Choice

1. c
2. d

3. a
4. a
5. c

Chapter 7 ☐ Answers to True/False

1. T
2. F
3. F
4. F
5. T
6. T
7. F
8. F
9. F
10. F

Chapter 8 ☐ Answers to Multiple Choice

1. a
2. b
3. c
4. c
5. b
6. b
7. d
8. a
9. d
10. a

Chapter 8 ☐ Answers to Matching

1. e
2. d
3. f
4. a
5. h
6. c
7. i
8. j
9. b
10. g

Chapter 9 ☐ Answers to Multiple Choice

1. c
2. a
3. d
4. b
5. c
6. a
7. d
8. a
9. c
10. b

Chapter 9 ☐ Answers to Discussion Questions

1. The patient who wants to avoid heroic measures must inform family and physician of intent. Terminally ill persons have choices if preparation is undertaken beforehand. Many states have "living will" legislation that offers guidelines and legal protection for health professionals when they participate in decisions about life and death. This patient must be advised to seek legal counsel in order to protect his or her rights.
2. Mr. Williams must be prepared to meet his wife's physical and emotional needs. He should enlist the help of his wife's physician in pursuing resources that will help him administer the necessary nursing care at home. A local area agency on aging, state health and welfare agencies, local hospitals, and Social Security Administration are some of the possibilities. Mr. Williams will have to be prepared for his wife's eventual death, and he should consider hospice alternatives that may be available in his community. Lastly, he will have to take measures to ensure his own health maintenance, rest, and emotional needs.
3. To be investigated by individuals in the states in which they reside.
4. The visitor must acknowledge that, indeed, the elderly relative is acutely depressed. She means what she says. She must be encouraged to express her concerns without fear of judgmental attitudes and remarks. The visitor must inform the nursing staff of the patient's request and follow up before the next visit to determine what action has been taken.

Chapter 10 ☐ Answers to Multiple Choice

1. c
2. b

3. c
4. b

Chapter 10 ☐ Answers to Matching

1. b
2. c
3. d
4. e
5. a

Chapter 10 ☐ Answers to Discussion Questions

1. The liquid shampoo generally used on white patients may not be suitable for the naturally dry, coarse, very curly hair of the black patient. A mixture of one part alcohol to four parts mineral oil can be massaged into the scalp and hair and toweled off.
2. Turning patients every 2 hours, using bed cradle to keep blankets off feet; use of alternating pressure pad, mattress; sheepskin, heel and elbow protector; therapeutically nutritious diet; maintaining skin cleanliness; lubrication of skin.
3. The skin of an elderly adult is less elastic, tends to be thin, dry. Pruritus is a common complaint. Nails are thick, brittle and growth is faster. Hair is dry due to scant sebum production. Brown spots may occur.
4. Meticulous skin care: washing, drying between each toe and cutting nails straight across. Scrupulously clean footwear. Regular podiatrist visits to care for corns, calluses.
5. Most elderly are on several medications for a variety of problems and drug-induced skin reaction must first be ruled out. Many systemic disorders, e.g., cancer and diabetes, show skin symptoms. In addition, grief and depression often cause skin eruptions, and emotional reactions may keep the patient from seeking treatment.

Chapter 11 ☐ Answers to Multiple Choice

1. c
2. d
3. b
4. c
5. c
6. b
7. c

Chapter 11 ☐ Discussion Questions

1. nasal cannula, nasal catheter, face mask, tent
2. intermittent positive pressure breathing
3. check equipment and supplies
4. trauma to mucous membranes, stimulate production of mucus
5. surgical aseptic technique
6. proper grounding of all electrical equipment, do not use electric razors, strict enforcement of no smoking rules, do not use equipment with frayed electrical wires, avoid use of any oils or flammable solutions, prevent static electricity
7. Oxygen is essential to life. Survival without oxygen is possible for only a few minutes. Insufficient supply impairs functioning of all body systems. Irreversible brain damage usually results from periods of prolonged oxygen deprivation.

Chapter 12 ☐ Answers to Multiple Choice

1. d
2. a
3. a
4. c

Chapter 12 ☐ Answers to Matching

1. c
2. g
3. h
4. j
5. d
6. e
7. i
8. b
9. f
10. a

Chapter 12 ☐ Answers to Discussion Questions

1. The signs of fecal impaction include oozing of liquid stool, smearing, diarrhea, abdominal distention. Headache, malaise and lack of appetite may also be present.

2. Peristalsis decreases in the aged. There is usually loss of teeth which interferes with proper mastication of food. Elderly persons often are taking medication that causes bowel problems. Diet may not have enough fiber and inactivity of the older adult will also contribute to bowel problems.
3. Establish a regular evacuation time (daily or on alternate days). Encourage exercise within limits and provide for maximum mobility. Maintain records; record all results observed. Encourage adequate fluids. Provide privacy, commodes, toilet extenders—anything needed to make the patient comfortable.

Chapter 13 ☐ Answers to Multiple Choice

1. b
2. a
3. d
4. b
5. c
6. a

Chapter 14 ☐ Answers to Multiple Choice

1. b
2. c
3. d
4. a
5. c
6. a
7. c

Chapter 15 ☐ Answers to Multiple Choice

1. b
2. c
3. c
4. d
5. a

Chapter 15 ☐ Answers to Matching

1. c
2. d

3. h
4. g
5. f
6. i
7. j
8. b
9. a
10. e

Chapter 16 ☐ Answers to Multiple Choice

1. d
2. b
3. a
4. b
5. c

Chapter 16 ☐ Answers to Matching

1. h
2. c
3. e
4. g
5. d
6. b
7. a
8. i
9. j
10. f

Chapter 16 ☐ Answers to Discussion Questions

1. The presentation should include the following information: Cerebrovascular disease is the third most common cause of death in the U.S. About 200,000 deaths per year are attributed to this disease. Some risk factors are race and sex. The risk of stroke in women is less than that in men *unless* smoking is a factor. Black men have a significantly higher incidence of stroke than do white men. Medical management of cardiovascular disease and diabetes, plus the cooperation of the patient, can help decrease the risk

of stroke. A diet that reduces weight and lowers blood cholesterol can prevent strokes. In addition, exercise, rest, relief from tension, and stopping smoking are valuable components in stroke prevention.

2. Hypertension (high blood pressure) is a persistent elevation of systolic blood pressure above 140 mm Hg and diastolic pressure above 90 mm Hg. Persistently elevated pressure and related symptoms (dull, early morning headache; nausea and vomiting; memory deficits; and epistaxis) will necessitate treatment. Conservative treatment will consist of a balance between rest and mild activity, weight reduction (if Mr. C. is obese), and salt restriction. Nursing measures will include explaining to Mr. C. the importance of compliance with diet, medication (if ordered), and reduction in stress. Mr. C. should be encouraged to learn that hypertension is a chronic condition that can be controlled.

Chapter 17 ☐ Answers to Multiple Choice

1. b
2. a
3. c
4. c
5. a
6. c
7. d
8. b
9. d
10. a

Chapter 17 ☐ Answers to Matching

1. g
2. a
3. f
4. e
5. i
6. d
7. h
8. j
9. c
10. b

Chapter 17 ☐ Answers to Discussion Questions

1.

PATIENT'S NAME __E. Webber__   PHYSICIAN __L. Jones, M.D.__
ROOM NUMBER __413__   DIAGNOSIS __L. leg vein ligation; diabetes__

Date		Nursing Problem Statements	Patient Goals	Nursing Intervention	Date Completed	Signed
3/18	1.	Knowledge deficit of diabetic diet and food exchange groups	Meal selection compatible with diabetic diet	Consult with dietician; have patient view video tapes on types of food exchanges; supply patient with diabetic nutrition pamphlets	3/22	
	2.	Potential infection related to lack of knowledge of appropriate skin care	Normal healing postop; maintenance of skin integrity	Teach signs of infection; teach diabetic foot care		
	3.	Possible activity deficit related to lack of knowledge of importance of exercise	Normal walking about house and neighborhood after discharge	Ambulate in corridor; discuss need for regular exercise arrange consultation with physical therapist		
	4.	Potential self-care deficit related to lack of knowlege of risk of not testing urine	Normal urine glucose and acetone levels	Provide guide for testing of urine; demonstrate urine testing		

2. Diabetes is a chronic disease characterized by a deficiency in insulin production. The aging adult has impaired ability to use glucose, and this glucose intolerance may be related to dietary factors. For example, excessive adipose tissue is associated with a resistance to the action of insulin. Therefore, where needed, weight reduction to appropriate levels is indicated. The most important aspect of dietary treatment of maturity onset diabetes is reduction of weight until ideal weight is reached. Many physicians prefer that their patients with this disorder achieve even slightly below ideal weight.

The client should be instructed in the exchange groups of foods *after* the physician establishes the needed energy and nutrient requirements. Emphasis should be on the six exchange food groups and the necessity to use exchanges within an individual food group.

Exercise is another important factor in the successful management of the elderly gentleman's diabetes. Some types of exercise can be devised for frail elderly even if there is a mobility impairment. Exercise can improve metabolism and mental attitude.

Lastly, if medication is a factor in the client's situation, the nurse would have to evaluate the client's ability to understand dosage and administration. If outside assistance is necessary, the nurse would contact the appropriate community agency to ensure successful health maintenance.

Chapter 18 ☐ Answers to Multiple Choice

1. c
2. a
3. c
4. b
5. d

Chapter 18 ☐ Answers to Matching

1. j
2. g
3. h
4. c
5. f
6. b
7. i
8. a
9. d
10. e

Illustration Credits

PART I   Courtesy of Ring Nursing Homes, Springfield, MA.

CHAPTER 1

Figure 1–1 Schrier, R.W.: Clinical Internal Medicine in the Aged. Philadelphia, W. B. Saunders, 1982, p. 3.

Figure 1–2 Schrier, R.W.: Clinical Internal Medicine in the Aged. Philadelphia, W. B. Saunders, 1982, p. 3.

p. 8   Breitung, J.C.: Care of the Older Adult. 1st ed. New York, Tiresias Press, 1981, p. 34.

p. 9   Courtesy of Ring Nursing Homes, Springfield, MA.

CHAPTER 2

Figure 2–1 Courtesy of Heritage Hall Nursing Home, Agawam, MA.

Figure 2–2 Courtesy of Heritage Hall Nursing Home, Agawam, MA.

Figure 2–3 Courtesy of Heritage Hall Nursing Home, Agawam, MA.

p. 21   Dennis, L.B., and Hassol, J.: Introduction to Human Development and Health Issues. Philadelphia, W. B. Saunders, 1983, p. 267.

CHAPTER 3

p. 41   Courtesy of Ring Nursing Homes, Springfield, MA.

p. 45, 49 Courtesy of Crescent Hill Nursing Center, Springfield, MA.

CHAPTER 4

Figure 4–1 Rambo, B.: Adaptation Nursing Assessment and Intervention. Philadelphia, W. B. Saunders, 1984, p. 77.

p. 64   Courtesy of Ring Nursing Homes, Springfield, MA.

CHAPTER 7

p. 103   Courtesy of Ring Nursing Homes, Springfield, MA.

p. 110   Courtesy of Ring Nursing Homes, Springfield, MA.

CHAPTER 8

Figure 8–1   Poleman, C.L., and Capra, C.L.: Shackelton's Nutrition: Essentials and Diet Therapy. 5th ed. Philadelphia, W. B. Saunders, 1984, p. 216.

PART II   Courtesy of Ring Nursing Homes, Springfield, MA.

CHAPTER 9

p. 148   Courtesy of Concern for Dying, 250 West 57th Street, Suite 831, New York, NY 10107.

CHAPTER 10

Figure 10–1   Jacob, S.W., Francone, C.A., and Lossow, W.J.: Structure and Function in Man. 4th ed. Philadelphia, W. B. Saunders, 1978, p. 77.

Figure 10–2   Leake, M.J.: A Manual of Simple Nursing Procedures. 5th ed. Philadelphia, W. B. Saunders, 1971, p. 40.

Figure 10–3   Rambo, B.J., and Wood, L.A.: Nursing Skills in Clinical Practice. Philadelphia, W. B. Saunders, 1982, p. 340.

Figure 10–4   Rambo, B.J., and Wood, L.A.: Nursing Skills in Clinical Practice. Philadelphia, W. B. Saunders, 1982, p. 340.

Figure 10–8   Talbot, D.: Principles of Therapeutic Positioning: A Guide for Nursing Action. Minneapolis, MN, Sister Kenny Institute, 1978, 1981, p. 107.

CHAPTER 11

Figure 11–1   Modified from Dugas, B.: Introduction to Patient Care. Philadelphia, W. B. Saunders, 1980, p. 373.

Figure 11–2   Kottke, F.J., Stillwell, G.K., and Lehmann, J.F.: Krusen's Handbook of Physical Medicine and Rehabilitation. 3rd ed. Philadelphia, W. B. Saunders, 1982, pp. 780–781.

CHAPTER 12

Figure 12–1   Dienhart, C.M.: Basic Human Anatomy and Physiology. 3rd ed. Philadelphia, W. B. Saunders, 1979, p. 184.

Figure 12–2   Howard, R.B., and Herbold, N.H.: Nutrition in Clinical Care. New York, McGraw-Hill, 1979, p. 351.

Figure 12–3   Rambo, B.J., and Wood, L.A.: Nursing Skills for Clinical Practice. Philadelphia, W.B. Saunders, 1982, p. 333.

Figure 12–5   Rambo, B.J., and Wood, L.A.: Nursing Skills for Clinical Practice. Philadelphia, W.B. Saunders, 1982, p. 534.

Figure 12–6   Rambo, B.J., and Wood, L.A.: Nursing Skills for Clinical Practice. Philadelphia, W.B. Saunders, 1982, p. 536.

CHAPTER 13

Figure 13–1   Jacob, S.W., Francone, C.A., and Lossow, W.J.: Structure and Function in Man. 4th ed. Philadelphia, W.B. Saunders, 1978, p. 150.

Figure 13–3   Rambo, B.J., and Wood, L.A.: Nursing Skills for Clinical Practice. Philadelphia, W.B. Saunders, 1982, p. 237.

Figure 13–5   Rambo, B.J., and Wood, L.A.: Nursing Skills for Clinical Practice. Philadelphia, W. B. Saunders, 1982, p. 359.

Figure 13–9   Courtesy of Ring Nursing Homes, Springfield, MA.

CHAPTER 14

Figure 14–1   Jacob, S.W., Francone, C.A., and Lossow, W.J.: Structure and Function in Man. 4th ed. Philadelphia, W. B. Saunders, 1978, p. 393; courtesy of David M. Spain, M.D.

Figure 14–2   Rambo, B.J., and Wood, L.A.: Nursing Skills for Clinical Practice. Philadelphia, W. B. Saunders, 1982, p. 416.

Figure 14–4   Rambo, B.J., and Wood, L.A.: Nursing Skills for Clinical Practice. Philadelphia, W. B. Saunders, 1982, p. 430.

Figure 14–5   DuGas, B.: Introduction to Patient Care. Philadelphia, W. B. Saunders, 1980, p. 583.

CHAPTER 15

p. 275   Courtesy of Mercy Hospital, Springfield, MA.

CHAPTER 16

Figure 16–2   Courtesy of Mercy Hospital, Springfield, MA.

CHAPTER 18

Figure 18–2   Gardner, G.: Hearing aids. Am Fam Phys, 15:94, 1977.

Figure 18–5   Carr, R.E.: Look them in the injured eye. Emergency Med, 9:53, 1977.

Index

Note: Numbers in *italics* refer to illustrations; numbers followed by t indicate tables.